U.C.H. HANDBOOK OF PSYCHIATRY

U.C.H. HANDBOOK OF
PSYCHIATRY

For Students and General Practitioners

Edited by

ROGER TREDGOLD
& HEINZ WOLFF

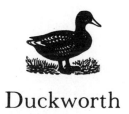

Duckworth

Reprinted 1979
Second edition 1975
First published 1970 (*as* U.C.H. Notes on Psychiatry)
Second impression 1971

Gerald Duckworth & Company Limited
The Old Piano Factory
43 Gloucester Crescent, London NW1

© Roger Tredgold and Heinz Wolff 1970, 1975

ISBN (*paper*) 0 7156 0569 0
        (*cloth*) 0 7156 0429 5

Typeset by
Specialised Offset Services Limited, Liverpool

Printed by Unwin Brothers Limited, Old Woking, Surrey.

Foreword to the first edition

The period spent in the Psychiatric Department is one of the most popular of the student appointments at University College Hospital Medical School. The reason is not far to seek. The department takes a great interest in its students who, attached singly or in pairs to one of the psychiatrists, often become involved in discussion with and management of patients. Informal discussions on patients' problems and seminars are held regularly and, at these, 'broadsheets' or notes on various aspects of psychiatry are distributed and discussed. This book arose from the collection of such broadsheets. It also includes a number of topics discussed with the students in their introductory clinical course as well as some additions to the regular broadsheets and it provides a simple, but fairly comprehensive, introduction to psychiatry with useful suggestions for further reading.

I am confident that it will prove most successful and that it will both add to the high reputation of the department and attract students to take a lively interest in psychiatry and some to become psychiatrists.

Professor of Medicine M.L. ROSENHEIM,
University College Hospital Medical School M.A., M.D., P.R.C.P.

Contents

viii

Preface to the second edition

This book was published in 1970 as a collection of contributions by many of our colleagues in this department and in the rest of the hospital. This edition is based on the same work, but we have thought it best, for reasons of continuity, now to edit and re-write most of the book on our own responsibility and to bring it up to date. There are, however, a few specialist parts of it which we have asked certain of our colleagues to provide, and we would like to express our thanks to them particularly for doing so: Miss Grace Rawlings (Sections 3 and 54), Professor Joe Smith (Sections 7 and part of 10), Dr. Max Glatt (Sections 22 and 23), Dr. Kitty Dalton (Section 35), and Dr. Jeremy Christie-Brown (Sections 58 and 59). The parts originally written by Dr. Gerald Stern (Section 8) and Professor Desmond Pond (Section 25) remain untouched. Drs. Colin Wilson, David Sturgeon, Michael Farthing, Julie Altschulova and Elizabeth Tylden have helped considerably with Sections 9 and 45, 20, 32, 34 and 42 respectively.

We should also like to thank Mrs. Mary Fisher, Mrs. Joyce Bruce and Miss Jean Mann for a great deal of typing and patient retyping.

Department of Psychological Medicine,
University College Hospital,   ROGER TREDGOLD
June 1975   HEINZ WOLFF

Preface to the first edition

The original versions of these notes were known as broadsheets and were handed out to U.C.H. students to supplement other methods of teaching these subjects — case demonstration, case taking, seminar or lecture. They were written over a number of years, spontaneously or less spontaneously, by many different members of the department and different people in the hospital and medical school; they were in many cases efforts to present particular syndromes or problems, from the different angles of the several persons involved. We are indeed grateful to all our colleagues whose initial work made up the major part of this book; their names are listed below, in alphabetical order. Their contributions ranged from several complete sections to a few helpful paragraphs.

As the number of broadsheets grew, various former students asked for copies, and we felt it worth while to present them together in a book. This has entailed a great deal of editing and, in many cases, of rewriting to bring the earlier broadsheets up to date and to present in a moderately uniform style. We are thus responsible for the existing views, and also for any errors. In the process of editing it occurred to us to add a number of new broadsheets, principally on the reactions of the individual to various stages and stresses of his life, and these form Part VI of the book; we also collected, as Part IX, some discussions on ethical problems. Overseas readers will understand that the psychiatric and social services described in Part VIII are those available in Great Britain.

Our thanks are due first to our hospital colleagues:

The Rev. John Barker, *Chaplain*
Dr. Patrick Hare, *Consultant Dermatologist*
Mr. Bernard Harries, *Consultant Neurosurgeon*
Dr. Peter Heaf and Dr. Monica McAllen, *Consultant Chest Physicians*
The late Professor Will Nixon, *Professor of Obstetrics*

Professor Joe Smith, *Professor of Morbid Anatomy*
Dr. Gerald Stern, *Consultant Neurologist*
Dr. Robert Trotter, *Physician in Thyroid Diseases*

and to Dr. I. M. Marks of the Maudsley Hospital for his contribution on Behaviour Therapy.

Secondly to all those past and present members of this department, psychologists, psychiatric social workers, psychotherapists and psychiatrists:

Dr. Bernard Adams, Dr. Julie Altschulova, Dr. Michael Balint, Dr. Dorothea Ball, Mrs. Irene Bloomfield, Dr. Camilla Bosanquet, Dr. Michael Browne, Dr. Sidney Carlish, Miss Mary Clark, Dr. Katharina Dalton, Dr. Gwen Douglas, Dr. Ernest Dunkley, Dr. David Enoch, Dr. Eleanor Farrell, Miss Irene Forstner, Dr. Brian Garvey, Dr. Max Glatt, Dr. Mary Hare, Dr. Sonia Holmes, Dr. Stanley Jacobs, Dr. Elizabeth James, Dr. Jangoo Kohiyar, Dr. Terry Lear, Mr. and Mrs. Moses Laufer, Mrs. Phyllis Mendoza, Dr. Margaret Morgan, the late Miss Eileen Morton, Dr. Jean-Claude Mougne, Dr. Desmond O'Neill, Professor Desmond Pond, Dr. David Prothero, Dr. David Pryce, Miss Grace Rawlings, Dr. Margaret Rich, Mrs. Adelheid Schweitzer, Dr. Paul Senft, Dr. Kenneth Soddy, Dr. Harold Stewart, Dr. Christopher Treves Brown, Dr. Elizabeth Tylden, Dr. Peter Whybrow, Mrs. Celia Williams.

Thirdly, to our secretaries: none of the original broadsheets for this book would ever have appeared were it not for the devoted work of the secretaries in the hospital and medical school, and especially of those in this department led by Misses Jean Mann, Ruth Strong, Joyce Dell and Eileen Rutter; their goodwill and patience in preparing and correcting these drafts has exceeded even that of the publishers and printers in coping with last-minute alterations.

We are indeed very grateful to them all.

Department of Psychological Medicine
University College Hospital   ROGER TREDGOLD
May 1969   HEINZ WOLFF

1 Background, aims and technique of the interview

THE BACKGROUND

In hospital

Students have already learnt how to take a history from a patient while on a medical firm: in many cases this has included questions about the patient's emotional reaction to his illness, about psychological factors in its onset, about his childhood, social interests, and work records, and his married life. Some assessment has been made of his personality, mental state and progress. Generally the student has learnt to make a good contact with his patient.

In spite of this, he is often perturbed at the idea of meeting his first 'psychiatric' patient, and fears the interview may be embarrassing to him or to the patient. If so, he will nearly always find that the same principles of genuine interest, friendliness and sympathetic listening which he displayed on his medical firm stand him in equally good stead here, and that the patient will talk more freely, and will be more relaxed at the end of the session. There are of course exceptions, such as the paranoid schizophrenic, or the manic, but these are rare.

The student will certainly need to allow a reasonable time, and privacy, for his first interview, and will no doubt have read whatever documents are available before he starts.

In a surgery

The situation is rather different from a psychiatric department. Many patients come to a surgery with complaints which sound as if they may be psychogenic. This provokes in the doctor a reaction according to his personality and skill; if he has little skill he may be puzzled, be irritated, or despair, none of which is very helpful to the patient (or to himself); but if he has some plan of campaign and uses his natural consideration and commonsense, he may find he can do a lot by simple measures.

The first essential is to arrange for a longer interview, either at once, or, more likely, at some convenient opportunity. The time spent profitably on this may well be less than the time otherwise spent *to no avail* on the same patient over the next months or years.

Ideally, both patient and doctor need to be relaxed (physically and emotionally). How this is best achieved must be left to the doctor's personality, and the circumstances. But two points must always be remembered: long waiting beforehand is a very bad beginning for the patient, and an atmosphere of 'rush' is most inhibiting, especially to a patient who is shy and is rather guilty at taking up the doctor's time.

AIMS AND TECHNIQUE OF THE INTERVIEW

The interview, whether by student or by general practitioner, has several aims which are often carried out simultaneously but must be considered separately here. It is important to realize that in any interview, even if primarily diagnostic, some simple, limited 'first aid' is being given. The aims are as follows:

Collecting information

There are certain rules: sympathy must be obvious, confidentiality assured, and no criticisms made or even implied if the doctor is to get the patient at ease, and ready to talk about things he is shy, guilty or fearful of. The patient may need the doctor's repeated reassurance that he is interested in him as a person, and prepared to care for him: that certainly he will not laugh at him, nor despise him.

Good listening avoids interruptions: essentially the patient will talk about what his problems are: and the listener can let him do so. Some guiding questions may however be required, for patients who are discursive or a little shy. It would certainly be a mistake to press someone too soon to discuss matters on which he is reluctant: these may include his views on sex, on religion, and on other people close to him: which, however important, may come out only when he feels confidence in his student or doctor.

The patient may express anger and hate, and these the doctor must tolerate, though he has not got to agree with the patient's views; it is easy enough if they are directed against a third party, less easy if the attack is on something the doctor approves of, or is identified with (e.g. the medical profession); least easy if it is on himself.

The whole history is not to be obtained at the first interview, since there may be no time, and in any case patients will talk more freely at a later interview.

Nevertheless, some skeleton plan (see p. 6) may be a useful guide for students to remember: it can gradually be completed if time permits, but hardly ever at one interview. The patient's reactions and behaviour during the interview should be carefully observed as they provide information about his personality and mental state (p. 10).

Physical examination should be done, unless satisfactorily and recently carried out by someone else, or unless temporarily contra-indicated, e.g. if thereby the patient's anxiety over somatic factors would be increased; it may, however, not be needed if the patient has come with a purely psychological or social problem, e.g. difficulties in personal relationships.

Diagnosis (in terms of personality reacting to stress, physical illness or both)

To reach this, the student or doctor should ask himself:

1 Is there physical illness? If so, to what extent does it account for the symptoms?

2 (a)   What sort of person *is* the patient, and what does he want to be?

   (b)   Why has he consulted me, with these symptoms now? What was happening in his life when the symptoms began?

   (c)   What is his feeling? Why is he feeling this way? Who is it that he feels this way towards?

(*d*)   Can his symptoms serve any useful purpose? And will he
       be better without them?

(*e*)   What does he expect from me? What can I expect from
       him? Is his attitude demanding, paranoid, rejecting?

(*f*)   What assets has he in his personality and environment?

3 What is my attitude? Am I understanding the situation from
the patient's point of view, or from mine alone? What is my
reaction to his behaviour?

Although it may be possible to provide a label of a diagnostic
syndrome, and of course especially in organically based illness,
in many other cases the student or doctor would do better to
try to understand the real causes of the patient's illness in terms
of the interplay of stress and personality, and may be helped to
do so by the above questions. There may be three factors
involved which, although emphasised by classical historians in
analysing the origins of war, are often not distinguished by
clinicians studying their patient's breakdown; these three are:—
the precipitating factor, which caused the moment of the
breakdown; the ostensible causes which were blamed for the
previous tension; and the basic underlying insecurities and
conflicts which led to this state and which must be resolved if
peace is to be regained. The latter two, and especially the last,
and most serious, are often missed; and it may of course be
impossible and sometimes unwise to search for them at the first
interview.

In any case, many patients will regain their adjustment on
their own, if given some help at a critical time.

First aid

The doctor must therefore consider what help he should give at
the first session; release of emotional tension may have already
begun by listening to the patient's story and is helped if the
doctor or student provides an appropriate reaction to emotional
tension, i.e. reassurance for anxiety, hope in depression,
tolerance of guilt and aggression. Above all, he must show that
he has understood the situation from the patient's own
viewpoint or these attitudes may seem insincere and antagonize
the patient.

Drugs are needed occasionally, (e.g. for insomnia) and diet should be adequate.

It is often difficult to realize at the time that many a patient may be adequately helped by first aid, and once tension is reduced, can solve his own problems and so need no further sessions. The doctor should therefore avoid taking too much action at this stage, and offer to see him later, to discover how he is then. If he is not better, further steps will of course be needed (see p. 307).

Clearly there will be some first interviews where a patient requires urgent action for medical or psychiatric reasons, e.g. if he is seriously threatening suicide.

INTERVIEWING THE RELATIVES

In a psychiatric department, great help may be given by the psychiatric social worker (besides her other functions: see p. 371) in obtaining a history from the patient's relatives: this is of course especially necessary in a children's department, but even with adult patients the account of husband or wife, or some other relative is often extremely valuable. The patient's consent must of course be obtained first. Often a very different view may be found, and so a much more comprehensive assessment of the whole picture can be made.

In general practice this may be less necessary, since the doctor may know the patient's relatives already: but even here, psychiatric or other social workers can be extremely useful. This is particularly so (in both situations) where the patient might feel that his relationship with the doctor would be impaired by any contact between the latter and possibly critical relations. In some cases it will be necessary for the psychiatrist himself to interview a relative, either alone or together with the patient, e.g. husband and wife or several family members, in a joint diagnostic interview.

FURTHER READING

Sullivan, H.S. (1954). *The Psychiatric Interview.* Norton, New York.

2 Outline of history taking and examination

Remember that this is not intended to be completed at every patient's first interview; and also that it may be helpful to get additional information from a relative or other informant. In that case note the informant's name, his relationship to the patient, and your impression of his attitude and reliability.

Patient's name   Age   Date of birth

PRESENT ILLNESS

Complaints in detail

Their nature, extent, duration and effect on the patient and his surroundings, especially his family: circumstances preceding their onset: patient's initial reaction and his later ones. A detailed sequence of the development of symptoms, their relation to the patient's life situation, and their effects should be made out.

FAMILY HISTORY

Mother

Her health, age, or age at death and cause of death: her personality, the patient's attitude and feelings towards her: her occupation.

Father

His health, age, or age at death and cause of death: his

personality, the patient's attitude and feelings towards him: his occupation.

Age of each parent at the patient's birth: if one or both parents are dead, the patient's age at the time of their death and his reaction to it.

Siblings

In order of age, with Christian names, personality, occupation, marital state, mental and physical health. Patient's reaction to birth of siblings, and miscarriages or stillbirths, if any.

Home atmosphere

Describe the social and economic position of the family and the emotional atmosphere in the home, including the emotional relationship between the parents and siblings, and the patient's attitudes towards each of them.

Familial diseases

Give details of mental illnesses, alcoholism, epilepsy or hereditary conditions in any of the relatives.

PERSONAL HISTORY *(in the form of a biographical account)*

Birth and early development

Mother's condition during pregnancy: normal or abnormal birth: feeding difficulties: health: milestones of development: habit training difficulties.

Behaviour and neurotic symptoms in childhood

Play and favourite toys: any periods of separation from parents and the patient's reaction to it: temper tantrums: night terrors:

bed wetting or soiling: nail biting: eating problems: stammering: model child.

School

Age of beginning and finishing: school refusal or truancy: standards reached: special abilities or disabilities: interests and hobbies: relationship to schoolmates: attitude to teachers, work and games: ambitions and day dreams.

Adolescence

Changes in attitudes to parents: relation to peers: reaction to puberty and bodily changes: attitude to sexuality, including masturbation: early heterosexual and homosexual experiences: fantasy life and new interests: drug taking: delinquency.

Occupation

Age of starting work: jobs held in chronological order and reasons for change: satisfaction in work and present earnings: ambitions: relation to work mates, colleagues, superiors and subordinates: service in the armed forces and experiences there.

Psychosexual history (see also adolescence above)

Introduction to facts of life and early sexual experiences: parental attitude towards sex. In girls age at first period: how regarded, regularity, duration, pain: psychic changes: date of last period.

Masturbation and sexual fantasies: homosexual and heterosexual experiences apart from marriage: abnormal experiences: emotional relationship to partners: previous marriages: present marriage: reasons for marriage: husband's or wife's age, personality, occupation: nature and degree of satisfaction in emotional and sexual relationships in the marriage: any sexual difficulties, e.g. impotence or frigidity: contraceptive measures: extramarital relationships and sexual fantasy life. Any menopausal symptoms and attitude to menopause.

Children

Chronological list of children, with ages and Christian names: miscarriages, still-births or death of a child: patient's reaction to these events, and his attitude to existing children: their mental and physical health.

Middle and old age

Attitude to getting older: reaction to children leaving home: retirement: failed ambitions: any impairment of memory: attitude to being alone and to dying.

Previous mental illnesses

All past psychiatric symptoms whether treated or untreated. Any past psychosomatic symptoms. Treatment received giving details of nature, place of treatment, and by whom. Any previous psychiatric disturbances or character changes noticed by relatives or friends.

Medical history

Illnesses, operations and accidents in chronological order: the patient's reactions to them.

PERSONALITY BEFORE ILLNESS

1 Social and intellectual activities, besides those already mentioned.
2 Mood: cheerful, despondent, anxious, worrying, optimistic, pessimistic; self-deprecating, satisfied, over confident; stable, fluctuating (in weeks or hours with or without reason); controlled, demonstrative.

3 Character: timid, sensitive, suspicious, resentful, quarrelsome, irritable, impulsive, jealous, selfish, egocentric, reserved, shy, self-conscious, strict, fussy, isolated, withdrawn.

4 Standards: moral, religious, social, economic, practical, aesthetic; attitude towards self, others, health, own body.

5 Energy, initiative, hobbies, ability for self-expression.

6 Fantasy life: daydreaming (frequency and content); dreams and nightmares (in detail); masturbation fantasies.

7 Habits: eating (fads), sleeping, excretory functions. Alcohol, tobacco, drugs (specify amount taken recently, and earlier; when, and why).

MENTAL STATE

Appearance and behaviour

Describe the patient's general appearance; his dress, whether cared for or not; his ability to talk and relate to the interviewer. Does he look ill, tense, anxious, agitated, depressed, angry or calm and composed? Is he in touch with his surroundings? Any unusual movements e.g. gestures or grimaces? Much or little activity, spontaneous or how provoked. Do real or hallucinatory perceptions seem to modify his behaviour? If inactive does he resist passive movements, or maintain a posture, or obey commands?

Talk

The form of the patient's utterances rather than their content is here considered. Does he say much or little, talk spontaneously or only in answer, slow or fast, hesitantly or promptly, coherently or discursively? Give sample of talk if significantly abnormal. Any evidence of thought disorder (see p. 116).

Mood

The patient's appearance may be described, in so far as it is indicative of his mood; is he anxious, sad, depressed or elated?

What are his answers to 'How do you feel in yourself?', 'What is your mood?'? Record the constancy of mood, the influences which change it, and the appropriateness of the patient's apparent emotional state to what he says.

Delusions and misinterpretations

Does the patient hold false beliefs (which are not in keeping with his social and cultural background) despite all evidence to the contrary and in the face of all rational arguments (delusions)? Does he misinterpret what happens and give it special meaning relating to himself (ideas of reference)? Does he blame himself or others? How firmly does he hold these views?

Hallucinations and other disorders of perception

Does he experience hallucinations, i.e. auditory, visual, tactile, or olfactory sensations without there being any corresponding external stimuli? When do they occur; when falling asleep ('hypnagogic' hallucinations, which are not of pathological significance), when alone or with people who do not hear or see what he does? What is their content? Does he misinterpret real external stimuli (illusions)? Does he feel that his self is unreal or not his usual self (depersonalisation), or that his environment is strange and unreal (derealisation)?

Compulsive phenomena

Obsessional thoughts, impulses or acts. Are the thoughts felt to come from without, or to be part of the patient's own mind? Does he repeat actions such as washing, to reassure himself? If so, does he realize that this is unnecessary while being unable to resist them?

Orientation

Record the patient's answers to questions about his own name and identity, the place where he is, the time of day, and the date. Is there anything unusual to him in the way in which time seems to pass?

Memory

This may be tested by comparing the patient's account of his life with that given by others, or examining his account for intrinsic evidence of gaps or inconsistencies. Where there is selective impairment of memory for special incidents, periods, recent or remote happenings, this should be recorded in detail and the patient's attitude towards his forgetfulness and the things forgotten specially noted. Record the patient's success or failure in grasping, retaining, and being able to recall spontaneously or on demand three or five minutes later a number, a name and address, or other data. Give him digits to repeat forward, and then others to repeat backward, and record how many he can repeat immediately after being told them.

Attention and concentration

Is his attention easily aroused and sustained or is he easily distracted or pre-occupied? To test his concentration ask him to tell the day or the months in reverse order or to do simple arithmetical problems requiring 'carrying over' (112-25), or subtraction of serial sevens from 100 (give answers and time taken).

General information

Tests for general information and grasp should be varied according to the patient's educational level and his experiences and interests.

Insight and judgment

What is the patient's attitude to his present state? Does he regard it as an illness, as 'mental' or 'nervous' or 'purely physical', as needing treatment? Is his judgment good? What does he propose to do when he has left the hospital?

Relationship between the patient and the interviewer

Was the patient co-operative? Suspicious, demanding, passive? Any change in the course of the interview? What were the interviewer's own reactions to the patient, e.g. did he feel sympathetic, irritated, frustrated, sad, etc? Did these change during the interview or later?

SUMMARY AND FORMULATION

Once the interview is over the student should do what he can to summarize the patient's history, in terms which indicate how he has reacted to particular stresses and why. He should discuss what he thinks is most likely to help the patient. For this he will need to know something of psychodynamics and psychopathology. An account of these is found in Part II.

FURTHER READING

Notes on Eliciting and Recording Clinical Information (1973). Department of Psychiatry, Teaching Committee, Institute of Psychiatry. OUP, London.

3 Psychological investigations

Psychology as a science is concerned with the study of behaviour and in particular the thought and feeling processes associated with it and motivating it. Clinical psychology is directed primarily to a study of the ways in which the behaviour of patients differs from that of individuals comprising the 'normal population', defined in statistical terms without reference to disease processes.

Departments of psychiatry are concerned with the diagnosis and treatment of mental disorders, discovering their aetiology, and assessing the results of treatment. Clinical research has to be undertaken in support of all these; and also teaching of students in the various professions involved — doctors, nurses, psychologists, social workers and others. This is collaborative work in all stages of which the contribution of the psychologist is derived from the application of his knowledge, methods and skills to various aspects of patients' problems and disabilities, to research design and to teaching.

First the psychologist may be asked for evidence on particular problems posed by the doctor, e.g. are there any signs of mental deterioration? Is the patient likely to respond to psychotherapy or behaviour therapy or both? The necessary investigations may take several interviews and involve the use of various methods of assessment including more or less structured interviews, standardised tests, and specially constructed experimental techniques. The principal methods of assessment used by psychologists aim to elucidate the patient's personality and functioning efficiency. They include:—

Cognitive tests

1 *Comprehensive scales*, best known as individual tests of intelligence, from which some measure may be made of the efficiency of a patient's present level of intellectual functioning. The scales normally include a variety of verbal and practical tasks designed to show whether a person has learned from his experience; whether he can reason and apply acquired knowledge in new situations, whether he can remember and how he controls and directs his mental functioning.

From the evidence which these tests yield some comparison can be made between the intellectual status of a patient and that of his peers; this comparison can be expressed in quantitative terms usually as an intelligence quotient (IQ) though this is now less often used. This term formerly expressed the ratio between a person's life age and his 'mental age' as shown by his responses to standardized tests. The use of this ratio to indicate measures of intellectual ability enabled comparisons to be made between people of different ages and between the positions of the same person on successive occasions! The IQ was found to have a fair degree of constancy due to the fact that the mentally subnormal develop more slowly than children of average intelligence and the intellectually able advance more quickly. This relationship was thought to apply consistently but more recent work has shown the need for caution in accepting it as a universal trend. Resolution of some statistical difficulties resulted in 'artificial' IQs based on the standard deviations of the test for the age groups tested, but there remain errors from other sources, in particular individual rates of change in growth and deterioration and the effects of early learning, influenced as it is by enriched or impoverished environments, on intellectual growth. The IQ as a measure of ability in adults is falling into disuse and in the case of children requires qualification and interpretation if it is to serve as a useful guide in education.

It may also be possible to form some opinion, based on these tests, of the relation between the patient's efficiency and his potential ability or between his present function and his former efficiency, but these opinions cannot always be expressed quantitatively or with the same degree of confidence as the estimate of his global intelligence. However, they are important observations and may be pointers to the need for further investigation. Also they will have refined the questions to be answered by additional investigation.

2 *Sub-scales and tests of specific processes*, e.g. of learning, of memory, of concept formation, yield more precise information on these functions and enable discrimination to be made, for example, between recall of material presented visually and that presented aurally, or they may throw some light on the patient's rigidity or flexibility of thought. Such data have relevance for the diagnosis of various psychiatric conditions as well as for the rehabilitation of patients in psychiatry and other branches of medicine.

Consequently, where there are complaints of intellectual difficulties, or impaired concentration or memory, which could be due to psychological or neurological causes, standardized tests of memory and learning ability, as well as intelligence tests, are used to assist in differentiating between them.

Children referred for investigation are always given intelligence tests, since the level of their ability affects their adaptive behaviour and their acquisition of skills. School backwardness is associated with many psychiatric problems in childhood, and it is important to know the level of a child's intelligence in order to have reasonable expectations of him, both as regards attainments and rate of progress.

3 *Tests of aptitudes or attainment*, e.g. of mechanical ability, of language skills, may provide a basis for educational guidance and vocational guidance and rehabilitation. Lack of adjustment between a person's abilities, achievements and aspirations is fertile ground for the development of personal and social maladjustment. Therefore information on their assets and deficits is often required before a sound programme for their treatment can be drawn up. While problems of this kind are frequently found in psychiatric practice they are by no means confined to it, nor even to a patient population. Such methods, as well as being used in clinical work, are also used by occupational and educational psychologists.

Personality tests

1 *Inventories, questionnaires and other direct methods* by which information about the patient's symptoms, attitudes, interests, experience, aspirations and relationships, are elicited and brought together in an orderly form — providing material which may be treated statistically. Data of this kind lends itself to comparative studies, e.g. of patients in different diagnostic categories, and also contributes to a body of knowledge on personality development and the probable associations between character traits and different symptom formations; e.g. the Maudsley Personality Inventory devised by Eysenck gives a measure of patients' neuroticism and extroversion.

2 *Projective techniques.* In these the material is presented to the patient, usually in pictorial form, e.g. inkblots in the Rorschach, human situations in the Thematic Apperception Test (T.A.T.), pictorial material in the Object Relations Test; it is comparatively vague, unstructured and ambiguous, so that he is led to interpret it in terms of his own unconscious attitudes and expectations, feelings, and fantasies. They thus provide

information about the patient which, often, could not be obtained either from interview or questionnaires.

Data of this kind are less susceptible to quantification but the techniques offer a holistic approach to the study of personality which often leads to further understanding of intra- and inter-personal stress, individual needs of a psychological nature and the ways in which a patient interprets and structures his personal environment. Thus projective techniques enable the psychologist to build up a picture of the patient's personality, and may be helpful in differentiating between various kinds of neurotic and psychotic disturbances and in gaining a picture of the major defence mechanisms used by the patient.

3 *Individual experiments.* Tests have been constructed and standardized for the assessment of many facets and features of human behaviour. Nevertheless, the clinical psychologist lacks techniques suitable for investigation of other questions which arise, as problems are differentiated. In order to refine his methods he then uses experimental devices of his own invention based on psychological principles. These can yield useful data, but in an unstandardized form until they become validated and their reliability is investigated. Problems which might require such methods of investigation include those of patients who have suffered a cerebral accident as a result of which they cannot easily express a conceptualized response, or patients with unusual combinations of handicaps or those from different cultural backgrounds for whom the tests and questions comprising standardized tests might have different meaning or relevance.

Links between investigation and treatment

The psychologist's investigation, by cognitive and personality testing, of the aetiology of a patient's symptoms is of interest beyond the diagnostic stage since the origin of symptoms may affect the kind of treatment chosen. More generally, the psychologist may help in assessing whether a patient by reason of his personality is suitable for one type of treatment or another; whether there is any likelihood of psychotic breakdown during psychotherapy; in what sense the personality is functioning effectively; and how the patient is likely to react to situations of stress.

Results of investigations are discussed with colleagues concerned with the patient, not only to help elucidate his problem
but so that the relevance of the finding to his treatment may be
considered. Some of the data is relevant to symptoms and
present issues, some to the ongoing personality growth and
adjustment of the individual. As discussed elsewhere (see p.
22) pathology cannot be studied apart from the person in
whom it occurs. At times communication about it can be
complicated, but doctors, nurses, occupational therapists or
whoever may be involved are likely to get a better response to
their treatment of the patient's pathology when they take
account also of his motivation, his abilities, skills and temperament which bear on his cooperation and their interpersonal
relationship.

Staff discussion is therefore essential to relate psychological
and other findings before a decision about treatment is reached.
Subsequently, when necessary, discussions at a different level
are held with those who have some further responsibility
towards the patient, e.g. relative, teacher, employer, to ensure
that maximum use is made of knowledge gained about the
assets and deficits of the patient's personality. For example, it is
common practice for psychologists to visit the schools of
children who become patients. It is helpful to learn from his
teachers something about the social and psychological climate
in which a child is working and to try to assess possible sources
of stress for him in his work or play; and by giving teachers
further insight into his difficulties and potentialities some
modification of his environment may result which is therapeutic
in its effect. Other aspects of the psychologist's role, in treatment and in research, are discussed on p. 336.

FURTHER READING

Anastasi, A. (1961). *Psychological Testing*, Macmillan, New York.
Bannister, D. M. and Mair, J. M. M. (1968). *The Evaluation of Personal
Constructs*. Academic Press, London.
Dixon, N. F. (1971). *Subliminal Perception: The Nature of a Controversy*.
McGraw Hill, London.
Hetherington, R. R., Miller, D. H., and Neville, J. G. (1964). *Introduction
to Psychology for Medical Students*. Heinemann, London.
Summerfield, A. (ed.) (1971) 'Cognitive psychology'. *Brit. Med. Bulletin*,
27, 3.

4 Basic principles

There are two main approaches to psychiatry, the organic and the psychodynamic (psychosocial) approaches, both of which play an important part in understanding and managing patients with psychiatric illnesses often in various combinations depending on the patient's personality and the nature of his particular disorder.

The organic approach, which like the rest of medicine is concerned with anatomical, physiological and biochemical abnormalities, deals with the physical basis of mental disease, either disorders of the brain itself (e.g. senile dementia and biochemical processes underlying mental disease) or cerebral dysfunction due to systemic disorders (e.g. myxoedema madness). In treatment the organic approach emphasises physical methods, e.g. the use of drugs or ECT.

The psychodynamic or psychosocial approach attempts to understand the patient's mental disorder in terms of his personality development, his present personality make-up and the way he reacts to stressful factors in his environment, especially his family, other close relationships, work situations and society in general; this approach applies particularly to the psychoneuroses and personality disorders. In treatment it emphasises the use of psychological methods, especially psychotherapy, and of social measures. The student will already be familiar with the basis of the organic approach, so more will be said here about the basis of the psychodynamic approach.

The field of psychodynamics in general is concerned with the study of the mental or psychological processes in health and disease, and tries to understand these in terms of personality development and the influence of personal experience. In psychodynamics these psychological processes are considered in their own right and no attempt is made to translate them into physiological terms, although all human psychological experience ultimately depends on cerebral function.

Dynamic psychopathology refers more specifically to the

study of the psychological processes responsible for abnormal mental states. Normal and abnormal psychodynamics overlap considerably and knowledge of the former is partly derived from clinical observation of patients undergoing psychotherapy. The methodology of the psychodynamic approach differs from that of the natural sciences in so far as it is only partly concerned with objectively observable and measurable phenomena such as behaviour. In so far as it deals with the detailed study of the development of individual personalities and their inner, subjective experience, including especially their feelings and fantasies, its approach often has to be biographical and descriptive and in these respects measurement and controlled experiments are sometimes not applicable.

HISTORICAL DEVELOPMENT

The systematic study of psychopathology originated with Sigmund Freud's work on hysteria (Breuer and Freud, *Studies in Hysteria*, 1895). Although greatly influenced by these early discoveries of psycho-analysis, especially the importance of unconscious mental phenomena and of childhood development, psychopathology has developed a great deal since. Freud's early emphasis on biological instincts (drives), especially sexuality and aggression, as the basis for understanding the human personality has become modified as the result of his own later findings and those of other psycho-analysts, psychotherapists and psychologists (see p. 308). There has been an increasing interest in the more conscious and rational aspects of the personality (ego psychology), especially under the influence of Anna Freud and Heinz Hartman, and in problems of human interaction and the influence of society. Melanie Klein has stressed the importance of very early developmental processes in infancy in relation to such objects as parts of the mother's body and later the whole person of the mother (object relationships). The Neo-Freudians have stressed the importance of the human personality as a whole functioning unit and its relationship to the culture in which it lives; Erikson has drawn attention to the process of identity formation, especially in adolescence, and existentialist psychiatrists have emphasised the need to understand the patient's actual experience and his mode of existence in the world in which he lives. Most psychiatrists now accept certain basic concepts, which can be summarized more or less as follows.

BASIC CONCEPTS

1 All psychological functions have their organic basis in the person's constitutional and acquired physical make-up but in psychodynamics we are concerned with the psychological phenomena themselves.

2 The personality develops as a result of biological maturation and is profoundly influenced by early childhood experiences in the family and later experiences in inter-personal relationships outside the family and in society.

3 The manner in which one handles one's sexual and aggressive drives influences to a large extent the function of one's personality in health and disease.

4 Knowledge of *unconscious* mental processes is essential for understanding normal and abnormal psychological functioning including, for example, dreams, slips of the tongue, and forgetting. Unconscious mental phenomena may be partly innate but they are in part the result of *repression* of ideas and affects which have once been conscious. The unconscious often finds expression in one's dreams and in neurotic symptoms in symbolic form (symbolism) (see p. 33).

5 Freud developed the concept of three aspects of human personality structure, the *id*, *ego* and *superego*; these are sometimes referred to as three parts of the 'mental apparatus'. However, it is better to think of these not as structural entities but as useful terms for describing certain aspects of psychological functioning. The *id* is a term used to describe the basic, inborn drives, especially sexual and aggressive impulses demanding immediate gratification (pleasure principle). The term *ego* is used to describe the more rational, controlling aspects, partly conscious and partly unconscious, of the personality which control the id impulses and adapt them to the demands of the environment (reality principle) and of the *superego*. The latter comprises our conscience and ideals, which are derived from parental and cultural influences through a process of introjection and identification from early childhood onwards.

APPLICATIONS OF PSYCHODYNAMIC CONCEPTS

1 Psychodynamic concepts help us to understand the nature of the human personality as a whole, including inner experience and outward behaviour in health and disease.

2 They throw light on the nature of human interaction, e.g. between parents and children, between marriage partners and in society in general.

3 A special case of this is the relationship between doctor and patient. Patients, whether suffering from physical or psychiatric disorders, tend to re-experience emotional reactions which are originally directed towards members of their own families, especially parents in childhood, in relationship to their doctors. Such *transference* phenomena occur in all human relationships but they are especially important in psychotherapy and psycho-analysis (see p. 309). Similar inappropriate reactions of the doctor to his patient are known as his *counter-transference*.

4 All psychotherapy, especially its major forms such as analytically orientated psychotherapy, is based on psychodynamic concepts.

5 The aetiology of the psychoneuroses (anxiety states, phobic states, conversion hysteria, neurotic depression and obsessional neurosis) and the meaning of psychoneurotic symptoms are best understood in psychodynamic terms.

6 The same applies to the personality disorders, e.g. immature, hysterical, obsessional and schizoid personalities, and sexual disorders.

7 The symptomatology of the functional psychoses (schizophrenic reactions, affective disorders) can often be understood in psychodynamic terms although a combination of organic, social and psychological factors may all play a part in their origin.

8 In patients with psychosomatic symptoms, i.e. physical symptoms in which emotional stress has contributed to the development of organic disease (e.g. irritable bowel syndrome, ulcerative colitis, peptic ulcer) the nature of the underlying conflicts is best understood in psychodynamic terms, although the mechanism responsible for the organic lesion has a physical basis (p. 173).

THE PSYCHOLOGY OF DREAMS

One of Freud's most important and original discoveries was his psycho-analytic theory of dreams. He found that by asking patients to free-associate about their dreams, repressed unconscious material could be brought back into consciousness; he thus called the analysis of dreams 'the royal road to the Unconscious'. In *The Interpretation of Dreams* (1900) he analysed many of his own dreams and formulated his theory.

Briefly, he considered that the dream expresses unconscious impulses and wishes, often using material from events of the previous day, the so-called day residue; but the unconscious or 'latent' dream content is modified or disguised by the so-called censor which converts it into the actual or 'manifest' dream. This process of converting the latent into the manifest dream he called dream work. This makes use especially of symbolization so that an object does not itself appear in the dream but is represented by a symbol; for example, a house might represent mother, or climbing a staircase and reaching the top may symbolize reaching a climax during a sexual relationship. The latent meaning may also be hidden by so-called displacement when, for example, an aggressive intention which is really the dreamer's own, is attributed to an unknown stranger in the dream; condensation is a third process observed in dreams and refers to the fact that several different meanings may all be represented by one dream image. Through free-association the latent meaning hidden behind the manifest dream can be rediscovered. Freud also stated that dreams are hallucinatory wish fulfilments, and by allowing wishes, which might otherwise wake him up, apparently to be fulfilled while the person is asleep, the dream acts as a 'guardian of sleep'.

Recent physiological studies have confirmed several of Freud's views (Hawkins 1966), namely that everyone dreams, that a great deal of what has been dreamt is repressed and hence forgotten, and also that dreaming is accompanied by motor inhibition, by diminished arousal and reduced awareness of external stimuli, while there is increased activity in the cortex and in the vegetative nervous system, and often sexual stimulation, depending on the dream content. Thus it has been shown by EEG studies (Dement and Kleitman 1957) during sleep that at regular intervals the individual enters a stage during which the EEG shows asynchronous, rapid, low voltage activity accompanied by rapid eye movements (stage 1, REM sleep); these stages occur approximately every 90 minutes several times during the night, and in an adult they occupy about 20% of the total night's sleep. If an individual is awakened during such a phase he will report vivid dreams but if he is woken some time after the REM sleep is over, a large proportion of the dreams will have been forgotten. Measurement of skin resistance and muscle tone have shown that arousal is usually diminished and that there is widespread motor paralysis during REM sleep, and in males there is often evidence of penile erection. The theory that the function of dreaming is to guard sleep is only partially true because, if an individual is woken up each time he enters a phase of REM sleep for several nights running, he will not only show signs of mental irritability during the day, but during the first night he is allowed to sleep undisturbed he will make up for the amount of dream or REM sleep lost by spending a proportionately longer part of the night's sleep in this stage. Similarly, the amount of REM sleep is reduced by drugs like barbiturates or dexamphetamine, and when the drug is stopped the deficit is made up in subsequent nights.

In other words, dreaming appears to be a necessary phenomenon in its own right in addition to preventing the individual from waking. Freud's original view that all dreams are wish fulfilments has also had to be modified in as far as dreams seem to have a wider psychological function, expressing many of the individual's conflicts and his attempts at solving them. It is also often possible to understand the meaning of a manifest dream without necessarily having to trace it back to an underlying latent content; and although symbolism undoubtedly plays a very important part in dreaming, and for that matter in many other human mental processes, one symbol may have many different meanings, depending on each individual's past and present experience and the culture he belongs to. In spite of these modifications of Freud's original dream theory it is remarkable how much of it still holds and has in fact received confirmation from modern physiological studies.

REFERENCES (*on dreaming*)

Dement, W. C., and Kleitman, N. (1957). 'Relation of eye movements during sleep to dream activitiy: an objective method for the study of dreaming'. *J. Exp. Psychol.*, 53, 339.
Freud, S. (1900). *The Interpretation of Dreams.* Standard edition, Hogarth Press, London (1955), vols. 4 and 5.
Hawkins, D. R. (1966). 'A review of psychoanalytic dream theory in the light of recent psycho-physiological studies of sleep and dreaming'. *Brit. J. Med. Psychol.*, 39, 85.
Oswald, I. (1966). *Sleep.* Penguin.
Oswald, I. (1970). 'Sleep, dreams and drugs', in Price, J. H. (ed.), *Modern Trends in Psychological Medicine* II, Butterworth, London.
Ratna, L. (1973). 'Psychophysiological aspects of dreaming'. *Brit. J. Hosp. Med.*, 9, 203.

For further reading see p. 36.

5 Personality development

INTRODUCTION

Personality development starts from the genetically endowed biological organism of the newly born infant and continues until this has been transformed into the adult personality under the influence of biological maturation and the formative influences of experience arising from human and social interaction.

Knowledge of personality development is important for the understanding of mental processes (psychodynamics); abnormal development may lead to pathological mental processes (psychopathology) which may, in combination with biological factors and environmental stress, lead to symptom formation and psychiatric and psychosomatic illness. Our knowledge of human personality development is based on several disciplines: direct observation of children (Piaget), prospective studies, learning theory and experimental psychology, psycho-analysis and related analytical schools, and on social and anthropological observations.

STAGES OF DEVELOPMENT

1 *Stage of absolute dependence of the infant on its mother*

This is the symbiotic phase or period of primary identification. There is no sense of separate 'self' as yet. Failure on the part of mother or mother-substitute threatens the baby with total annihilation. Compare symptoms of extreme dependence, severe anxiety ('existential anxiety') and depersonalization in psychiatric disorders, confusion of identity in schizophrenia and the effects of drugs (LSD), toxic states and sensory deprivation.

2 *Gradual development of a sense of separate existence (self)*

Persistent dependence on parents now gives rise to fear of loss of security and affection, so-called *separation anxiety*. Children at this stage normally get attached to soft toys, like a teddy bear, a rag, blanket or doll which they insist on having with them; so-called transitional objects (Winnicott 1971) which take the place of parts of mother or of their own thumbs. Ill effects occur from separating children from their mothers, e.g. by hospitalization (Bowlby): infants separated from their mothers for more than a day or two pass after a period of protest and acute despair into apathy and depression (hospitalism). On rejoining their mother they fail to recognize her and become anxious, clinging children. These effects are most marked if separation takes place between six months and three years but harmful results may occur in older children up to the age of five or six. Institutionalization has similar immediate and long-term effects on personality development. *Maternal deprivation* is, however, not necessarily due to physical separation but is often experienced by children whose mother is not sufficiently affectionate or consistent (Rutter, 1972). Whatever its cause, maternal deprivation may lead to neurotic symptoms like bed-wetting, nightmares and disturbed behaviour at the time, and then to developmental, including intellectual, retardation, asocial behaviour, delinquency or to increased liability to anxiety states and depressive reactions in later life. Similar observations have been made in animal studies by separating newly born monkeys from their mothers and following their behaviour and development (Harlow 1961).

3 *Mother and father experienced as either 'good' or 'bad'*

The infant experiences the good mother who pleases him as separate from the bad mother who displeases him. *Introjection* of good experiences lays the basis for future trust, of bad, disappointing or painful experiences for future mistrust. Both are inevitable in childhood but a preponderance of good experiences is essential for future healthy development. The child's aggressive feelings directed against the frustrating mother also lead to fear of punishment and rejection (*persecutory anxiety*). *Projection* of these early experiences on to others influences our future relationships. Compare, for example, neurotic fears, paranoid delusions and marital maladjustment.

4 *Emergence of a sense of concern for others*

The good and bad aspects of the parent (mother) are now experienced as belonging to one and the same person. This leads to feelings of love and hate directed towards the same person (ambivalence) with resultant feelings of concern for the person who is loved and needed, and guilt feelings on account of associated angry feelings or actions, real or phantasied. An exaggerated sense of guilt (superego), usually the result of excessive disapproval or punishment by the parents, may lead to future psychiatric illness, especially depression or obsessional neurosis.

5 *Special importance of feeding experiences in the mother-child relationship (oral stage)*

Feeding is not only a means of satisfying hunger but is also a pleasurable activity. The mother's attitude towards the child at this stage profoundly affects the child's relationship to her. Satisfactory oral experiences lead to pleasure in which the mouth is the main organ for pleasurable contact with mother, associated with passive receptiveness and active taking in (sucking). This lays the basis for a trusting, accepting relationship to mother and good, trusting relationships in later life. Frustrating experiences lead to demandingness and angry biting and screaming attacks, or to food refusal. Such early reactions may adversely influence future character formation or lead to symptom formation. Note e.g. greed, demandingness and compulsive over-eating in some depressive patients and anorexia and withdrawal from all human contact in others. Note also the influence of emotions on gastric function as in 'nervous indigestion', hysterical vomiting and in the development of peptic ulceration (see p. 183).

6 *Special importance of excretory functions and toilet training in the mother-child relationship (anal stage)*

The child now develops an interest in its own excretory products, in the processes of retaining and expelling and in gaining control over these functions. Simple encouragement and approval on the part of the mother allows the child to attain such mastery over his sphincters at his own pace by a process of identification based on the natural wish to please her and get her affection and approval. Too rigid and controlling an attitude on the part of the mother makes the child rebel and it may use its excretory functions as weapons in a battle against her (*battle for autonomy*), e.g. constipation, soiling or bed-wetting. These early experiences may also affect future character formation. Compare adult character traits of obstinacy, or of extreme submissiveness and compliance. The wish to make a mess may survive in later life or may be suppressed with resultant obsessional tidiness and perfectionism (reaction formation). Note the concept of unconscious fixation at, and regression to the anal stage in patients with obsessional symptoms. Note also the effect of emotions on adult bowel function as in constipation, functional diarrhoea and the irritable bowel syndrome (see p. 184). The child's need to develop and fight for its own autonomy is, however, by no means only experienced in relation to toilet training but applies at least as much to other activities like eating, playing, talking, motor activity and other forms of self expression.

7 *Increasing interest in genital organs and sexual fantasies (autoerotic activities)*

An attitude of acceptance on the part of parents of these normal interests and of auto-erotic activities in childhood lays the basis for future positive attitudes to sexuality. A punitive, puritanical parental attitude leads to fear of punishment for forbidden sexual pleasure, to anxiety and guilt feelings associated with sexual activity. Note 'castration anxiety' in boys and corresponding anxieties concerning their feminine attractiveness and sexual and reproductive functions in girls. Girls may also develop envy of the male role, so-called penis envy, especially in families and cultures in which there is a marked preference for the male members of society. Hence arise such later symptoms as masturbation guilt, impotence, frigidity, difficulties in accepting one's sexual role, or compulsive promiscuity to prove one's ability to attract the opposite sex and to function adequately in sexual relationships (reaction formation). Anxieties may also get attached to other pleasurable activities endowed with sexual significance.

8 *The Oedipal stage (age 3 to 5)*

Strong sexual feelings towards the parent of the opposite sex lead to competition with, and jealousy of the parent of the same sex. Persistent feelings of love and affection towards the latter lead to ambivalence and fear of rejection or punishment, which in the boy may cause castration anxiety. Sublimation, postponement of gratification and identification with the parent of the same sex leads to resolution of the Oedipal conflict and thus to further strengthening of one's own biological, sexual role. Failure of such identification, or identification with the parent of the opposite sex, may lead to uncertainty about one's sexual role and homosexuality. Persistent fixation on the parent of the opposite sex may interfere with the choice of a satisfactory partner outside the family in later life.

9 *Increasing importance of social influence outside the family (so-called latency period)*

A growing sense of identity and healthy self-image arises out of further satisfactory identifications, now with persons outside the family, teachers, friends, etc. There is a need for encouragement and sense of achievement in personal, educational and athletic activities. Excessive pressure or criticism by parents and teachers and the imposition of alien or contradictory expectations ('double binding') may interfere with identity formation and lead to withdrawal into a fantasy life, the adoption of false roles and social isolation, often with feelings of depression (schizoid personality).

10 *Adolescence* (see also p. 242)

The physiological changes associated with puberty lead to important new problems in development. These include the following. Sexuality becomes a practical reality leading to capacity for orgasm, masturbation, and a desire for sexual relationships, homosexual or heterosexual. The problem of fusing tenderness and affection with sexuality arises. How these sexual needs are dealt with depends to a large extent on previous experiences at earlier stages of development and the attitude of the parents and society towards the adolescent. At the same time there arises a struggle for independence from parents, often in conflict with persistent dependency needs. The struggle for independence leads to rebellion, rejection of past values and identifications derived from the family, and to the need to be an accepted member of one's peer group instead, and to experiment with new values and identifications. The outcome of these developments is a growing awareness of an independent identity of one's own. Failure may lead to an adolescent crisis, often marked by depression, disturbed behaviour and sometimes by an overt psychiatric illness.

11 *Concept of healthy adulthood (not a final achievement but subject to further progressive and retrogressive changes)*

The following are some of the characteristics of a healthy adult which arise from satisfactory experiences at earlier stages of development: a satisfactory sense of identity and self-image; a capacity for adaptation to society without undue conformity; concern for others, and an ability to tolerate frustration, losses, sadness, conflict, anxiety and guilt without the breakdown of defences and the development of psychiatric illness; a capacity to fuse affection with sexuality, to show anger and to make reparation, and to express one's potentialities in work and pleasure.

For further reading see p. 36.

6 Symptom formation and mechanisms of defence

Symptoms are liable to develop when psychological conflicts are in danger of disturbing the dynamic equilibrium necessary for the normal functioning of the personality within its social setting. Conflicts often arise from stressful situations in relation to other people or to society but such *external conflict* situations lead to *internal conflicts* and it is the latter, often reinforced by past conflicts reawakened by the present situation, which may cause a breakdown of defences and symptom formation. Such intra-psychic conflicts may exist between opposing instinctual (*id*) impulses such as love and hate directed towards the same person (object), or between one's instinctual wishes, the id, and one's conscience or superego. Such conflicts are often partly or wholly unconscious but they give rise to anxiety which acts as a danger signal. How such conflicts are dealt with depends largely on the person's ego strength. Normally the underlying conflicts, if sufficiently conscious, and the accompanying normal anxiety are dealt with by realistic action, by sublimation, by postponing gratification and by tolerating normal degrees of frustration, anxiety, guilt and depression. This is helped by favourable factors in the environment including the support of others.

If these methods fail, as may be the case in people whose personality development has been disturbed or if present day stresses are excessive and insoluble, the anxiety may persist and become excessive, and symptoms of an *anxiety state* may develop, often accompanied by somatic manifestations of anxiety such as palpitations, sweating, trembling, diarrhoea or insomnia and these may lead to secondary anxiety. If the anxiety is repressed the patient may develop symptoms of *conversion hysteria* or of an *obsessional neurosis* instead. If the anxiety has followed a loss or is due to guilt feelings associated with aggression a *neurotic depression* may develop. In practice several of these psychoneurotic manifestations may co-exist in the same patient e.g. an anxiety state with depression or a mixture of hysterical symptoms and anxiety, so called anxiety-hysteria. Persistent unresolved intra-psychic conflict may also lead to *psychosomatic disease* with organic pathology. Withdrawal from the painful reality situation into the world of fantasy may lead to *psychotic states* with delusions and hallucinations.

The details of psychological symptom formation are sometimes best understood in terms of the so-called *mechanisms of defence* employed by the ego in its effort to deal with the threatening inner conflicts. These defence mechanisms should be regarded as descriptive terms referring to observable psychological phenomena. They play a part in normal mental functioning but their excessive or inappropriate use or their failure may give rise to psychiatric symptoms. For example, some degree of repression of sexual wishes is normal, too great a degree may lead to neurotic inhibition, complete lack of repression may lead to uninhibited expression of sexual wishes and socially unacceptable behaviour. The following are some of the *ego mechanisms of defence* that have been described. They are not mutually exclusive; they are not always successful.

Repression

Being totally unconscious of such inner impulses as wanting to be aggressive, sexually promiscuous, etc. The repressed impulse may find symbolic expression in the patient's symptoms, e.g. in conversion hysteria where the symptom may represent in symbolic form both the repressed wish and the defence against it, e.g. a patient with a hysterical paraplegia may simultaneously draw attention to the sexual, lower half of her body while at the same time indicating the complete absence of any sensations or movements in this part of her body. (In contrast to repression, suppression means being conscious of inner impulses but controlling their outward expression.)

Denial

Consists of being unaware of an external reality situation, e.g. denying that a close relative has actually died as in psychotic states. It is also used to describe the tendency to deny feelings and thoughts of which one is in fact almost, if not entirely aware.

Displacement

Displacing an affect from one object to whom it originally belonged on to another, e.g. no longer being aware of feeling angry with one person but being angry with someone else or damaging an inanimate object instead.

Isolation

Isolating a thought from its appropriate affect, e.g. having aggressive thoughts without the expected accompanying feelings of anger.

Magic undoing

If, for example, someone believes that his aggressive thoughts could magically lead to someone else's death, magic undoing would consist of having a loving thought or carrying out some ritual instead in the belief that this would magically protect the object of one's aggressive thoughts from danger. Commonly seen in the obsessional neuroses but also in superstitions and primitive religious ceremonials.

Reaction formation

Behaving in a manner which is the opposite to forbidden, repressed desires, e.g. being excessively clean and perfectionist as a reaction against the wish to make a mess, or being non-aggressive and submissive as a reaction against the repressed wish to destroy and dominate.

Introjection

Dealing with the loss of someone's affection by introjecting his attitudes and personality, e.g. feeling that one has acquired the characteristics of a close relative who has died, thus making oneself feel that one has not completely lost him.

Identification

A similar process but extending further to actually becoming like the other person. This plays an important part in normal personality development but also leads to neurotic symptoms, e.g. in hysterics who develop someone else's symptoms by identification. This process also plays a part in normal mourning and in depression following a bereavement when the patient feels identified with the deceased.

Projection

Attributing one's own feelings and thoughts to someone else, e.g. being unaware of feeling angry but attributing one's angry feelings to someone else so that one feels persecuted by him, as in paranoid states.

Fantasy

Day dreaming is often used as a compensation for feelings of inadequacy or disappointment.

Regression

Regressing to earlier childlike stages of development and reacting and behaving accordingly; e.g. a child of eight may under stress wet his bed and revert to thumb-sucking.

Rationalization

Explaining one's actions and attitudes by distorting the facts and by producing false intellectual excuses, i.e. being dishonest with oneself, a common mechanism in every day life; e.g. by finding high-sounding reasons for why one has lost one's temper.

Sublimation

Attempting to deal with one's socially unacceptable aggressive or sexual wishes by developing socially more acceptable outlets, e.g. sport as an outlet for aggression or male friendships as a sublimation for homosexual wishes.

Reparation

Being helpful and constructive to make up for one's destructive impulses. This may be a source of creative activity.

Although these mechanisms of defence are useful in our understanding of some normal and abnormal psychological phenomena they have descriptive rather than explanatory value and sometimes symptom formation is better understood in terms of disturbance of the whole personality, e.g. failure of identity formation, adoption of false roles under external pressure, alienation from one's 'true self' or from one's personal or cultural background, withdrawal from one's inner experience leading to a sense of inner emptiness and depersonalization, or withdrawal from reality into a compensatory fantasy life or a psychosis.

FURTHER READING (sections 4, 5 and 6)

Bowlby, J. (1965). *Child Care and the Growth of Love.* Penguin.
Bowlby, J. (1969). *Attachment and Loss I: Attachment.* Hogarth, London.
Brown, J. A. C. (1961). *Freud and the Post-Freudians.* Penguin.
Cameron, N. (1963). *Personality Development and Psychopathology: Dynamic Approach.* Houghton Mifflin, Boston.
Erikson, E. H. (1950). *Childhood and Society.* Norton, New York.
Freud, A. (1936). *The Ego and the Mechanisms of Defence.* Hogarth, London.
Freud, S. (1949). *An Outline of Psycho-analysis.* Hogarth, London.
Harlow, H. F. (1961). 'The development of affectional systems in infant monkey's. In Foss, B.A. (ed.), *Determinants of Infant Behaviour*, Methuen, London, p. 75.
Laing, R. D. (1959). *The Divided Self.* Tavistock Publications, London.
Rutter, M. (1972). *Maternal Deprivation Reassessed.* Penguin.
Winnicott, D. W. (1959). *The Family and Individual Development.* Tavistock Publications, London.
Winnicott, D. W. (1964). *The Child, the Family and the Outside World.* Penguin.
Winnicott, D. W. (1965). *The Maturational Processes and the Facilitating Environment.* Hogarth, London.
Winnicott, D. W. (1971). *Playing and Reality.* Penguin.

PART THREE   THE PHYSICAL BASIS OF MENTAL
ACTIVITY

7 The development of the brain*

The last part of this book gave some account of the human
being's psychological development, and the various healthy and
unhealthy reactions which might occur under stress. These
reactions are associated with physiological changes; although
the precise relationship of mind and body is still the subject for
argument, it is obvious that gross physical defect or disease
affects psychological growth and function. While the central
nervous system is not the only physical system involved, it is
the most important and its development and function are
therefore briefly described next.

Man shares with other animals a genetic system which
involves diploidy in the cells of the body, reduction of the
chromosome number during the formation of gametes, and
sexual union of gametes to produce a fertilized egg in which the
chromosome number is again diploid, one half being derived
from each parent. In the differentiation of the egg these same
chromosomes pass into every cell, irrespective of tissue. The
development of all the varieties of cells and tissues must involve
the simultaneous and co-ordinated operation of large numbers
of genes and circular interactions between genes and cytoplasm,
by which the former determine the specificity of protein
molecules being synthesized in the cell, while the cytoplasm is
immediately responsible for deciding which complexes of genes
shall be active (Waddington 1956). In this system we have every
reason to suppose that other epigenetic factors as well as genes
are important in man although they have only been demonstrated in animals. They are fundamental in the establishment
of the neural plate on a particular site of the early embryo, the

* (The following account consists of extracts from Professor J. F.
Smith's 'Development of the brain', published in Tredgold's *Textbook of
Mental Deficiency*, Eleventh Edition, edited by R. F. Tredgold and K. Soddy,
Baillière, Tindall and Cassell, London, 1970. We are very grateful to the
author, publishers and editors for permission to quote from it here.)

esssential thing being an ability of the ectoderm to respond to, or be induced by, an underlying chordomesoderm. In this *organization* two factors are recognized: an active chemical substance or *evocator* and certain gradients in the responding tissues which are referred to as *individuation fields*.

The neural plate first appears in man in the late presomite stage; with the appearance of somites it has formed a groove and by the 7-somite stage (3 weeks) the groove has become a neural tube, the cephalic two-thirds of which will form the future brain. Glucksmann (1951) has observed that in this process there is not only cell proliferation but numerous cell degenerations and deaths. At 20 somites the anterior end of the tube has closed and its brain part shows three dilatations, the cavities of the fore-, mid- and hind-brains. Diverticula from the forebrain are the optic vesicles, which by the 5 mm stage have become optic cups. Soon after this the cerebral or telencephalic vesicles appear on either side of the forebrain and the flexures between the main parts become more accentuated. At 15 mm (6 weeks) medulla oblongata with caudal cranial nerves, primordium of cerebellum and cerebral hemispheres are recognizable. As the latter expand they grow backwards over the diencephalon and mid-brain so that their caudal ends approximate to the developing cerebellum but are separated from it by a condensation of connective tissue which forms the tentorium cerebelli. By 50 mm (12 weeks) the future lobes of the cerebrum can be roughly identified while a depressed area in the lateral aspect is the future insula.

Meanwhile the primitive medullary epithelial lining of the neural tube has differentiated into three zones — an inner marginal or ependymal layer, an intermediate mantle or nuclear layer, and an outer marginal zone which is at first devoid of cell nuclei. Some medullary epithelial cells remain attached to the inner limiting membrane of the tube and form ependymal lining cells of the central canal of the spinal cord and the ventricular system; others remain attached for a time by cytoplasmic processes to inner and outer limiting membranes of the tube and develop into spongioblasts which later will divide to form astrocytes, the supporting cells of the nervous tissue. Other medullary cells lose their attachment to both limiting membranes early and form the so-called germinal cells which can give rise to generations of cells which by subsequent differentiation may become either definitive nerve cells or further supporting cells.

At the 50 mm stage described above there has already been a complex development of nervous tissue lining the cavities of the brain to form the beginnings of such masses as the pons, mid-brain, thalamus and basal ganglia as well as a migration of neuroblasts from the mantle layer outside the marginal layer to form the cortical grey matter. At the 50 mm stage this sheet of cells extends over the entire hemisphere. In the later months of foetal life these neuroblasts differentiate into neurones and become arranged into the layered pattern of the adult, eventually forming 6 layers, the outer two of which constitute the neopallium, being peculiar to the higher mammals.

PATHOLOGICAL PROCESSES AND REACTION PATTERNS

The formation, development and maturation of the brain can be disturbed by abnormalities in the genes of the parents, by changes in the chromosomes as they disperse and reunite in the fertilized egg, by distortion of other epigenetic factors (i.e. the causal processes of normal development), and through a variety of environmental agents. The latter may act not only in foetal life but also in the natal and post-natal period, for the brain is not biologically mature until at least the end of the second year. (Maturity in terms of behaviour is more difficult to limit.)

The operation of the abnormal factors indicated in the preceding paragraph may lead to gross malformation of the brain, to damage of the developed organ or to a combination of these things. Such lesions are present perhaps only in a quarter of institutionalized mental defectives (Berg 1959), but occur in the vast majority of cases with severe defect (Crome 1954).

It is not possible to draw up an accurate time scale and indicate from the nature of the morbid anatomical change the time at which the damage occurred. This is because some factors cause a gradual retardation of growth and not a sudden cessation of development. Furthermore, the capacity for repair varies at different periods of development – this has been brought out clearly by study of the lesions produced in embryos by X-ray injury. However, certain points can be made, and an upper limit for the development of some lesions can be given. Thus an absence of cortical gyri — so-called pachygyria or lissencephaly — indicates an abnormality occurring before the end of the fourth month of foetal life when gyral formation is well under way.

Injury to the early embryonic brain is likely to cause malformation or suppression of growth but significant residual scarring is exceptional. This may be because the glia cells are not fully developed or because immunological tolerance is present. Furthermore, the existence of 'morphogenetic degeneration' of nervous tissue during early development indicates some mechanism for disposal of dead tissue without leaving any trace of it. Most of the investigations from which this paucity of residual reaction in the early embryo is deduced are on animal experiments with X-rays, hypoxia and other agents. It is unfortunate that detailed descriptions of the brain damaged by rubella in the second to fourth months of foetal life are scanty. Here the clinical history and the associated cataract (lens formation at second month) or deafness (organ of Corti at third month) enable the time of injury to be dated.

More significant scarring is seen in late foetal and neonatal life. If the cause of damage to nervous tissue is hypoxic or ischaemic the reaction is mainly by mononuclear phagocytes which take up lipid and pigment and by astrocytes which can form areas of gliosis. Such injury is rare in the late foetal period but can be important at the time of birth or in the early neonatal period (see p. 56). If the brain is damaged by an infective agent, inflammatory cells such as lymphocytes and plasma cells can appear in the nervous tissue and meninges. Rare causes of this in the late foetal period are toxoplasmosis and cytomegalic inclusion disease. In infancy and childhood, viral infections, brain abscess and meningitis are conditions in which such reaction can develop.

It is probable that there are many errors in development which are not solely determined by genes, but by the interaction of other factors and genes. Waddington (1956) used the term epigenetics to cover the study of these. The major phenomena of development comprise the three processes of regionalization, histogenesis and morphogenesis. The analysis of these involves a consideration of such things as the position in the fertilized egg, gradient rhythms and induction effects with the genes, which explain many facts of experimental embryology, but not as yet maldevelopment of the human nervous system.

REFERENCES

Berg, J. M. (1959). 'Discussion on the aetiology of mental defect'. *Proc. Roy. Soc. Med.*, 52, 789.

Crome, L. (1954). 'The morbid anatomy of epilepsy in mental deficiency'. *Proc. Roy. Soc. Med.*, 47, 850.

Glucksmann, A. (1951). *Biol. Review*, 26, 59.

Jacobziner, H. (1966). 'Poisonings in childhood'. *Advance in Paediatrics*, 14, 55.

Lorber, J. (1971). 'Results of treatment of myelomeningocoele'. *Devel. Med. Child Neurol.*, 13, 279.

Moncrieff, A. A. et al. (1964). 'Lead poisoning in children'. *Arch. Dis. Child.*, 39, 1-13.

Smith, J. F. (1974). *Pediatric Neuropathology.* McGraw Hill, New York.

Waddington, C. (1956). *Principles of Embryology.* Allen and Unwin, London.

8 Cerebral function and its relation to psychiatry

In this section certain aspects of psychology, physiology and neuro-anatomy which bear a direct relationship to the practice of psychiatry will be briefly reviewed. In addition reference will be made to the effects of organic disease of the nervous system upon mental functions and upon associated disorders of perception, memory and emotion.

THE NEUROLOGICAL BASIS OF EMOTION

The possible anatomical substratum of emotions has been a controversial subject throughout human history. Descartes favoured the pituitary and more recently — often with equally unconvincing arguments — other specific parts of the brain have been incriminated. For example, Henry Head favoured the optic thalamus but this was refuted by Lashley who concluded that the thalamus was not related to emotional feelings but might be concerned with patterns of motor expressions of emotion. Bilateral lesions of the anterior nuclei of the thalamus produce no change in behaviour in monkeys but similar lesions in the dorso-medical nuclei provoke restlessness, loss of fear and distractibility. Experiments on cats have shown that destructive lesions rostral to the hypothalamus lead to 'sham rage' whereas hypothalamic lesions were accompanied by abnormal tranquillity. However, while there is good evidence that the hypothalamus coordinates and influences neural and hormonal mechanisms of emotional expression, it is improbable that a governing mechanism exists in this portion of the brain.

The relationship between the temporal lobe and certain emotional responses is supported by an impressive accretion of clinical and experimental observations. Earlier work suggested that the cingulate, anterior insular and temporal pole cortex primarily served olfactory functions but more recently the possibility of profound alterations upon emotional behaviour has been claimed. (On the medial surface of the cerebral hemispheres the brain stem and the interhemispheric commisures are surrounded by a great arcuate convolution, the dorsal and ventral halves of which are called the cingulate, 'limbic' and hippocampal gyri. The entire two arcuate convolutions were earlier designated the limbic lobes.) Ablation experiments have shown that removal of temporal lobe cortex produced profound effects on monkey behaviour and in particular hypersexuality and loss of normal fear reactions. Among the numerous psychological disturbances that may occur in the course of a temporal lobe attack are profound fear or a sensation of impending death. Papez proposed that the hypothalamus, the antero-thalamic nuclei, the cingulate gyri, the hippocampus and their inter-connections constitute the essential anatomical substrata for emotional responses. It is true that evidence from laboratory animals indicates a relationship with primitive elemental emotional responses but it is by no means established that these structures are concerned in higher psychic functions underlying human emotional responses. A more diffuse and generalized brain response must be concerned.

MEMORY

Lesions of the temporal lobe are known to cause disturbances of memory and Penfield's classical observations on temporal lobe stimulation in humans have shown that past experiences can be vividly revived. Amnesia for recent events has been produced by electrical stimulation in the posterior part of the middle temporal gyrus, and amygdaloid stimulation in man frequently produces confusion, disturbances of awareness and amnesia for current events. This suggests that amygdaloid stimulation may interfere with memory recording mechanisms and processes influencing conscious perception. The mamillary bodies and the mamillothalamic tracts have also been implicated among the anatomical lesions associated with defects of memory. The amnesia and confabulation occurring in Korsakov's syndrome are associated with lesions at this site.

The similarity between the pathways, damage to which causes loss of recent memory, and those postulated by Papez as the anatomic basis of emotion is worthy of comment. It has been suggested that the amnesic defect may be due in part to the loss of an emotional factor necessary for the embedding of experience.

The fact that these structures appear to be essential to the storage and evocation of memories does not mean that they are also the site of storage. It is much more probable that memory storage — the engram — is a complex function involving extensive areas of the brain.

THE FRONTAL LOBES

It has long been held that the frontal lobes play an important part in mental and emotional life. In animals, experimental damage to frontal cortex affects the ability of the animal to solve problems which depend primarily upon the use of past experience. In man, extensive experience with frontal lobectomies and leucotomies has shown defects of abilities to perform planned initiative tasks. In general disturbance of mood is quantitative rather than qualitative. Diminished inhibition, affective responses, euphoria and, less often, depression have been recorded. The more automatic aspects of intelligence tend to be preserved with attention and memory, but higher forms of reasoning, judgment and conceptualization are disturbed.

In man, the prefrontal regions appear to be concerned with foresight, imagination and awareness of the self. On the whole the functions of the prefrontal lobes are concerned with adjustment of the personality to future contingencies. Imagination — rather than pure intellectual abstract thought in the sense of analysis, synthesis and selectivity — does not appear to require integrity of the frontal and prefrontal areas. Destruction of the dorso-medial nuclei of the thalamus which project to the frontal cortex, has been shown to produce similar effects to frontal leucotomy. Selective prefrontal leucotomies aim at the relief of emotional tension with minimal impairment of other aspects of mental life (see p. 344).

CONSCIOUSNESS AND SLEEP

Consciousness — the awareness of environment, sensation, emotions, memories, ideas — depends upon activities of the cerebral cortex and thalamus in the limited sense that destructive lesions of these structures may alter the content of experiences without significantly altering the state of alertness. Other structures, particularly the central reticular formation of the brain stem, profoundly influence the level of consciousness. The cortex receives at least two kinds of afferent impulses — those which alter the activity of the greater part or the whole of the cortex and those which activate specific projection areas. Destruction of the reticular-hypothalamic system does not appear to interfere with the specific projection system but tends to eliminate the tonic impulses which affect the cortex as a whole. There is evidence that drugs which produce unconsciousness, such as anaesthetics and hypnotics, selectively depress the central reticular formation of the brain stem or at least that part which is known as the ascending reticular activating system which extends from the lower border of the pons to the ventro-medial thalamus.

Sleep may be regarded as a rhythmical depression of those parts of the brain concerned with consciousness. The electro-encephalogram indicates that as sleep deepens there is a transition from alpha rhythm through a phase of bursts of more rapid waves finally to the development of slow random activity. Dreams have been associated with bursts of alpha activity in the second stage of sleep. Barbiturates produce similar EEG changes to those seen accompanying normal sleep. Sleep has been regarded as the consequence of withdrawal of afferent impulses leading to reversal depression of the alerting system which normally activates the cerebral cortex.

PSYCHOPHYSICAL RELATIONSHIPS

More study is needed of how psychological processes find expression through transient or enduring changes within the body and how psychological processes influence bodily function and structure. Increasing interest and attention has been paid to a group of illnesses in which no cause, other than psychological factors, can be found to explain symptomatology. Fatigue, headache, palpitations, nausea, backache and indigestion are among the commoner presenting complaints, and there are certain illnesses in which there may be tissue changes of a reversible or sometimes irreversible nature. Such disorders in which psychological factors are considered to be of significant aetiological importance include urticaria, neurodermatitis, migraine, asthma, peptic ulcer, ulcerative colitis and possibly rheumatoid arthritis. These and other psychosomatic conditions and the neuro-physiological mechanisms involved are discussed in section 28 (p. 173). In general the central mechanisms sub-serving the emotions or the 'neural chassis' — hypothalamus, midbrain, cerebral cortex and limbic system — have all been implicated and so have the mechanisms through which the central nervous system exerts a direct influence on peripheral organs through the pathways of the autonomic nervous system and through the hypothalamic-pituitary axis.

FURTHER READING

Brain, Lord (1964). 'Psychosomatic medicine and the brain-mind relationship'. *Lancet*, 2, 325.
Eccles, J. C. (ed.) (1966). *Brain and Conscious Experience.* Springer, Berlin.

Herrington, R. N. (ed.) (1969). *Current Problems in Neuropsychiatry. Brit. J. Psychiat.* Spec. Pub. No. 4.

Oswald, I. (1966). *Sleep.* Penguin.

Wolf, S. G., and Wolff, H. G. (1943). *Human Gastric Function.* OUP, London.

9 Classification and incidence

Table I: Classification

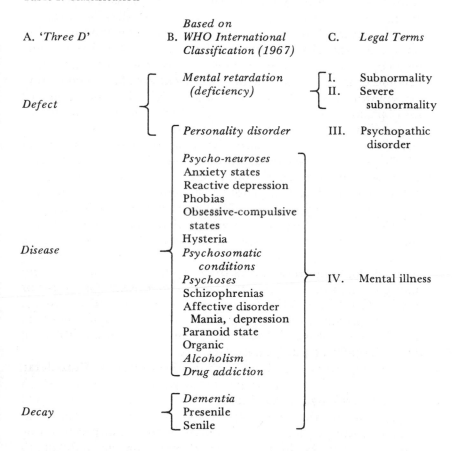

A. *'Three D'*	*Based on* B. *WHO International Classification (1967)*	C.	*Legal Terms*
Defect	*Mental retardation (deficiency)*	I. II.	Subnormality Severe subnormality
	Personality disorder	III.	Psychopathic disorder
Disease	*Psycho-neuroses* Anxiety states Reactive depression Phobias Obsessive-compulsive states Hysteria *Psychosomatic conditions* *Psychoses* Schizophrenias Affective disorder Mania, depression Paranoid state Organic *Alcoholism* *Drug addiction*	IV.	Mental illness
Decay	*Dementia* Presenile Senile		

Note: Both depressions are discussed below under the heading of depressive illnesses (see p. 75).

Even in the 3D classification there was doubt as to whether personality disorder was a defect or a disease: hence the bracket overlaps.

The classification of psychiatric conditions presents many difficulties, and many systems of classification have been evolved in their time. Attitudes are constantly changing; for instance in the past psychoneuroses were regarded as conditions in which there was an exaggeration of a normal reaction, anxiety or depression, whereas psychoses were regarded as totally different, with a lack of insight, detachment from reality, and bizarre symptoms such as delusions and hallucinations. Such a distinction was based on studies of advanced cases of either. But with improvements in understanding and in treatment, this sharp borderline between the two has become blurred, and distinction between early cases of either has become quite difficult. Further, many patients have a collection of symptoms, some 'neurotic', some 'psychotic', and do not fit into pigeon-holes. They will be understood in terms of personality reacting to stress rather than in a too rigid classification. There are also the 'psychosomatic' illnesses, in which psychological stress has contributed to somatic disease: and the 'somatopsychic' conditions — when primary organic illness has produced psychological symptoms. In many the precise relationship of body and mind is difficult to define.

Difficulties in classification and statistics also arise from the fact that psychiatrists differ in ascribing specific psychiatric diagnoses to their patients; e.g. American psychiatrists use the label schizophrenia more often than psychiatrists in Britain, who may give the same patients the label of depressive psychosis or mania (Kendell, 1971). Nevertheless, titles are still necessary, both to provide some arrangement of clinical syndromes, in descriptions, and even in students' examinations. A classification must therefore be put forward (see Table I).

The simplest is the 'three D' shown in column A. More detail is given in column B which is based on the WHO list. A complete *aetiological* classification is not possible yet, and what is given is for the most part a symptomatic one. However, genetic, early and late environmental factors, and precipitating causes (i.e. those influences that make up an individual's psychopathology) do justify a separation of mental abnormalities along these lines. In column C are shown the legal terms of the Mental Health Act (1959) and the way they (roughly) correspond with the others.

INCIDENCE

In Britain

Statistics of the incidence of psychiatric patients and of the numbers admitted to hospital often give misleading impressions on account of the lack of any agreed criteria on diagnosis, and because admissions may depend on the ability of the medical and social services to look after patients in the community. Nonetheless the mass of the problem can be recognised by broad figures: until recently some 43% of all hospital beds in Britain were occupied by the mentally ill or retarded, the bulk being chronic psychotics. Although the number of inpatients in mental hospitals on any one day decreased from 152,000 (3.44 per thousand population) in 1954 to 110,000 (2.25 per thousand) in 1971, this has been mainly because more patients were discharged after a briefer stay in hospital: many of them, however, required re-admission. In fact, re-admissions in 1969 were treble those in 1952. The fall in the number of resident inpatients was mainly in the middle age group while there was an increase in those under 15 and over 75. There is still a large number of chronic inpatients: in 1971 64% had been in hospital for over 2 years, 40% over 10 years and 26% over 20 years (Bransby, 1974).

There are of course many psychiatric patients who are never admitted. The incidence of those with various psychiatric disorders and emotionally determined symptoms in the population is difficult to assess. There are several reasons for this; many people with minor emotional disturbances or psychosomatic symptoms never consult their doctors; surveys carried out by general practitioners vary according to the particular doctor's interest in and skill at diagnosing psychiatric illness, and on whether they restrict themselves to formal psychiatric disorders or whether they include patients with minor stress disorders and psychosomatic symptoms. Thus Hopkins (1956) considered that 43% of all patients seen in his practice had symptoms which were wholly or partly emotional in origin; 11% suffered from a formal psychiatric illness and 32% from a variety of 'stress disorders'. Other practitioners have given much lower figures. In a recent study by Goldberg and Blackwell (1970) it was reported that a general practitioner especially interested in psychiatric aspects of patient care found that 20% of consecutive attenders in his practice showed evidence of psychiatric morbidity but when the same patients were seen by a psychiatrist as well a further 10% were found to be psychiatrically ill, making a total of 30%; however, only 8% were suffering from purely psychiatric illnesses. The figure of 30% is similar to that of 34% found by Watts (1962) who published figures on behalf of the College of General Practitioners.

In order to get information on the incidence of psychiatric illness in the population at risk, as opposed to patients actually seen, Shepherd et al. (1966) studied 12 general practices in the London area. They found that of all patients registered in these practices 14% consulted their doctor at least once during the survey year with some form or other of psychiatric illness or emotionally determined symptom not readily classifiable under one or other of the categories of psychiatric disorders ('psychiatric associated conditions'). When the total figure of 14% is broken down it is seen that 9% suffered from psychoneuroses, 3% from psychosomatic conditions and only 0.6% from psychoses. The remainder of the 14% included personality disorders (0.5%), mental subnormality (0.2%), dementia (0.1%), organic illness with psychiatric overlay (1.5%) and psychosocial problems (0.8%). Some patients had to be counted more than once as they suffered from more than one psychiatrically determined condition. It is of interest to note that the corresponding figure for respiratory diseases is 25%, and that for gastro-intestinal diseases 9% of the population at risk.

The most striking conclusion from these studies is that psychiatric illness in the population, of sufficient severity to make the patient consult his doctor, amounts to about 30% of patients seen by general practitioners; but the vast majority of these suffer from either a psychoneurosis or from psychosomatic symptoms. It should also be noted that in almost all categories there is a striking preponderance of females over males; thus in the case of psychoneuroses, the commonest disorder seen, the sex ratio of females to males is approximately 2:1; but possibly women consult their doctors more readily than men do.

Studies of the incidence of neurosis in industry (see p. 271) show that a quarter to a third of sickness absence is due to psychiatric illness.

The GP in Britain, therefore, is likely to see a high proportion of anxiety states, depressive states, psychosomatic disorders, and exaggeration of organic conditions; with far fewer schizophrenics, obsessionals, alcoholics and gross hysterics; but an increasing number of psychiatric symptoms related to old age. However, symptomatology changes for reasons which are not clear; thus in World War I vast numbers of soldiers suffered from shell shock, generally hysterical (see p. 281), while very few did so in World War II, when anxiety states or psychosomatic conditions were far commoner in Europeans.

The above picture is probably representative of any heavily industrialized country and reports suggest a further increase of neurosis in countries as they industrialise. Other cultures may show different pictures.

Incidence in Africans

Detailed studies have been made for example in Africans and the commonest type of psychiatric illness seems to be organic. Lamont and Bignault (1953) reported that 40% of admissions to their South African Mental Hospital were suffering from organic states. German and Arya (1969) stated that in Uganda in 1967 46% of patients were in this category and 75% of those were below 40 years old. Severely disturbed behaviour is often a feature of these organic states and they are usually attributable to alcohol which is used for medicinal rather than social purposes. Delirium tremens is very common in Africans.

Schizophrenia in West Africans has been extensively studied by Lambo (1968). The incidence seems to be the same as elsewhere in the world and it occurs at all levels in the community; acute attacks of sudden onset are common with florid hallucinations, usually visual, delusions, generally magical or religious, and extreme behavioural disturbance. The prognosis is good. Manic-depressive psychosis is almost as common in Africans as in Europeans, but mania is three times as common as depression, unlike the pattern seen in Europe; maybe the manic patient is more often noticed than the withdrawn depressive. Depression is more commonly recorded among town dwellers; suicidal attempts are rare.

Anxiety states are common in Africans but the anxiety is usually focused on a particular area of the body. Hysterical states also occur frequently; Herzberg (1964) stresses that the essential difference is that the African internalizes the concept of depression and says 'I have a pain in my chest' rather than 'I am so depressed my heart is aching'; whereas the European would say 'I am depressed'. It was also observed in World War II that less educated African and Indian troops were still subject to gross hysterical attacks which were due more to the loss of traditional patterns of communal and religious life than to the stress of war. Similar observations have been made about Africans moving from tribal to urban surroundings.

When seen in Britain, the symptoms of Africans, West Indians and Asians are greatly complicated by the fact that they are expatriates, with all that that entails (see p. 284).

It is thus clear that cultural factors play a part, not only in the amount, but also in the nature of psychiatric syndromes. Halliday has pointed out that certain psychosomatic illnesses (see p. 173) occur for a period and then diminish remarkably, e.g. effort syndrome. Wider studies have been contributed by Wittkower and Murphy at the Institute of Transcultural Psychiatry in Montreal.

REFERENCES

Bransby, E. R. (1974). 'The extent of mental illness in England and Wales'. *Health Trends*, 6, 56.

German and Arya, D. P. (1969). *Brit. J. Psychiat.* 115, 1323.

Goldberg, D. P. and Blackwell, B. (1970). 'Psychiatric illness in general practice'. *Brit. Med. J.*, 1, 439.

Herzberg, I. (1964). 'African students in English universities'. 1st. Internat. Congress of Social Psychiat.

Hopkins, P. (1956). 'Referrals in general practice'. *Brit. Med. J.*, 2, 873.

Kendell, R. E. (1971). 'Psychiatric diagnosis in Britain and the United States'. *Brit. J. Hosp. Med.*, 147.

Lambo, T.A. (1968). Deuxième colloque africain de psychiatrie. Association Universitaire pour le Developpement de l'Enseignement et de la Culture en Afrique et à Madagascar. (Paris).

Lamont, A. and Bignault, W. J. (1953). *S. Afr. Med. J.*, 27, 637.

Shepherd, M., Cooper, B., Brown, A. C. and Kalton, G. W. (1966). *Psychiatric Illness in General Practice.* OUP, London.

Watts, C. A. H. (1962). 'Psychiatric disorders'. In *Morbidity Statistics from General Practice*, III: *Studies on Medical and Population Subjects*, No.14, HMSO, London.

10 Mental subnormality or retardation

Such patients are seldom seen by students; the higher grade cases may not be recognized, and the lower grades tend to be looked after in distant hospitals, which students do not visit.

Yet the problems posed by the individual child to its parents, and so to the GP, are extreme: and there are great stresses on the community. Again, the detection of certain failures of development has contributed information about normal psychological and physical growth and the intricate co-ordination needed between these two. For all these reasons, the subject is of profound interest.

TERMINOLOGY

The terminology is unfortunately confused. The older term mental deficiency (of which mental defect and amentia — and in North America oligophrenia — and now mental retardation, are synonyms) was originally both a clinical and a legal term: it was defined as 'a condition of arrested or incomplete development of mind existing before the age of 18 years, whether arising from inherent causes or induced by disease or injury' (Mental Deficiency Act, 1927).

Further there were three grades of this: (1) idiots, who could not guard themselves against common physical dangers; (2) imbeciles, who could not be taught to manage themselves or their affairs; (3) the feeble-minded, who required some care, supervision or control or could not benefit from instruction in ordinary schools.

In the Mental Health Act, 1959, two new *legal* terms were used: these were (1) severe subnormality — a state of arrested or incomplete development of mind, which included subnormality of intelligence so that the patient could not lead an independent life or guard himself against serious exploitation: and (2) subnormality (not amounting to severe subnormality) which requires or is susceptible to medical treatment or other special care or training. It will be seen that (1) is based on a social criterion and (2) depends on medical possibilities: and that there is no term to cover (1) and (2). But the old terms mental deficiency etc. are often still used *clinically*: and idiocy and imbecility roughly correspond to severe subnormality. The term mental retardation then gained ground, but mental handicap is now increasingly used.

CRITERIA

There has also been much controversy on the criteria required for diagnosis. At first mental defect was equated with intellectual defect, but it was pointed out that high intelligence could exist with grave social incompetence. Later, E. A. Doll suggested that six criteria must apply:

1 Social incompetence;
2 mental subnormality;
3 mind developmentally arrested;
4 obtaining at maturity;
5 of constitutional origin;
6 essentially incurable.

But this excludes conditions not considered to be constitutional; and the fact that medical treatment has been able to improve certain cases, e.g. of cretinism and phenyl pyruvic acid defect, has made the criterion of incurability out of date.

Educationally subnormal (ESN) children form an administrative, not a diagnostic category: it includes those whose emotional instability or lack of drive accentuates the effect of their subnormality.

INCIDENCE

Various attempts have been made to assess the incidence in Britain and elsewhere: but consistent standards are difficult. The total figures in the population are probably about 3 per 1000: but in certain age-groups, the proportion is higher, e.g. 3·61 severely subnormals per 1000 in the 10-14 groups: for naturally their expectation of life is less. Some factors diminish the number, e.g. the diminution of syphilis and better ante-natal and obstetric care: other factors, e.g. maternal rubella, may increase it.

AETIOLOGY

There are of course a multitude of causes for developmental failure: and the nature and extent of the latter depends on the severity, time of onset and duration of the cause. Moreover the original deficiency may itself provoke secondary reactions in the patient or in his family, which hinder development still further. Thus most cases are in practice the product of more than one cause.

An aetiological classification can be attempted on the basis of the major factors involved.

1 *Developmental*, where some internal factor has prevented normal development. Three groups can be described.

   (*a*) Genetic. These include many types: disorders of lipoid metabolism, in neurones or elsewhere may give rise to physical defects as well as mental: e.g. amaurotic idiocy; there are several disorders of carbohydrate metabolism, notably galactosaemia and gargoylism; disorders of amino-acid metabolism are increasingly recognised, phenyl-ketonuria (see p. 59) being the best known; neurological faults, e.g. tuberous sclerosis, with adenoma and epilepsy; angiomatosis producing skin naevi; and demyelination of various types.
   (*b*) Chromosomal errors: e.g. Down's Disease (mongolism) (see p. 59).

(*c*) Anatomical. This term is used to include malformations of which the cause is unknown. The most important is the Arnold Chiari in which hydrocephalus is associated with myelomeningocoele. Until recent years most cases were fatal in early life if not stillborn and the condition was of more pathological than clinical importance. However, the successful use of atrioventricular shunts in management of the hydrocephalus has led to treatment of large numbers of infants, some of whom are left with neurological and mental defect. The medical and moral problems arising from this situation are complex.

2 *Environmental*, where trauma, infection, neonatal jaundice, hypoxia, therapy, toxicity or deprivation cause the defect.

(*a*) Traumatic: mechanical trauma to the brain at birth is now less common, e.g. subdural haematoma following tentorial tear is rarely seen in places where obstetrical care is good but may be important in other places. Even in so-called civilized communities mechanical trauma to the infant and young child is either more common or recognized more frequently — battered babies and road traffic accidents. The brain may be damaged by subdural or other haemorrhage.

(*b*) Infective: Rubella may damage the early embryo (p. 40) as a result of transplacental infection, or the newborn infant — the rubella syndrome in which the virus is still active. Immunization of mothers not previously affected by rubella has reduced its incidence. Other viruses which may rarely cause brain damage are measles, mumps and cytomegalovirus. Modern therapy has decreased the significance of bacterial meningitis, but it is still liable to cause brain damage in infancy.

(*c*) Hypoxic: this is an important cause of cerebral 'birth injury' and in the early neonatal period. At the time of birth of the full term baby respiratory arrest, e.g. from meconium aspiration may be accompanied by cardiac arrest or the latter may occur independently, e.g. from cord compression. This is a rare cause of severe brain damage which may be fatal or lead to the survival of a vegetable-like child or to one with mental retardation and/or spasticity.

Modern medicine has led to the survival of large numbers of low birth weight infants who develop normally. These are also liable to hypoxia at the time of birth and in neonatal life from such conditions as hyaline membrane disease. The most important cause of serious brain damage in this group is, however, subependymal plate haemorrhage with extension into the ventricles. Most cases are fatal; in a few a slow leak from the plate haematoma can cause destructive hydrocephalus; minor haematomas may cause no permanent damage. However, the brain of the premature baby may show normal maturation after quite severe hypoxic injury and the incidence of mental and physical defect is low in those who have optimal management.

(d) Therapeutic. Immunization against smallpox and whooping cough is occasionally complicated by an encephalopathy. The recognition of this has led to revision of immunization programmes.

(e) Toxic. Lead encephalopathy. Jacobziner (1966) found lead responsible for·1704 cases of lead poisoning under 20 years of age in New York between 1953 and 1963. The majority of these were under 5 and many had encephalopathy, which has a high mortality and permanent sequelae, cf. Moncrieff et al. (1964).

(f) Deprivative: where some physical lack occurs, e.g. of thyroid tissue in cretins: and more common where psychological stimuli fail to reach the child, either because of sensory loss, or because of institutionalization, or lack of stimulation in an unfavourable family or social environment.

(g) Bilirubin encephalopathy (Kernicterus) due to neonatal jaundice, caused either by rhesus incompatibility or prematurity, is another cause of retardation. Prophylactic treatment of rhesus negative mothers and exchange transfusion of the newborn infant have diminished its incidence.

3 *Primary (or Simple)*. This group still includes the majority of defectives: who fail to develop fully for no apparent reason and with no gross physical defect. They may be regarded as the lower end of the curve of normal distribution of intelligence; but it is likely that as our knowledge increases, more of these will be found to have a specific biochemical fault.

CLINICAL PICTURE

This naturally varies according to the extent of the deficiency: from the helpless, inarticulate idiot to the high-grade doing a useful steady job. Gross physical deformities are sometimes present as a result of the cause which produced the mental defect: these are much more common in the lower grades, e.g. hydrocephalus, spasticity, naevi and various deposits of lipoids or carbohydrates in various organs.

The defective child is not always recognizable at birth: it is his falling behind in his developmental landmarks, and later the contrast with his contemporaries which attracts concern, and his IQ can be measured to reveal his disability. Besides this his awareness is limited, his tolerance to frustration is poor, he fails to perceive the social significance of behaviour, or to deal with* more than one subject at once, or to plan for long term satisfactions. His emotional control is slow to develop, but he can make personal relationships and these can certainly be used to encourage him to learn some skill.

Unfortunately, his retardation or its effects on the attitude of others, especially his parents (see below), often deprive him of their support in making the normal stages of development, and he overreacts to stress, fails to gain control of his instinctual drives, and provokes further hostility — and so is further isolated, or behaves worse.

Many subnormals, supported by tolerant patient parents, have reached adult life and succeeded in holding down jobs requiring some skill, reliability and persistence. The trouble is likely to come if this support is withdrawn, or under unaccustomed stress in the environment, e.g. by a strike, a new bullying superior, or serious physical illness. Once such people may lose jobs they may find it hard to get others. The success of unarmed companies in the Pioneer Corps in World War II is well known: they contained many high-grade subnormals, who were not only kept from breakdown but did excellent work under the control of flexible, if somewhat unmilitary superiors.

Four syndromes are important enough to warrant special accounts.

Mongolism (Down's disease)

After much research the cause is now known to be an extra chromosome in pair 21 (hence the name 'Trisomy 21'). Rarely, in 10% of cases, the extra may be attached to another chromosome by translocation, usually to pair 15. This extra is caused by the chromosome's failure to separate, and why this happens is still obscure, but hormonal disturbance, infection, or irradiation have all been blamed. If the mother has a Mongol child her risk of a second one is greater, the earlier she had the first. Advancing maternal age is a significant factor.

The appearance of the Mongol is distinctive, with a small, round head, downward sloping palpebral fissure and epicanthic fold, a small nose with a small bridge, a transversely furrowed tongue and typical hands with a square palm and single crease.

Mentally, Mongols are generally cheerful and given to mimicry, and often musical.

The condition may range from severe subnormality to higher grades with few physical features (sometimes known as Mongoloid).

Hydrocephalus

Hydrocephalus may be due to adhesions at the base of the brain after meningitis. These obstruct the circulation of the cerebrospinal fluid and if severe enormous enlargement of the head occurs, with spasticity of the limbs and gross mental retardation; death is likely from intercurrent infections.

However, in milder cases, a balance may be found between the absorption and secretion of the CSF and life may be prolonged. Surgically, a Spitz-Holter valve has been used as a shunt between the ventricular and vascular systems and has so far proved a success in some cases for some years.

Phenylketonuria

In phenylketonuria an enzyme deficiency prevents conversion of phenylanaline into tyrosine. The raised blood level of phenylanaline is the basis of a screening method in early infancy;

alternatively phenyl pyruvic acid, a degradation product of phenylanaline, can be detected in the urine but this is less reliable. A diet low in phenylanaline started as early in infancy as possible prevents the development of mental retardation (Smith and Wolff 1974).

Galactosaemia

Here enzyme failure causes accumulation of galactose-1-phosphate resulting in mental retardation, liver enlargement and cataracts. Treatment consists of exclusion of lactose from the diet.

DIFFERENTIAL DIAGNOSIS

Disorders of relationship formation can occur from adverse factors at any stage of development, and may be mistaken for subnormality (see below). It is easy to miss deafness in a small child.

PARENTAL REACTIONS

Few parents find it easy to accept the presence of a defective child: guilt may be intense but repressed; some deny an obvious fact, and so expect the child to develop normally; some blame the other parent for having produced an abnormality; some blame the doctors who break the news, at least for their inability to cure the condition; some over-compensate with exaggerated affection, to the neglect of other, normal children.

None of these attitudes is a good start to the patient collaboration of parents, and others, which is needed to give the defective child the best chance. The GP or specialist can do much to produce a healthier attitude by explaining to the parents that it is not their fault, and how best the child can be helped. He should recognize the various ways in which this guilt or helplessness can be displayed.

ADMISSION TO HOSPITAL

Clearly the presence of a gravely subnormal child can be a tremendous strain on the whole family who can give little special care. Hence, a hospital with specially trained staff and special facilities may help the child more: and the results of special training, by very skilled staff, have been remarkable, even for imbeciles (Tizard and O'Connor 1950, 1951). Unfortunately such units are rare, for staff is short, and admission to an over-crowded hospital may deprive the child of even the little individual affection his mother can give. Most hospitals in any case have long waiting lists, and the staff shortage gets worse.

Advice to parents about admission must therefore depend on a consideration of all sides of the local position in home and hospital, as well as on the degree of defect.

THE DEFECTIVE IN THE COMMUNITY

The local health authorities provide training or occupational centres for defectives outside hospital. Again, staff is short. The education authorities provide ESN schools.

Thus at present, there are many people who need more skilled help and supervision than they can get. Their social inadequacy and irresponsibility leads them into situations which gradually increase the stress on them, e.g. crime, VD, unemployment, and pregnancy, legitimate or illegitimate; thus they will produce children likely to be deprived of adequate parental care and occasionally cursed with hereditary defect, who thus become a burden on the more socially responsible members of the community (who limit their own families). As the latter in any case are getting increasingly unable to look after their own elderly relatives and chronic sick, the social problem is very serious. The policy which followed the Mental Health Act led many to be discharged from hospital, but only to break down into illness, crime, or poverty, as they could not survive without more adaptability and more support.

TREATMENT AND TRAINING

Recent research in biochemistry and genetics have led to the hope that more can be done by diet and drugs for certain types of defect, and in those due to metabolic errors, e.g. phenyl pyruvic defect, results have been achieved by early and persistent treatment. But in general, so far the most effective help has come from (*a*) special types of training in hospitals and (*b*) some attempts to diminish the stress on defectives in the community so as to allow them to earn a living; this includes the provision of hostels, the decrease of popular prejudice against them, and the support of social services.

But none of this is yet comprehensive, and in many areas it does not meet the demand. Education is needed: the doctor's influence can play a part in this. Meanwhile, he can support the parents of defective children.

FURTHER READING

Earl, C. J. C. (1961). *Subnormal Personalities.* Baillière-Tindall, London.

Heaton-Ward, W. A. (1967). *Mental Subnormality.* Bristol.

Jacobziner, H. (1966). 'Poisonings in childhood'. *Advance in Paediatrics,* 14, 55.

Moncrieff, A.A. et al. (1964). 'Food poisoning in children'. *Arch. Dis. Child.,* 39, 1.

Penrose, L.S. and Smith, G.F. (1966). *Down's Anomaly.* Churchill, London.

Smith, G. F. and Berg, J. (1974). 'The biological significance of mongolism'. *Brit. J. Psychiat.* 125, 537.

Smith, I. and Wolff, O. H. (1974). 'Natural history of phenylketonuria and influence of early treatment'. *Lancet,* 2, 540.

Tizard, J. (ed.) (1974). *Mental Retardation: Concepts of Education and Research.* Butterworth, London.

Tizard, J. and O'Connor, N. (1950 and 1951). *Amer. J. Mental Deficiency,* 54.5 and 55.1.

Tredgold, R. F. and Soddy, K. (1969). *Mental Retardation.* London.

W.H.O. Working Party (1974). 'Malnutrition and mental development'. *W.H.O. Chronicle,* 25, 95.

11 Autism and late onset childhood psychosis

These conditions are sometimes mistaken for mental deficiency but there are certain differences which set them apart. The infants or children affected show bizarre, psychotic features and behaviour. Kanner (1943) first described the condition and called it infantile autism because the condition was present at birth or started in the first year of life; but since then children have been described in which psychotic features developed later in childhood after a period of apparent normal development. It seems best to distinguish two groups (Kolvin, 1971):

1 Early childhood autism in which the disturbed behaviour is noticed early in the first year up to the end of the third year of life.

2 Late onset childhood psychosis where the condition appears during the early school period, usually after the age of 5.

EARLY CHILDHOOD (INFANTILE) AUTISM

This is characterised by profound withdrawal, and an inability to make contact with the mother and other people resulting in severe disturbances in relationships. The child shows a 'desire for sameness' and becomes acutely disturbed by any changes in its environment, which produce attacks of terror and aggressive behaviour. It avoids eye to eye contact, and speech development is severely impaired, occasionally to the point of mutism. Motor behaviour may be monotonous, bizarre, and repetitive, and the child treats people and toys like objects, and lacks a normal child's curiosity and ability for imaginative play.

The strain of having an autistic child in the family puts a heavy burden on the mother, father and siblings so that residential care may become necessary if only to relieve the parents of the burden. Although there may be some improvement in speech, personal relationships and learning ability as the child gets older, the majority remain severely handicapped; only a small proportion improve sufficiently to find limited employment in adult life. Those with relatively high intelligence have the better prognosis, especially if they are given special education and skilled care and attention.

AETIOLOGY

It seems likely that both organic and psychological factors play their part but the view previously held that it is caused by the parents' failure to give the child sufficient affection and understanding can no longer be accepted, certainly not as its sole cause. Soddy (1969) has stressed the importance of disturbance at the various stages of relationship formation. He considers the condition can start either at the stage of the first interpersonal relationship formation, especially with the mother, or at the stage of instinct modification in relationship extension. Brain damage may play its part; abnormal EEG findings and the occasional appearance of epilepsy support the view that organic factors are of importance. There is no conclusive evidence that genetic factors are involved, and the incidence of autism in the siblings of an autistic child is not significantly higher than the incidence in the general population; in this country the incidence is 4/10,000 children of school age, boys being affected about 4 times as often as girls. The condition is commoner in children of families of higher socio-economic class.

Treatment

The less severely affected children can be kept at home if the strain on the rest of the family is not too great. Others will require residential care. All of them need special education and skilled individual attention; support and counselling for the parents is essential.

LATE ONSET CHILDHOOD PSYCHOSIS

This condition develops at a later age, usually after 5, following a period of apparently normal development. The condition resembles adult schizophrenia; thought disorder, hallucinations and delusions may appear as the disease progresses and the children often show unpredictable and chaotic behaviour. Unlike autistic children they may respond to phenothiazines, and institutional treatment is often required.

FURTHER READING

Kanner, L. (1943). 'Autistic disturbances of affective contact'. *Nerv. Child*, 2, 217.
Kolvin, I. (1972). 'Infantile, autism or infantile psychoses. *Brit. Med. J.*, 2, 753.
Rutter, M. (ed.) (1971). *Infantile Autism: Concepts, Characteristics and Treatment*. Livingstone, Edinburgh.
Rutter, M. (1974). 'The development of infantile autism'. *Psychological Med.*, 4, 147.
Soddy, K. (1969), in Tredgold, R. F. and Soddy, K., *Mental Retardation*. Baillière-Tindall, London.
Stone, F. H. (1970). 'The autistic child'. *Practitioner*, 205, 313.
Wing, L. (1970). 'The syndrome of early childhood autism'. *Brit. J. Hosp. Med.*, 4, 381.

12 Psychopathic disorder, or pathological personality

DEFINITION

In the terms of the Mental Health Act, 1959, Section 4, psychopathic disorder means persistent disorder or disability of mind (whether or not including subnormality of intelligence) which results in abnormally aggressive or seriously irresponsible conduct on the part of the patient and requires or is susceptible to medical treatment. The terms pathological and psychopathic personality are used practically synonymously.

Most psychiatrists prefer to assert that they can recognize psychopathic disorder more easily than they can define it, though various attempts have been made at a definition. It seems best to restrict the term to a particular type of personality which is characterised by aggressive and antisocial behaviour without proper concern for others. The psychopathic personality should be distinguished from other personality disorders such as: schizoid (see pp. 22, 30), hysterical (see p. 100), obsessional (see p. 95) and cyclothymic (see p. 78) personalities.

AETIOLOGY

Various theories have been proposed:

1 *Emotional deprivation.* Bowlby has suggested, in a series of studies, that lack of a secure and affectionate relationship between the infant and one person seems to be significant in the production of a psychopath. The person is generally, but not necessarily the mother. If she is prevented by poor home circumstances, poverty, or her own emotional problems from providing this, and no substitute is available, the risk of psychopathy is increased; psychopathy in the father may also predispose to psychopathic behaviour.

2 *Heredity.* James Lange found that in 10 out of 13 cases the uniovular twin of a criminal was himself criminal. Moreover the actual type of crime and the age of manifestation were similar. In another series of 17 binovular twins, however, there were only two cases in which both were criminal. Modern writers stress environmental rather than hereditary factors.

3 *Chromosomal abnormality.* A higher incidence of a 47XYY chromosomal abnormality in men in maximum-security hospitals than in the general population has suggested that this abnormality may be an aetiological factor; but psychopathy also occurs in the normal population, especially the emotionally immature, and men with this chromosomal abnormality not necessarily psychopathic.

4 *Brain damage.* Psychopathy is sometimes seen following trauma to the brain. Birth injury, encephalitis, meningitis,

chorea and congenital syphilis are all mentioned as aetiological factors in some cases, and others occurred after the earlier drastic forms of leucotomy.

It is often difficult to assess the relative value of these factors. The weight of current opinion is behind (1) above but biological and psychological factors may co-exist.

CLINICAL DESCRIPTION

Obviously the condition may take many forms, but the following facets of personality appear to occur with considerable frequency and indicate immaturity in one or other field of development:

1 A tendency to seek immediate gratification at whatever cost.
2 An inability to form lasting or close relationships and a tendency to exploit associates for short term ends.
3 A difficulty in conforming with the dictates of society and a lack of response to social training.
4 Emotional lability, expecially with quarrelsomeness and violent temper which may be extremely dangerous and destructive.
5 An absence of guilt, shame or remorse.
6 Occasionally some superficial charm.
7 Alcoholism or addiction to other drugs may occur as a complication, especially to drugs which produce some immediate, if temporary, pleasure.

Because of the above tendencies, patients frequently come in conflict with the law and are well known to prison and probation officers. They are likely to disrupt social groups and are thus most difficult to treat in psychiatric hospitals and need separate units.

DIFFERENTIAL DIAGNOSIS

The clinical picture drawn above sounds distinctive enough. But it must be remembered that some of the symptoms are seen as temporary phenomena in psychoneurotics, and even in phases of 'bloody-mindedness' seen in 'normal' people. It is therefore essential to take as accurate a life-history as possible, from relatives as well as from the patient.

EEG STUDIES

Abnormalities have been found in the EEG's of 55% of aggressive psychopaths and the tracings have resembled those of difficult children. As the patterns of EEG's in children differ from adults, it has been postulated that the psychiatric abnormality shown by behaviour disorder of early adult life, i.e. psychopathy, may be related to emotional immaturity.

TREATMENT

1 *Inpatient units.* There is a special unit for psychopaths in Henderson Hospital, Sutton, Surrey, which was started by Dr Maxwell Jones. Patients work together, are given some responsibility for the hospital routine and for each other and have regular discussion groups. The atmosphere is very informal and the medical staff are encouraged to be permissive. The results are not conclusive as to the value of this form of treatment but are more encouraging than attempts to cope with psychopaths in mental hospitals. Obviously considerable 'acting-out' may occur.

2 *Outpatient clinics, etc.* A degree of support can be given to psychopaths at outpatient clinics, social clubs, probation offices, etc., especially to the inadequate type. This will require much patience and often be disappointing, but may save the behaviour of the patient from deteriorating. Any professional worker involved must expect to be let down again and again.

Psychopaths often land in prison; or under the Mental Health Act they may be transferred compulsorily to a psychiatric hospital if they are under 21 years. This compulsory detention lapses at the age of 25. Though an advance this step will not be very effective until there are more special units to deal with these patients.

COMPLICATIONS

Psychopaths certainly constitute one class of drug addicts (see p. 139) and may develop alcoholism (see p. 132). Drugs of any kind should therefore be used with great caution.

FURTHER READING

Gunn, J. (1971). 'Forensic psychiatry and psychopathic patients'. *Brit. J. Hosp. Med.*, 6, 260.
Henderson, Sir D. K. and Gillespie, R. D., revised by Batchelor, I. R. C., (1969). *A Textbook of Psychiatry*. OUP, London. See especially Chapter 13.
Jones, Maxwell, (1968). *Social Psychiatry in Practice*. Penguin.
Lancet (1974). 'What becomes of the XYY male?'. p. 1297.
Pitcher, D. R. (1971). 'The XXY syndrome'. *Brit. J. Hosp. Med.*, March, 379.
Whiteley, J. S. (1970). 'The psychopath and his treatment'. *Brit. J. Hosp. Med.*, 3, 263.

13 Anxiety and anxiety states

NORMAL ANXIETY

Normal anxiety has been felt by all. Stressful reality situations, e.g. oral examinations, provoke in most of us tension, difficulty in relaxing mentally and physically, difficulty in concentrating and in remembering, some emotional instability (a tendency to weep, laugh or 'snap' without due cause) and occasionally physical accompaniments, such as a dry mouth, anorexia, dyspepsia, diarrhoea, frequency, headache, palpitations, due to over-activity of the autonomic nervous system.

Such symptoms are sometimes embarrassing in the stress of 'vivas' but they have a biological value in animals and human beings exposed to danger, when alertness or physical action is required. They disappear if action is adequate and appropriate.

ANXIETY STATES

An anxiety state — a form of psychoneurosis — is, by *definition*, anxiety without apparent cause or out of proportion to its cause in intensity or in time. This entails a concept of a 'normal' reaction which, like the law's example of a reasonable man, is useful though it cannot be defined with precision.

The symptoms are similar to those of normal anxiety, but they may be carried to extremes, are present most of the time and produce secondary symptoms. The patient is mentally and physically tense, can't relax, fidgets and feels on edge, cannot get off to sleep, with consequent fatigue. His concentration is poor, so that his memory and judgement become impaired and he is preoccupied with constant worries. He becomes depressed; anorexia may lead to loss of weight, and other physical symptoms, such as nausea, diarrhoea or palpitations, may produce further anxiety about possible physical illness, thus setting up a vicious circle. The effect of an anxiety state on a responsible, intelligent person, e.g. an executive, is even greater in that he begins to fear for his job. Moreover, it is still thought to be somewhat beneath him to admit to any form of mental inefficiency or illness.

These symptoms, especially in an appealing person, are almost 'infectious' in that they provoke action in those around, including the doctor; and if action is impossible or in vain, relatives and doctor may both feel helpless, impatient and annoyed, which in turn increases the patient's anxiety.

SEQUELS

Anxiety may be partly or entirely controlled by certain ego defence mechanisms, which may themselves lead to symptoms if exaggerated. Repression or denial, for example, may produce a superficial mood of calmness or 'belle indifférence', as in hysteria, even under marked stress or shock — a reaction which should make the observer wonder. Similarly, obsessions and compulsions may arise as an attempted defence against anxiety, as in an obsessional neurosis. Phobic states may arise if the anxiety is displaced on a particular object or situation. In a particular patient several of these psychoneurotic symptoms may co-exist.

Anxiety may lead to feelings of inferiority and self-consciousness and inhibit all action; it may induce activity which is quite inappropriate to the situation or may lead to actions appropriate in kind but grossly excessive, e.g. a panic. This may also be 'infectious', affecting several people.

AETIOLOGY

In the majority of cases disturbance of the patient's basic personality is an important pre-disposing factor, usually as the result of abnormal personality development, e.g. if he has been left with a great deal of separation anxiety due to early emotional deprivation. Genetic constitutional factors may also play their part. The following may act as precipitating factors.

Psychological

1 If severe anxiety under stress has no physical or mental outlet, because it is barred by circumstances or by inhibitions due to upbringing or by both, an acute anxiety state may develop.
2 Conflict between opposing psychological forces, e.g. love and hate, may be conscious or, if repressed it may leave the patient with anxiety and tension, worse if circumstances play on the underlying area of conflict. If the conflict persists a chronic anxiety state may develop.

Physical

Physical exhaustion and fatigue and physical ill-health such as virus infections may precipitate the development of anxiety states.

DIAGNOSIS

Good history-taking and physical examination should assess these factors and differentiate physical conditions such as hyperthyroidism (see p. 206). Spasmodic attacks of anxiety, unrelated to any external factor, may occasionally be due to a phaeochromocytoma.

TREATMENT

1 Superficial treatment begins from the doctor's first contact with the patient, in that his attitude, here more than ever, will affect the patient's ability to express his anxiety. If he senses or imagines contempt and impatience, he is likely to suppress it. Full history-taking may in some cases itself provide enough relief, and the patient may regain his adjustment without realising the help he has been given.

2 Reassurance on specific anxieties and explanations about the cause of symptoms is valuable.

3 More prolonged formal psychotherapy (see p. 307) will be required for chronic or severe anxiety states and for the underlying personality disorder and emotional conflicts.

4 Drugs may be useful for symptomatic relief and to check vicious circles, described above. In general, drugs are far more useful for tiding patients over acute anxiety and tension than for the treatment of long term cases. They may be used as daily sedatives or tranquillizers or as hypnotics by night.

SEDATIVES

Tranquillizers

Chlordiazepoxide (Librium) 10 mg t.d.s.
Diazepam (Valium) 2 mg or 5 mg t.d.s.
Trifluoperazine (Stelazine) 1 mg t.d.s.
Oxazepam (Serenid-D) 15-30 mg t.d.s

These are the safest drugs to use for the control of anxiety; they can either be used to control an acute anxiety attack, or can be taken regularly for a long period.

Barbiturates (to control anxiety)

e.g. Amylobarbitone (Amytal) 50 mg t.d.s.

These may be used for short periods in hospital, but for outpatients they should be avoided because they cause addiction, and are often used for suicidal attempts. Sudden withdrawal may cause epileptic fits. If drugs are needed to control anxiety it is, therefore, safer to use one or other of the tranquillizers mentioned above.

Hypnotics

For the same reasons it is safer to use a non-barbiturate, e.g.:
　　Dichloralphenazone (Welldorm) 650-1300 mg at night
　　Glutethimide (Doriden) 500 mg at night
　　Mogadon 5 mg at night

Barbiturates are still used occasionally, e.g.:
　　Amylobarbitone (Amytal) 200-400 mg
　　Quinalbarbitone (Seconal) 100-200 mg at night
　　Pentobarbitone sodium (Nembutal) 50-100 mg at night

Side effects must be remembered: rashes, potentiation with alcohol, transient disorientation in elderly patients, habituation, addiction, withdrawal fits, and the risk of suicide.

Patients should be warned not to place their supply of drugs at the bedside because of the danger that, if drowsy, they may take further doses of the drugs which could be fatal.

PANIC ATTACKS

Panic attacks generally occur as part of an anxiety state but have special importance, being at times most disabling in preventing the patient from leaving home or work.

Generally they arise from some repressed emotion, such as anger, sexual feelings, anxiety or guilt connected with past experiences, fantasied or real, and re-awakened by the present environment. Fear of losing control over such feelings may precipitate an attack.

Apart from the use of a tranquillizer or sedative to control the acute attack such cases need psychotherapy to deal with the underlying causes. Occasionally abreaction, e.g. under pentothal, may be useful for dealing with particular panics.

PHOBIC ANXIETY STATE

In ordinary anxiety states the anxiety is diffuse or generalized and more or less continuous so that the patient is worried most of the time; instead the anxiety may be experienced in relation to certain specific situations or objects only, so-called *phobic anxiety states*. Common examples are a fear of being in closed spaces (claustrophobia), fear of going out unaccompanied (agoraphobia), fear of travelling, e.g. by tube or by air, fear of heights, fear of sharp objects like knives, or fear of thunder. These symptoms may exist in association with other psychoneurotic symptoms such as depression, anxiety, obsessionality and depersonalisation.

The patient may remember the first occasion on which he experienced anxiety in a particular situation and, usually after an interval, he begins to dread having to face the same situation again. From then onwards his fear increases and he avoids the anxiety-arousing situations altogether. This may seriously interfere with his work or personal life with the result that he gets depressed and even more anxious than before. There is often a history of disturbed childhood development, e.g. of maternal deprivation in patients with agoraphobia. Stress in present day inter-personal relationships is almost always an important feature of the condition. These patients often have difficulty in expressing anger, and psycho-sexual problems are very common. The phobia may express an unconscious fear in a symbolic manner, e.g. the fear of travelling and of not being able to control the external situation may be related to the fear of not being able to control inner feelings of anger or sexuality. In other cases the anxiety may have resulted more from an original anxiety-rousing experience followed by re-inforcement; but it seems unlikely that a severe phobic anxiety state ever arises without some underlying psychological conflicts being present as predisposing, if not causative, factors.

The best *treatment* is psychotherapy but even prolonged and intensive treatment may fail to relieve the phobic symptom in some cases. Behaviour therapy, using desensitization directed towards relief from the specific phobic symptoms, may in such cases by helpful (p. 327), especially if prior psychotherapy has succeeded in resolving some of the psychological conflicts and difficulties in inter-personal relationships. Desensitization may also be useful if the patient has few problems other than the phobia itself or is unsuitable for psychotherapy for other reasons. Tranquillizers or sedatives may be of some help symptomatically to allow the patient to face the phobic situation if he has to, e.g. before having to travel by air, but are of little help in relieving the phobic anxiety state as such.

FURTHER READING

Freud, S. (1949). *Inhibition, Symptoms and Anxiety*. Hogarth, London.
Gelder, M. G., Marks, I. M., and Wolff, H. H. (1967). 'Desensitization and psychotherapy in the treatment of phobic states'. *Brit. J. Psychiat.*, 113, 53.
Lader, M. M. and Marks, I. M. (1973). *Clinical Anxiety*. Heinemann, London.
Marks, I. M. (1969). *Fears and Phobias*. Heinemann, London.
Rycroft, C. (1968). *Anxiety and Neurosis*. Penguin.

14 Depressive illnesses

DEFINITION

Feeling depressed is a normal mood change in reaction to certain circumstances, especially bereavements and other serious losses and disappointments. It is pathological and hence regarded as a depressive illness either when no obvious cause for depression can be detected in the patient's recent life experience, so-called endogenous depression (see below), or when its degree or duration is out of proportion to its cause, so-called reactive depression. Melancholia is an old term for depression, dating back to the theory that black bile caused the condition.

SYMPTOMS

The patient's depression varies from mild gloom, an inability to enjoy anything and a feeling that the future holds little to look forward to, to utter misery and despair. He cannot concentrate except on woes, cannot take an interest in what he is doing or is supposed to do, and cannot cope with his daily work and ordinary chores. His appetite is poor so that he loses weight; however, some depressed patients get some temporary relief from compulsive over-eating; sexual interest is diminished or absent and a man may become impotent, a woman frigid. Sleep is disturbed and the more severely depressed he is the earlier he wakes, feeling at his worst when he does. He tends to oppose offers of help or advice by producing apparently sound reasons for doing so; he feels that life is not worth living and he wants to escape from it, so that he may attempt suicide or successfully kill himself. In severe cases he may develop delusions of guilt, unworthiness, persecution or bodily illness, often supported by hallucinations (psychotic depression), and he believes himself to be a complete failure in this world, responsible for all evil, and doomed to eternal punishment in the next. This condition may last for weeks or months and is one of the most terrible illnesses known.

Mental retardation is often marked, thinking is obviously slow and requires effort. Physically the pulse may be slow, constipation may occur, movements are slowed down, and in severe cases he may no longer be able to cry. Some patients, especially those of middle age, may exhibit a different picture with intense agitation and restlessness (agitated depression).

Depressed patients usually show evidence of anxiety as well and may ask constantly for reassurance but seem to get no help from it; their repetition of complaints tends to antagonise their relatives and so can lead to further isolation and misery.

CLASSIFICATION

Three types of depression are described:

(a) Reactive or exogenous; (b) Endogenous; (c) Involutional.

This classification has often been criticized and many believe that depressive illnesses form a spectrum, with endogenous depression at one end, and clear-cut reactive depression at the other (Kendell 1968). These may be difficult to distinguish by a study of their symptoms, but their causation is very different.

AETIOLOGY

At one end of the range lie patients with endogenous depression in whom genetic predisposition plays an important part and psychological factors very little. Twin studies have revealed a higher concordance rate in monozygotic than in dizygotic twins, and a family history of manic-depressive psychosis (see p. 89) is common in these illnesses. At the other extreme lie the reactive depressions in which heredity plays little or no part and in which psychological factors are predominant. Between these extremes lie the majority of cases in which both physical and psychological factors and their inter-action are important.

Apart from genetic predisposition there is other evidence for a physical basis of depression. This is strongly suggested by its physical accompaniments and by its frequent response to physical treatment but there is as yet no proof of any consistent biochemical change associated with depression; physiological changes which have been reported, such as electrolyte changes and alterations in steroid function may be the effect rather than the cause of the depressive mood. It is, however, known that physical causes can produce a depressive illness; thus virus infections, hepatitis and drugs, e.g. sulphonamides or reserpine, can cause depression. One hypothesis which has considerable experimental support is that depression is associated with reduction of available catecholamines at the synapses in the CNS: reserpine which lowers the catecholamine level can cause depression and the mono-amine oxidase inhibitors, by increasing this level, relieve depression (Granville-Grossman 1971). The periodicity of endogenous depression and manic-depressive psychosis also suggests a biochemical basis (see also p. 89).

On the psychological side, there is evidence that disturbed development in childhood, e.g. loss of, or separation from a parent early in life, may lead to a vulnerable personality, and in such cases emotional stresses in later life more easily lead to a depressive illness. Psychoanalytic studies have stressed the similarity between depression and prolonged mourning or grief reactions after bereavements (Freud 1917) and the importance of the loss of love objects in general; marked discrepancies between what one feels oneself to be (actual self) and what one would like to be (ideal self), aggression turned against oneself, exaggerated guilt feelings, and regression to early, especially oral, stages of infantile development are other aspects stressed by psychoanalysts; but to what extent these are causes of depression or its effects is often difficult to decide in the individual case. Social factors may also be important; Murphy and others (1964) hold that 'depression is not related to a specific culture, or to religious views or to social class or residence, but to the level of cohesion in the community'.

The study of the previous personality and precipitating stresses and their interaction is therefore essential.

On the one hand, the personality in so-called *endogenous depression* is prone to mood swings (cyclothymic), sometimes associated with a pyknic build (Kretschmer). The patient may have displayed phases of previous depression, mild overactivity or hypomania, or mania (see p. 89). This condition is known as *manic-depressive psychosis*. There is often also a family history of depression or mania. No precipitating cause may be apparent in endogenous depression, but sometimes a minor stress may have triggered off the attack.

On the other hand, the personality in *reactive depression* is often inadequate and dependent, with too little security and affection in childhood. To this has often been added the inculcation of high ideals and strict standards; the patient may have developed a facade of a polite social manner; he may even have learnt to conceal his depression. Nearly always there has been a major precipitating cause such as bereavement, failure, loss or disappointment or, more often, a concatenation of these stresses, with inadequate emotional outlet. Aggression, aroused by stress and repressed in a rigid or fearful personality, may well lead to depression in which suicide is a serious risk. Poor physical health may add to depression. Social isolation, so common in big cities, is certainly a major factor; and is generally more painful to bear on festive and sentimental occasions such as Christmas. In involutional depression the frustrations and disappointments of late middle age, with little left to look forward to, are obvious factors, with the additional hormonal changes in women at the menopause.

Bereavement is naturally a major factor in many depressions (Parkes 1972). There are circumstances which make prognosis poor. They are low socio-economic status, short terminal illness with little warning of impending death, previous conflict and ambivalence towards the deceased, e.g. in a marital relationship. Certain reactions to bereavement, including anger or self-reproach, or failure to mourn and adequately to experience and express feelings of grief, also worsen the prognosis.

These correlations were found whether single or multiple correlation methods were used and they enable a predictive questionnaire to be derived which could be of value to doctors, clergy, nurses, social workers or others whose work brings them close to people at times of bereavement.

It seems likely, therefore, that in depression physical and psychological changes constantly interact; psychological factors may initiate a depressive reaction which in turn has its somatic counterpart; if the depressive mood persists or if there is an associated and constitutional basis, persistent physical changes may develop which, by setting up a vicious circle, may further aggravate the depression which could then be said to have entered a biological phase; conversely, physical causes may initiate a biological state of depression and the resulting depressive mood may in turn aggravate the physical features of the depression. In either case, depressive posture may be maintained, whether it started on a psychological or a physical basis or both (Hill 1969).

DIAGNOSIS

Depression is generally easy to recognise, unless masked, as described below, but the doctor must do more than recognise it; he must try to understand fully the interactions of stress and personality which have caused it. In so doing he will be better able to provide appropriate help.

He should, however, remember that there do exist certain cases of endogenous depression in which attacks occur acutely or insidiously with no stress or with a very minor trigger; they present the same pattern of symptoms each time. Attacks of mania or hypomania (see p. 89) may also occur at other times in the same patient who in between attacks is normal, rational and competent.

Besides this, three points should be remembered:

1 Depressive attacks may occur as early symptoms of insidiously developing schizophrenia; or, in later life, an organic disease such as GPI or dementia.

2 The patient may mask his depression by insistence on physical complaints, either those which are themselves symptoms of it, e.g. anorexia, insomnia, impotence, or frigidity, or those which arise coincidentally and which act as a focus for the depression, such as bodily pains; with a complaint of any of the above, e.g. physical pain which cannot be accounted for on an organic basis, or impotence, beginning in middle age, depression should always be considered.

3 The patient may also mask his symptoms by denial and apparent normality or even cheerfulness. This is especially common in adolescents and younger age groups.

COMPLICATIONS OF ANY DEPRESSIVE ILLNESS

1 Suicide is a real risk in any severe depression (see p. 85).

2 Alcohol or stimulant drugs provide easy relief from depression, for a time: a habit may thus be formed, which is most difficult to treat (see p. 132).

TREATMENT

General principles

Treatment is essential in every case, since in the acute case the symptoms are intolerable and the risk of suicide is ever present.

1 Simple psychotherapy: reassurance, hope and support, which must be continued, even if the patient seems impervious. In particular a bereaved patient may be helped if he is given a chance to express his feelings to a sympathetic listener and thus work through his grief reaction.

2 Symptomatic drugs and diet for lack of sleep and appetite.

Barbiturates should be avoided as they are often used for suicidal attempts.

3 Always consider the risk of suicide, and arrange for adequate supervision, if necessary. This may entail admission to a psychiatric unit. But admission to horrifying surroundings may be the last blow to the patient's self-respect. Seek a second opinion if in doubt. Patients in single rooms often get more gloomy. The risk of suicide is less if rapport has been established with a doctor, nurse, or relations (see also p.88).

4 The attitude of relatives, the environment, and some occupation can all influence the patient more than appears at first sight. The former will need help and advice themselves from the doctor if they are to persevere. They can be a most important factor in the patient's recovery. Isolation will diminish his chance of recovery.

5 Anti-depressant drugs have proved their use, and are generally necessary, and effective in lifting some of the patient's depression. But this should not make the doctor neglect to consider whether some form of deeper psychotherapy is also required as is likely in reactive depression; even if a patient is at first inaccessible this should again be considered as he improves (see p. 322).

6 ECT or surgery (see pp. 326 and 341) should be considered for those who do not respond to the above.

Anti-depressant drugs

There are four groups: The two longest established are:—

(*i*) *Tricyclic compounds.* Imipramine (Tofranil): increase gradually over one to three weeks from 25 to 50 to 75 mg. t.d.s. Little effect is seen until 10 to 14 days.

Side effects: dryness of the mouth, sweating, dizziness due to postural hypotension, urinary retention, raised intra-ocular tension, cardiac arrhythmias, tremor and Parkinsonism, agitation, confusional states, especially in elderly patients. Toxic effects: skin rashes, agranulocytosis, hepatitis.

Amitriptyline (Tryptizol) in the same dosage has fewer side effects, but may cause drowsiness, and after a time increased ocular tension, retention of urine, and constipation. Usually it produces some hypotension for the first two or three days and it is therefore best given as 25 mg b.d., increasing on the third day to t.d.s., and then a week or so later to 50 mg t.d.s.; some people are helped to sleep better by giving the bulk of the daily dosage at night, though in a few people sleep may be disturbed by doing so.

Other Tricyclics are: Nortriptyline (Aventyl), Protriptyline (Concordin) and Trimipramine (Surmontil). Each has its uses, and seems to suit certain patients best. The choice depends on a knowledge of the effects of previous drugs and finding by degrees the most effective and the correct dosage.

Anafranil (Clomipramine Hydrochloride) can also be given orally or by injection and has special value in patients with phobic and obsessional states associated with depression.

Prothiaden (Dothiepin) 25-50 mg t.d.s. produces a quicker lift of depression in some patients; Sinequan (Doxepin Hydrochloride) 10-100 mg t.d.s. is effective in others.

(*ii*)   *Mono-amine oxidase inhibitors*:
　　　Phenelzine (Nardil) 15 mg t.d.s.
　　　Nialamide (Niamid) 25-30 mg t.d.s.
　　　Isocarboxazid (Marplan) 10 mg t.d.s.
　　　Tranylcypromine (Parnate) 10 mg t.d.s.

The first three usually take 10 to 14 days to act; tranylcypromine acts more quickly but side effects are more likely.

If the depression is accompanied by much anxiety the anti-depressant may usefully be combined with a mild tranquillizer, e.g. Librium 10 mg t.d.s. or Valium 5 mg t.d.s. which can be given together with a MAOI or one of the tricyclic compounds. Parnate is sometimes combined with stelazine in the form of parstelin (parnate 10 mg and stelazine 1 mg).

Side effects of all the MAOI include hypertensive crises with severe headache and occasionally an actual subarachnoid haemorrhage. They are precipitated if food containing tyramine is taken by a patient who is on MAOI. He must therefore be warned to avoid cheese, marmite, bananas, strawberries, beer and high meat. Certain drugs, especially the tricyclic compounds, amphetamine, pethidine and morphia must not be given to a patient on a MAOI and the patient should carry a card to this effect. If a patient is to be changed over from a MAOI to one of the tricyclic compounds or vice versa, an interval of 10 to 14 days should be allowed.

(*iii*) *Stimulants.* These are now largely replaced by the preceding drugs but still used exceptionally to give a brief temporary lift, or to meet a specific non-recurrent event. Dexamphctamine (dexedrine), 5 mg t.d.s., is the stimulant of choice but must not be taken after 4 p.m. Side effects include tension and overactivity, sudden lowering of mood when the effect of the drug has worn off after a few hours, addiction especially in teenagers: and amphetamine psychosis after prolonged addiction.

It is important to remember that in a severely depressed and apathetic patient the partial lifting of his depression by any of these drugs may remove his apathy and induce him to action. As a result if a patient has been contemplating suicide but has been too apathetic to do it, he may become actively suicidal as his depression is lifting under treatment.

OTHER METHODS OF TREATMENT

ECT (see p. 326) still has a higher rate of success in severely depressed patients than any one drug. It should therefore be used if relief from severe depression has not been produced by anti-depressant drugs. Relapses, however, are common.

Formal psychotherapy can be very helpful if reactive factors predominate; a few successes have been recorded in endogenous depression, but severe mood swings often prevent co-operation. Hence drugs or ECT are the best forms of treatment in severe endogenous depression.

Restricted orbital undercut (see p. 344) has given considerable relief to chronic reactive and involutional depressives when all other treatment has failed: either by a direct effect, or by allowing the patient to be more amenable to psychotherapy and drugs. It has also been shown to remove the tendency of endogenous depression, and mania, to recur. Yttrium implantation has similar successes.

Thus it is clear that the decision what treatment or combination of treatments, e.g. drugs and psychotherapy, to use is very delicate and depends on the severity of the risk of suicide, the extent of his reliability (to avoid cheese and alcohol), the co-operation likely from those around him and the efficiency of psychiatric help available.

PROPHYLAXIS

Lithium Carbonate, though more commonly used to control manic states (see p. 93), may in some patients with recurrent endogenous depression prevent extremes of mood swings and thus help to prevent a further attack of depression. It is best given as Priadel in a single daily dose of 400 to 1600 mg. The serum Lithium level should be checked at intervals and kept between 0.6 and 1.5 m Eq per litre. Tremor of the hands is a common side effect, and impaired renal function contra-indicates its use. Lithium appears to act by affecting the adenyl cyclase activity of brain tissue (Dousa and Hechter 1970).

Modern forms of leucotomy (see p. 342) have also prevented the recurrence of depressive and manic attacks.

Intensive formal psychotherapy, if successful, may reduce the risk of further depressive attacks, especially of the reactive type.

REFERENCES

Dousa, T. and Hechter, O. (1970). 'Lithium and brain adenyl cyclase'. *Lancet*, 1, 834.

Freud, S. (1917). *Mourning and Melancholia.* Standard edition, Hogarth, London, vol. 14.

Coppen, A. and Walk, A. (1968). 'Recent developments in affective disorders'. *Brit. J. Psychiat.*, Special publication No. 2.

Granville-Grossman, K. (1971). *Recent Advances in Clinical Psychiatry.* London, J. & A. Churchill.

Hill, D. (1968). 'Depression: disease, reaction or posture'. *Am. J. Psychiat.*, 125, 445.

Kendell, R. E. (1968). 'The problem of classification'. *Brit. J. Psychiat.*, Special publication No. 2, 15.

Kretschmer, E. (1936) *Physique and Character.* Routledge, London.

Murphy, H. B. M., Wittkower, E. D., and Chance, M. A. (1964) 'Cross-cultural factors in depression'. *Transcultural Psychiatric Research*, 1, 5-21.

Parkes, C. M. (1972). *Bereavement.* Tavistock Publications, London.

Schildkraut, J. J. (1965). 'The catecholamine hypothesis of affective disorders'. *Am. J. Psychiat.*, 122, 509.

FURTHER READING

John Bunyan's *Pilgrim's Progress* (1673), though written in allegorical
terms, describes his own attack of depression very graphically.
Marris, P. (1974). *Loss and Change*. Routledge, London.

15 Suicide and attempted suicide

PREVALENCE

The published figures of suicides are probably below the actual,
since the coroner may give the patient the benefit of the doubt.
Sainsbury (1973) has collected figures, split by age and sex,
from 1900 to 1970 in England and Wales. There were peaks in
the period of unemployment in the thirties, and troughs in the
two World Wars. There is surprisingly a slight general decrease in
men, with a major decrease among those over 45, but an
increase in females over this time. The totals still run at over
4000 a year, which is much commoner than many people
realise, being the cause in Britain of nearly as many deaths a
year in men as road accidents, while more women kill
themselves than die on the roads. Besides this, a rough estimate
is that seven times as many attempts are made as succeed,
though these are not by any means all sincere attempts. On the
other hand, some road accidents are probably suicides. The rate
is said to be higher in spring. Sadly, one in every 50 doctors kills
himself.

Elsewhere in Europe the highest suicide rate is in Scandinavia
and Berlin, and the lowest in Eire. Various reasons, none
entirely convincing, have been adduced (the 'welfare states'
smother enterprise and the desire to live; the climate in
Scandinavia; personality traits; the strong religious prohibitions
in Eire; or possibly that statistics in Scandinavia are more
thorough).

REASONS

Many suicides have occurred without psychiatric disability: for example for personal honour (Japanese hara-kiri, or until recently, an RN captain going down with his ship); to save relations the trouble of long nursing; to avoid torture and betrayal of comrades; to curtail prolonged illness; to bear witness to one's faith; to save someone else's life. This has of course the sanction of the New Testament; it also occurred in many pagan cultures, where the willing sacrifice of the king, or his substitute, was made for the sake of the people (there is evidence that William Rufus and Anne Boleyn were examples). Nonetheless there is still some stigma attached to suicide: on religious grounds (especially Roman Catholic); on out-dated legal grounds (the citizen's body was not his property, but the king's); in terms of life assurance (so that one can not gain money for one's heirs) and in some countries' immigration laws (which punish people if their relatives have committed suicide).

Until recently attempted suicides could be (but seldom were) charged by the police in England (but not in Scotland). The law has now been altered, but the survivor of a suicide pact may be charged with murder if his partner dies.

Psychiatric illness is today by far the commonest cause, as follows:

1 Depression of any type is the commonest syndrome, so that the risk of suicide must be considered carefully in any case, whether the depression is mainly of endogenous or of reactive origin; suicide is more likely in the latter if the patient sees that the precipitating stress will increase. An early history of maternal deprivation is often a factor and so are recent bereavements and other losses or disappointments.

2 Schizophrenia: suicide may occur, especially in a depressed phase.

3 Compulsions to jump over cliffs, or in front of trains, result in many deaths a year; the individual realizes how foolish this is, but cannot always oppose his compulsion indefinitely.

4 Acute anxiety states may lead to suicide, as the only way of escape from an intolerable position.

5 Hysteria: it is not true that 'hysterics' never kill themselves;

death may occur from a panic gesture in a threatened and hopeless patient, or from a dramatic attempt (not intended to succeed), which goes wrong and succeeds by accident. Nonetheless, an attempt at suicide occurs often as a gesture which demands help and must be treated accordingly. Failure to do so may lead to despair, and a genuine attempt.

6 Confusional states may lead to death, which is more likely to be due to mistakenly taking an overdose, but sometimes is a genuine suicide, once drugs or alcohol have diminished the patient's control and contact with reality.

7 Chronic alcoholism arising from, and increasing depression.

In all these, loneliness is an important factor. It must be remembered that there are many socially isolated people in big cities, especially London; this isolation is increased by the above illnesses, and by poverty, housing difficulties and old age.

Many of these syndromes occur in inadequate dependent people, especially if rejected or isolated.

METHODS AND THEIR CONTROL

Methods vary enormously with the opportunities and social customs prevailing. Since 1948 self-poisoning with barbiturates has become the commonest method of attempting suicide in this country. Aspirin is another drug used for this purpose; turning on the gas is nowadays less common, and natural gas is of course ineffective.

Hetzel (1971) records the easy availability of barbiturates in Australia as a major factor in the high incidence there, and the easy access to drugs for doctors may be one reason for their high rate. Although it is practically impossible indefinitely to prevent a person determined on suicide, it is clear that by diminishing the opportunities (e.g. by making drugs hard to come by) one can prevent many patients from an attempt.

On the other hand it is clear that severely restrictive measures (such as exist in prisons or in old mental hospitals) can make mild depressions worse, and drive some people to suicide. Restrictions which consist of removing scissors, etc., after 10 p.m. at night and on Sunday are obviously ludicrous, but still exist (as do their counterparts in other fields). Good unobtrusive supervision which does not impair the patient's self-respect is most valuable.

THE GENERAL PRACTITIONER'S TASK

Faced with such risks, the general practitioner has a difficult task to decide what to do, and in particular whether to leave the patient at home, or persuade him to go to a psychiatric unit. He can compel admission by using Sec. 25 or 29 of the MH Act, if he feels suicide is likely (see p. 390).

His decision will be made by assessing:

1 The state of the patient's mind, i.e. the depth of his depression, the strength of his control, his ethical standards, his views on life after death, whether he intends or fears suicide, whether he will co-operate with the doctor, and his aggressiveness. The more overtly aggressive he is towards others the less likely is he to turn the aggression against himself in a suicide attempt. The doctor need not fear that he is likely to put ideas into his patient's mind by discussing it with him; on the contrary, the more openly it is discussed, the better.
2 The degree of loneliness of the patient and the support and understanding relatives can give him.
3 The facilities available in the local psychiatric unit.

A patient contemplating suicide is not likely to be deterred by the general practitioner expressing horror. But a discussion of his motives for suicide may help and, above all, the general practitioner's inculcation of some hope. Further treatment clearly depends on the psychiatric condition.

At times the risk must be taken not to admit to hospital, if it is likely to do more harm than good. If in doubt, a psychiatrist's opinion certainly should be sought urgently. Even if delay is inevitable the fact of an appointment being made gives hope. The sudden swing down of the autogenous depression is always difficult to prevent.

The Samaritans are a voluntary body founded by the Rev. Chad Varah, in London, and now active in other cities. They answer telephone calls for help from people who are anxious and depressed, and have certainly saved some from attempting suicide and induced them to seek medical advice (compare Alcoholics Anonymous).

FURTHER READING

Hetzel, B. (1971). *Life and Health in Australia.* ABC, Sydney.
Kessel, N., and McCulloch, W. (1966). 'Repeated acts of self-poisoning and self-injury'. *Proc. Roy. Soc. Med.*, 59, 89.
Sainsbury, P. (1973). 'Suicide: opinions and facts'. *Proc. Roy. Soc. Med.*, 66, 579.
Stengel, E. (1964). *Suicide and Attempted Suicide.* Penguin.
Williams, G. (1955). *The Sanctity of Human Life and the Criminal Law* (London, Faber), has an excellent chapter on suicide.

16 Mania

Endogenous mania is one phase of *manic-depressive psychosis* — being the counterpart of endogenous depression (see p. 78). A milder form is known as hypomania.

THE PREVIOUS PERSONALITY

The previous personality is generally cyclothymic and there may have been previous attacks of hypomania, mania and/or depression, which are sometimes of marked regularity. Patients include a high proportion of professional people.

AETIOLOGY

This is uncertain. Biochemical and psychological causes have both been suggested and changes in electrolyte balance have been recorded. As with recurrent depression, relatives may be affected. According to psycho-analytic theory mania occurs as a defence against underlying depression. Depression under treatment may swing into mania, either spontaneously, or in response to ECT or drugs; presumably because biochemical changes have been reversed (see p. 317).

SYMPTOMS

An actual description of the manic's impression of his own state, which he referred to as mental integration, ran as follows:

'Mental integration produces a healthy mind in a healthy body. The skin loses its sensitiveness to grit and dirt, and its liability to injury by abrasion. There is a delicious feeling of physical fitness and well-being throughout the whole body, and great joy and elation. Both physical and mental energy seem inexhaustible. The man can sleep anywhere, even amid noise, when he needs sleep. The whole world becomes indescribably beautiful, even things and persons that seem positively ugly to others. Heat, cold, pain, hunger, and thirst are all much more easily borne than before, and are often scarcely noticed. The sun and the frost both cease to harm the skin. Alcohol ceases to intoxicate. The man is practically immune to every kind of disease, including the common cold. Accidental infections are overcome very quickly. Skin troubles, such as psoriasis and 'nervous' dermatitis, disappear.

'The memory is complete. One idea calls up a host of related ideas without effort. The man cannot but consider every question of judgment or conduct in all its aspects simultaneously, and he sees the right answer at once. He has no mental conflicts, and ceases to be capable of fear and doubt. Everything seems an occasion for sheer merriment.

'He has unbounded faith, courage, patience, tact, resource, wit and humour, and what less fortunate persons regard as will-power.

'He is filled with an overpowering feeling of benevolence towards every other human being, animal, and thing; and they in turn all seem and are well-disposed towards him. They simply cannot help being so. He can thus control horses, charm snakes, tame lions, etc. The whole world seems suffused with friendliness, kinship, and significance. He realizes as never before that he belongs to it; that this is his true home; and that he is merely a part of the living whole. He loses all capacity for anger, hate, contempt, guilt, anxiety, suspicion, and the other disturbing emotions. Everything in nature, literature, and art takes on a new and richer meaning.

'He can solve any kind of problem immediately, by a kind of intuition. He will never change his mind merely to please another person, but he may change it in the light of fresh knowledge or at a new turn in the situation.'

Later, however, the benevolence mentioned by the writer passed, and he became aware of opposition, attributing it to stupidity or deliberate persecution; the major religions of history and their founders were dismissed and his own writings were extolled. Nevertheless he was still capable of putting his finger with considerable shrewdness on the weak spots of contemporary political and religious leaders.

Such a patient can be seen by an observer to be elated, to feel (and often to look) very well, to be very over-active physically and mentally and to need very little sleep. His judgement is by no means as good as he believes. But he will at once produce plausible reasons for making what is an impulsive decision, which overrides his usual standards; and shows no consideration for others. Pressure of thought, flight of ideas and delusions of grandeur (and later of persecution, if thwarted) are common, but hallucinations are rare. In the extreme case, the patient may believe he is almighty and omniscient; in milder forms, he is over-confident, cocksure and managing and brooks no opposition. The acute case may ruin himself financially or be violent if opposed, and his extravagances in matters of money, sex and drink may place an intolerable strain on his wife and children. The realisation of what he has done will be an additional stress to the patient in his next normal or depressed phase.

All grades exist between this and cheerful, busy optimism.

Spontaneous recovery is common. But some cases become chronic and considerable harm may be done to reputation, relationships and bank balance meanwhile. The behaviour of the manic patient is a tremendous stress on his family, friends and associates. Perhaps at times the latter can enjoy his good spirits; but the former are worn out by his egocentricity and pace of living.

DIFFERENTIAL DIAGNOSIS

A severe case is unmistakable, but delusions of grandeur and failure of judgment may occur in cerebral tumour, GPI, encephalitis and alcoholism.

Reactive mania

Since endogenous mania is clinically the opposite· of endogenous depression, it has been asked if any condition may occur as the counterpart of reactive depression, i.e. reactive mania. This is contradicted by the psychoanalyst's theory that manic behaviour may in fact be a defence against underlying depression; which certainly is borne out by some case studies. However, another clinical picture has been described as mania as a reaction to a particular and prolonged emotional and physical stress which was then suddenly removed; those concerned were largely highly responsible people with no previous cyclothymic tendency (Tredgold 1947).

TREATMENT

This must vary considerably with the severity of the condition. The typical case will not feel ill, nor agree to treatment. Nor can he be compelled to have it. But tactful advice may be accepted, while dogmatic opinions will provoke antagonism. While the patient in a mild phase may realize he is 'going up' again and be aware of his own internal drive and so accept advice, this amount of insight and co-operation is lost as his mood rises. Extreme patience is therefore required on the doctor's part.

Drugs: Haloperidol (serenace) 1-3 mg t.d.s. is most useful; it may lead to symptoms of Parkinsonism, which can be controlled by orphenadrine (disipal) 50 mg with each dose. Lithium carbonate, in doses of 750 mg q.d.s. for three days, may be used for an acute attack; and then reduced. It should be stopped at once if severe tremor develops. It should only be given in the absence of renal disease and under close supervision. Sedatives should be used at night to produce as much sleep as possible.

In cases of severe mania the patient may have to be restrained and compulsorily detained. Intermediate cases may accept drug treatment as out-patients. The most difficult to handle are those, generally professional, people who act on impulse — often disastrously — but sober down at once if compulsorily restrained, and so have to be discharged.

ECT: Has been used but is seldom necessary with modern drugs.

The effect of a manic patient on his relatives has been described; they will also need much support.

PROPHYLAXIS

The use of lithium for acute manic attacks led to the hope that smaller doses (250 mg t.d.s.) might prevent recurrences both of mania and depression (Schou et al. 1971) and in view of the severe disability of the illness this certainly should be tried; again under careful supervision of blood levels (Crammer 1974). Unfortunately not all patients can tolerate it, and some who can do not respond.

There is evidence that surgery (see p. 345) has prevented the recurrence of attacks of either mania or depression in people previously prone to either.

REFERENCES

Crammer, J. L. et al. (1974). 'Blood levels and management of lithium treatment'. *Brit. Med. J.*, 2, 650.

Maggs, R. (1963). 'Treatment of manic illness with lithium carbonate'. *Brit. J. Psych.*, 109, 56.

Schou, M., Amdisen, A. and Baastrup, P. C. (1971). 'The practical management of lithium treatment'. *Brit. J. Hosp. Med.*, July, 53.

Tredgold, R. F. (1947). 'Manic states in the Far East'. *Brit. Med. J.*, ii, 522.

17 Obsessive-compulsive neurosis

Under the name of obsessive-compulsive neurosis, or 'obsessional neurosis' in short, are included a number of conditions characterized by compulsive thoughts, doubts, repetitive actions or rituals and compulsive fears accompanied by such actions. These phenomena are isolated from the rest of the patient's mental activity; he knows them to be irrational but cannot resist them in spite of all efforts to do so, and may despise himself for his weakness.

CLINICAL FEATURES

The compulsive thoughts are often aggressive, sexual or obscene in nature. The patient realizes that they originate from within his own mind and he feels ashamed and depressed on account of their presence and disturbing nature. He may believe that, as it were by magic, these thoughts could give rise to real consequences such as the death of someone; or he may try — usually in vain — to replace these thoughts by more pleasant ones, or to ward off the imagined ill effects by repetitive actions, so-called rituals, in the belief that in this way the harmful effects can be prevented (so-called magic undoing).

More often, compulsive actions, singly or in series, occur without the patient being aware that they have any relation to aggressive or sexual thoughts, which have been completely repressed. To him, therefore, they seem nonsensical, which is a further source of shame, guilt or anxiety. Actions are generally either danger-avoiding, e.g. turning off gas-taps, locking doors, or expiatory, e.g. washing hands. Preventing the ritual causes great anxiety, performing it only temporary relief. Frequent, persistent and complicated rituals, e.g. taking several hours getting undressed and into bed, may completely ruin a patient's life and produce acute depression.

The condition usually develops on the basis of a pre-existing obsessional personality characterized by being rigid, controlled, meticulous and perfectionist. Having high standards these people are conscientious, reliable workers but they tend to suffer from being anxious if they cannot live up to their own or others' high expectations and are given to doubt their own decisions and actions. In a minor form these characteristics are useful attributes but if excessive and if they lead to compulsive need to check work and other activities repeatedly, the condition may become a handicap and verge on an obsessional state.

The illness usually starts in the early twenties, sometimes earlier. Occasionally it is symptomatic of a depressive or schizophrenic illness but in most cases obsessional and depressive symptoms, if co-existent in the same patient, are both expressions of related psychological conflicts. Sometimes the symptoms clear up spontaneously but most cases tend to become chronic and the longer the condition has been present the less likely are the chances of recovery without, and often even with, treatment.

AETIOLOGY

Although constitutional factors may play a part, the basis for the development of an obsessional neurosis usually lies in a disturbance of personality development related to interaction between the patient and his family. The inculcation of too high ideals and too strict a conscience by parents and other influences, such as too strict a religious upbringing, are important factors as they will lead to exaggerated guilt on account of aggressive and sexual impulses. Many of these patients have been overcontrolled and handled too strictly and punitively in childhood, and, according to psychoanalytic theory, fixation at, and regression to, the anal stage of infantile development plays an important part in the development of an obsessional personality and neurosis. However, similar observations also apply to many other psychiatric conditions and our understanding of the origin of this condition is still incomplete.

TREATMENT

Obsessional neuroses are notoriously difficult to treat but the following are the main therapeutic approaches available.

1 *Superficial psychotherapy*

This will be the method first used by the GP. Although unlikely to lead to the disappearance of the obsessional symptoms it will be aimed at making the patient feel that he is being understood, that his fears are unrealistic but can be seen to have some meaning in terms of exaggerated guilt feelings, and that if he could begin to pay a little less attention to his symptoms without fighting them too hard they might gradually interfere less with his life and diminish in intensity. As in all other superficial psychotherapy, the GP must be prepared to listen and to discuss the patient's problems with him; he must at all costs avoid antagonizing the patient by telling him to 'pull himself together'. The patient knows better than the doctor what useless advice this is as he has already tried desperately but unsuccessfully to resist his compulsive thoughts and rituals, and he is already impatient enough with himself without getting further impatience from his doctor.

2 *Formal psychotherapy*

If the patient is sufficiently intelligent and motivated to undergo analytical psychotherapy or psycho-analysis, and if such treatment is available, this is the treatment of choice even though it may take a long time and a successful outcome cannot be guaranteed. By helping the patient to discover the unconscious meaning of his symptoms and to work on them in a secure psychotherapeutic relationship he will not only get the satisfaction of being taken seriously in all the aspects of his illness and underlying problems but he may gradually find that his symptoms become less of a pre-occupation for him, and ultimately his rigid, obsessional personality may change as well. The main difficulty is that obsessional patients tend to rationalize, and instead of changing in the course of psycho-therapy they may incorporate the insight gained into their obsessional thinking and pre-occupation.

3 *Behaviour therapy*

Planned behavioural techniques which prevent the patient from carrying out his rituals can be helpful in some cases; however, where the symptom is thus removed, underlying problèms in interpersonal relationships may come out into the open and require psychotherapy (see p. 322).

4 *Drugs*

These have little to offer in the treatment of obsessional neurotics but occasionally, if the symptoms are part of a depressive illness, they may respond to treatment with an anti-depressant drug. Similarly, if much anxiety is associated with the patient's symptoms tranquillizers may give some relief and may make the patient more amenable to psychotherapy.

5 *Leucotomy*

If all other methods have failed this may be worth considering in patients who are seriously disabled by their symptoms, who show much anxiety and tension but whose previous personality has been reasonably stable. Again, results are unpredictable and in any case the operation should be preceded by establishing psychotherapeutic contact and regarded as a step to diminish tension and the force of established habits and so allow further psychotherapy: without the latter, relapse is likely (see p. 345).

FURTHER READING

Pollitt, J. (1969). 'Obsessional states'. *Brit. J. Hosp. Med.*, 2, 1146.

18 Hysteria

Hysteria is not a clear-cut clinical entity, but a term which covers a variety of reactions, shown by many people from time to time to a greater or lesser degree; they are regarded as unhealthy if extreme or habitual. Unfortunately, this is often not realized, and the word 'hysteria' is used as a term of abuse and arouses prejudice; the whole subject has thus become complicated by many misconceptions, set out below. It is of historical interest that it was Freud's work with patients suffering from hysteria which led to his fundamental discoveries of unconscious mental processes and hence to psycho-analysis (see p. 308). In World War I a large number of cases at first labelled 'shell shock' were later found to be hysterical, and much more was learned from them. They were fewer in World War II, being replaced by anxiety and depressive states, and psychosomatic conditions.

SYMPTOMATOLOGY

1 Symptoms are manifold and include a variety of complaints: common *physical* (conversion) symptoms are motor (fits, tremors, faints, paralysis of one or more limbs, difficulty in walking and aphonia); sensory (anaesthesia of glove or stocking distribution, and blindness); or visceral (e.g. hysterical vomiting or urinary retention). *Mental* (dissociative) disturbances include amnesia, and fugue states when complicated actions like travelling from one place to another are carried out in a state of mental dissociation. Gross conversion symptoms are less frequent nowadays and hysterical exaggeration of organic ailments is much more common.
2 Although the physical conversion symptoms do not correspond, in nature and extent, with any organic lesion, they do correspond with an idea in the patient's mind, based on information he has (though this may be erroneous).

3 Hysterical symptoms aim at some gain but unconsciously. It may be (*a*) 'primary gain' (Freud's term) through repression which gives relief from an intolerable intrapsychic conflict, and (*b*) 'secondary gain' arising from the symptoms and demanding help or allowing escape from a stressful situation. Often, however, the total loss to the patient exceeds any short-term gain.

4 There may be anatomical discrepancies in the symptoms, e.g. a selective disability, but this again will not be realized by the patient.

5 Classically the hysteric is calm (*belle indifference*) because there is dissociation of feeling from an underlying painful conflict, the anxiety having been 'converted' into the symptom ('conversion hysteria'). But this may not be completely so, and then some anxiety persists (anxiety-hysteria). Again, there may be some anxiety over the symptoms which have developed, though this is generally less than they might be expected to provoke.

6 If he meets suspicion, as he nearly always does, the patient will dramatize and exaggerate his symptoms; he will make unreasonable demands, make statements which are unlikely to be true, and tend to manipulate his environment and so infuriate his family and his GP. The latter's reactions will lead the patient to exaggerate still further.

7 In particular, pain is a common complaint; although in the hysteric it is usually dramatized, it still puts the doctor in a dilemma, for he is rightly afraid of missing some organic complaint, and yet he knows that excessive investigations may simply focus the patient's attention more firmly on his own symptoms. The middle course must be chosen, of as full and as early a physical examination as the symptoms warrant, coupled with a full psychiatric assessment (see p. 36); and he must then consider the probabilities of either diagnosis.

But even well-established hysterics do develop organic illness; and an incipient carcinoma, say, may be missed. The chances of this tragedy will be less if any marked *change* in the nature of the patient's symptoms is taken as an indication for further psychological and physical investigation.

8 Under severe stress, the patient may react acutely in one of several ways:

    (*a*) Panic and flurry, when he may damage himself and others, like a bird trapped in a room.

(*b*)Mimicry, when he imitates symptoms and behaviour of those around him — whole groups may at times do this ('chameleon-like'), e.g. in schools. This is usually due to unconscious identification.

(*c*) Inhibition of normal reactions, such as fight or flight, and so paralysis, or even stupor ('opossum-like').

9 Suicide is often threatened, and sometimes attempted; in general, it is a demonstration, or an appeal for help, and is not meant to succeed; but it may be fatal, by accident; and occasionally, from a desperate gesture. The risk must be accepted, for if not, the patient may blackmail all around him by his threat.

DIAGNOSIS

Diagnosis has in the past been made too often by the exclusion of organic illness; this is wrong. Positive psychiatric indications must be found in the history, symptoms and appearance; in particular:

1 There has previously been some threatening situation or emotional conflict, often connected with aggression or sexuality; this may well now be repressed, so that the patient will see no connection between its occurrence and his illness; but sometimes this can be elicited by a careful history from the patient and if possible, relatives; or it may emerge only in the course of psychotherapy when the patient's defences are gradually being overcome.

2 There may also be a clue as to the nature of the symptoms in a history of a chance accident, or of a purpose served; often the symptom represents the underlying conflict in a symbolic manner e.g. paralysis of the right arm if the patient wants, but fears, to hit someone.

3 There have generally been similar symptoms under past stress.

4 Usually there is evidence of an underlying *hysterical personality* as shown by selfish, evasive, irresponsible, immature, exhibitionist, attention-seeking and suggestible characteristics. These tendencies are learned, not hereditary.

5 There may be behaviour which indicates regression to infantile dependence.

6 According to classical psycho-analytic theory unresolved Oedipal problems may play an important causative role.

If a positive diagnosis of hysteria is made, further questions must be asked: Why did these symptoms occur when they did? Will the patient be happier without them, or better? What effect are they having on other people, including the doctor? The answers to these indicate whether further treatment is needed, or whether the patient is better left with his symptoms and the partial adjustment he has reached. The GP may also get some insight through his own reactions. Hysterical behaviour may make him feel helpless and angry, and so inclined to criticize. No doubt some misconceptions arise in this way.

Hysteria should be distinguished from conscious simulation of illness, i.e. malingering, which is generally carried out for purely selfish aims, but may be for patriotic reasons, e.g. a soldier escaping from a prison camp. In some patients hysteria and malingering may of course co-exist: they are hard to separate, especially if either, or both, are superimposed on an organic ailment or injury.

Münchausen's syndrome

A remarkable example of this is Münchausen's syndrome, entertainingly described by Asher (1951). Patients simulate an acute illness supported by a dramatic history, just plausible and perhaps based on truth which leads to extensive investigation and sometimes surgery. They tend to move from hospital to hospital, creating first interest, then suspicion and finally triumph on the part of the doctor, who unmasks the patient and discharges him with ignominy, and unfortunately with the reasons for his complaints still undiscovered, and his emotional needs unsatisfied. This may be because they have by now been replaced by the sheer pleasure of a war with the doctors and the syndrome has become a fairly harmless hobby; but in other cases there is considerable misery and isolation on the patient's part and frustration on the doctors', which could have been prevented by an earlier effort to understand its psychological basis.

Korsakov's syndrome (see p. 134) can generally be distinguished by detecting its underlying memory failure.

If the GP is in doubt on the diagnosis, or on the questions above, or if specialist treatment seems indicated, he should seek psychiatric advice. Here, it is vital that his letter referring the patient should be full, and give his assessment of the history, the present state, and the results of any treatment he has already done. Personal contact between GP and psychiatrist is most helpful.

COMMON MISCONCEPTIONS

The common misconceptions are worth listing — each with the facts in brackets:

1 'Hysteria occurs only in adolescent girls.' (In fact, it occurs in both sexes at all ages.)
2 'It is the same as malingering.' (Malingering is conscious simulation of ailments the owner knows he has not got; hysteria is unconscious, and the patient believes he is ill.)
3 'It is entirely despicable.' (Patients are not to blame, and contempt increases their symptoms.)
4 'It is always socially damaging.' (Sometimes it is, but at others it solves social problems.)
5 'It is treated best by pulling oneself together.' (Pressure of circumstances does sometimes check hysterical tendencies, but being told to pull himself together only makes the patient worse.)
6 'It is untreatable.' (Many cases respond to psychotherapy.)
7 'It consists of violent or wild behaviour.' (This is rare.)
8 'Diagnosis is by the exclusion of any physical lesion.' (The physical state needs to be carefully assessed, but hysteria also has positive psychiatric indications.)

TREATMENT AND THE GP's PART

Psychotherapy is the treatment of choice but progress is likely to be slow. During it, narco-analysis and hypnosis may be used. It is necessary not only to remove symptoms (which may be easy, and gratifyingly spectacular, but unfortunately temporary), but also to educate the patient away from habits of selfishness and evasion which have lasted for years, and to aim at resolution of the underlying conflicts. If the patient will co-operate, psycho-analysis or analytically oriented psychotherapy are often indicated, the aim being not only to remove the symptoms but to bring about changes in the patient's personality so that he learns to express his problem more openly instead of using his symptoms as an indirect means of communication.

The first step in treatment is to understand the patient's present symptoms in terms of his relations with others (see questions above). This offers a constructive approach to the real situation; to label him 'a hysteric' and leave it at that leads nowhere, except to a stalemate.

The next step is to give the patient insight into his behaviour and the meaning of his symptoms; but as his resistances are tackled he is likely to get angry with whoever does so; nonetheless, this can indeed be valuable, if he sees that anger can itself be used constructively and safely, and that he is being offered help in this real situation, rather than in his attempts to escape from it. Reproof or rejection will harden his repressions.

If the patient is being treated by formal psychotherapy the GP still has a part to play between psychiatric sessions. If he feels he has not enough advice on this from the psychiatrist, let him say so. He must understand that he too may be made angry or helpless by the patient, and this may lead him into critical attitudes and misconceptions — conscious or not. Certainly he can do valuable work, in collaboration with the psychiatrist, but he must remember that patients tend to drive wedges between their helpers, and beware of falling into this trap.

It is a truism that both patient and doctor demand more from treatment of psychological than of physical illness; that is, both find it more difficult to accept residual disabilities. Yet many cases of hysteria are not fully curable. The GP must all the same be prepared to do what he can, with psychiatric help, and this may make a considerable difference to the adjustment of the patient and his relatives.

Total amnesia, i.e. inability to recall any event of one's past life, is much less common than a decade ago; but it still occurs and generally represents some very traumatic experience, the memory of which is intolerable. Hypnosis or pentothal abreaction may recover the memory, but release great anxiety and depression which obviously needs urgent treatment.

Unfortunately some cases develop hysterical symptoms as the only way out of an intolerable situation; thus gastric pain which occurs under the stress of a too demanding job may persist as an escape from it. Unconsciously determined 'accidents' may serve the same purpose (see p. 274). Treatment here is unlikely to succeed for the secondary gain cannot be given up.

REFERENCES

Asher, R. (1951). 'Münchhausen's syndrome'. *Lancet*, 1, 339.
Breuer, J., and Freud, S. (1895). *Studies in Hysteria*. Standard edition, Hogarth, London, vol. 2.
Carter, A. B. (1972). 'A physician's view of hysteria'. *Lancet*, 2, 1241.
Guze, S. B. (1967). 'The diagnosis of hysteria: what are we trying to do?'. *Amer. J. Psychiat.*, 124, 77.
Kretschmer, E. (1961). *Hysteria, Reflex and Instinct*. Owen, London.
Reed, J.L. (1971). 'Hysteria'. *Brit. J. Hosp. Med.*, 237.
Szasz, T. S. (1972). *The Myth of Mental Illness*. Paladin.
Walshe, F. M. R. (1965). 'Diagnosis of hysteria'. *Brit. J. Hosp. Med.*, 237.

19 Psychosexual disorders

GENERAL INTRODUCTION

Problems in sexual behaviour and conflicts relating to sexuality are so common that everyone is likely to be affected at some time or another in his life, but only a minority are sufficiently troubled by them to need help, and even fewer are willing to seek it. General practitioners, doctors working in hospitals or family planning clinics, psychiatrists and others can make it easier for those who come to them to talk about these problems if they themselves feel free to introduce the subject when they sense that it may be relevant to do so. Much sexual behaviour that used to be regarded as abnormal, and led to fear and shame, is nowadays more widely accepted.

The commonest difficulties encountered in adult life are impotence and frigidity; others include various degrees of sexual disharmony, or even unconsummated marriages; exhibitionism which may have brought the patient in conflict with the law; sadomasochism, fetishism, transvestism (the desire to wear clothes of the opposite sex, often in order to get sexually aroused), and trans-sexualism (the desire to change sex). Homosexuality in men and in women (lesbianism) is so common that it should no longer be regarded as abnormal in itself, but difficulties arise if the person concerned is unable to adjust to it (which may be made more difficult by the attitude of society), if he wishes to change his sexual orientation or if it is associated with a personality disorder which prevents him from making meaningful and lasting relationships; the same, however, applies equally to many of the problems associated with heterosexual behaviour. Homosexuality will be discussed separately (see p. 242).

In general, psychosexual problems are usually the result of environmental factors leading to disturbed personality development, although genetic and endocrine factors have been considered as possible predisposing factors. In the latter respect it is of interest that if androgens are administered to animals, including guinea pigs, rats and rhesus monkeys at certain critical periods during pregnancy, female offspring will be born with masculinised external genitalia, and will, as they mature, behave more like males than females. Conversely, if an anti-androgen (Cyproterone acetate) is given to the pregnant female her male offspring will be born with feminised external genitalia and behave like females rather than males. There is, however, no evidence that this is relevant to humans. In fact, in human infants whose sex is uncertain or misdiagnosed at birth, e.g. in pseudohermaphroditism due to the adreno-genital syndrome where female infants are born with masculinised external genitalia, their future sexual behaviour and their subjective sense of sexual identity (gender role) is determined by whether they are brought up as boys or girls. In monkeys, too, social factors are influential in determining sexual behaviour. Environmental factors certainly remain the most important ones to consider in humans.

Freud (1905) drew attention to the influence of early childhood experience on sexual development (see p. 29) but later experiences in life are also of importance. In fact, psychosexual problems are usually only one aspect of more widespread personal and emotional problems and should be considered in the context of the person as a whole and his interpersonal relationships rather than as isolated phenomena.

Sexual behaviour is always directed towards an object which is sexually arousing, and is profoundly influenced by the strength of the individual's sexual drive, i.e. the activity that leads to sexual excitement and gratification; outward sexual behaviour is usually accompanied by sexual fantasies which determine the nature of the object sought and the type of activity preferred.

At the earliest, infantile stages of development, oral activity like sucking is a source of pleasurable excitement, followed later by pleasure associated with excretory (anal) functions, before the child's genitalia become the main source of sexual (auto-erotic) activity. These pleasures remain part of normal, adult sexual behaviour, but are often inhibited or repressed, by guilt feelings caused by the attitudes of parents and society; alternatively, fixation at these early stages may interfere with and limit psychosexual development. At the Oedipal stage (see p. 29) failure to identify with the parent of the same sex, or incestuous guilt feelings, may again lead to uncertainty about one's sexual role; some degree of bisexuality is, however, universal and social factors, such as living in an exclusively male or female environment, may determine whether the sexual partner chosen is of the same or the opposite sex. Conscious or unconscious confusion between sexual and aggressive impulses may lead to sado-masochistic behaviour, or to inhibition with resultant impotence or frigidity; fear of doing damage or of being damaged during intercourse (castration anxiety) is particularly important here.

Any of these problems and more widespread difficulties in forming interpersonal relationships often prevent the person from combining sexual activity with the ability to love and care for the sexual partner; this may lead to excessive promiscuity or to the absence of any meaningful sexual relationships. On the other hand love and sexuality do not always co-exist, and to insist that they should is to set an ideal that may be unrealistic for many people, and so lead to feelings of inadequacy and sexual inhibition.

Some of the common psychosexual syndromes will be considered next.

IMPOTENCE

Definition

The inability in the male to achieve and maintain an erection, so that he can not perform sexual intercourse with orgasm and emotional satisfaction. If the man has never been able to achieve this he is said to be suffering from primary impotence. More often it is intermittent or develops only later on in certain situations (secondary impotence). It may present as:

1 A total lack of sexual desire.
2 An inability to obtain an erection even though desire is present.
3 An inability to maintain an erection.
4 Premature ejaculation, either before or immediately following penetration.
5 An inability to ejaculate.
6 Ejaculation without physical satisfaction.

Aetiology

The disturbance is nearly always emotional in origin but rarely it may be associated with some endocrine abnormality, e.g. hypopituitarism or diabetes, a neurological disorder or severe systemic disease. It also occurs as a complication of treatment with such drugs as hypotensive agents and anti-depressants, especially the mono-amine oxidase inhibitors. The majority of impotent males suffer from some form of anxiety state but impotence may be an early symptom of a severe mental illness, e.g. depression, schizophrenia, organic psychosis, drug addiction, alcoholism.

This anxiety state often develops after the first attempt at sexual intercourse, when excessive sexual excitement or anxiety about the unknown may lead to failure; this then causes additional anxiety about failure at subsequent attempts and the setting up of a vicious circle of failures. Fears of contracting venereal disease, of pregnancy, of being too aggressive, or even of the possibility of being impotent, may all affect performance. The mistaken belief that masturbation could cause physical harm and impotence may be another factor. Feelings of excessive respect, or of disgust for the female, may also lead to failure. It is sometimes observed that a husband is impotent with his wife, whom he respects, and yet is potent in extramarital relationships with women he despises. Impotence is often only a temporary phenomenon, due to fatigue or unsuitable circumstances for making love or the wrong sexual partner. Although impotence is commoner in men of advanced age this is often due to fear of losing one's potency rather than of physiological origin; potency is often preserved although it may take longer to achieve an erection and orgasm.

Common aetiological factors involved in this condition are:

1 Guilt feelings associated with sex due to adverse familial or social, including too rigid religious, influences.
2 Emotional and sexual incompatibility with the partner is a common cause of secondary impotence.
3 An unconscious incestuous fixation on mother or sister with associated anxieties and guilts which have not been surmounted.
4 Castration fantasies and fear of women, which may lead to preference for male company and the adoption of a passive, feminine attitude, and conscious or unconscious homosexuality.
5 It may be a symptom of general lack of assertiveness and fear of being too aggressive, in an inadequate personality.
6 Excessive self-love and self-regard which makes for an inability to love another person (narcissism).

Treatment

1 In mild cases, it may be sufficient for the patient to have discussion with his doctor about his anxieties and ideas about sexual intercourse and receive education on these topics if he is ignorant or has erroneous ideas. However 'ignorance' is often used as an unconscious defence against sexual conflict. Superficial interpretive psychotherapy may be enough. The female partner may also need to be told not to ridicule or shame the

man about his impotence but to help with sympathetic understanding of the difficulty. It may even be the female partner who needs help for her conflicts about intercourse, as they contribute to the impotence of the male.

2 In more severe cases, more formal psychotherapy may be necessary to eliminate and resolve the unconscious conflicts giving rise to the symptom.

3 Masters and Johnson (1970) have developed a behavioural technique in which both partners are instructed how to help each other at the various stages of intercourse starting with stimulation of sensitive areas to increase sexual desire, right up to penetration and orgasm.

4 If severe mental illness is present, this will need its appropriate treatment. Impotence arising for the first time after 40 may well be part of an incipient depression.

FRIGIDITY

Definition

This is the female equivalent of impotence and consists of an inability to achieve an orgasm during sexual intercourse. It may take several forms:

1 Total lack of sexual desire.

2 Sexual excitement may be felt during external genital stimulation but orgasm is not achieved.

3 Orgasm can be reached during external stimulation but not during penetration.

4 Penetration does not lead to sexual excitement or it may be experienced as painful (dyspareunia), or both.

5 Penetration is accompanied by various degrees of sexual excitement but orgasm is not achieved.

Aetiology

As with impotence in males so frigidity may on some occasions be a symptom of mental illness, especially depression; it is likely to occur when the woman is ill due to some general organic disease; occasionally, especially if there is dyspareunia, it can be due to a local gynaecological abnormality which requires physical treatment.

In the large majority of cases, however, it is of psychological origin, due to some disturbance in psychosexual development. In many societies, including our own, the view used to be held, mainly by men, that sexual pleasure was not an essential experience for women; it was even thought that it was improper for respectable women to enjoy sex so that girls were made to feel guilty, and denied or dissembled their sexual desires and feelings with the result that they were frigid when they became sexually mature. Only in relatively recent years has the attitude of society begun to change; it is now recognised that frigidity is as much a symptom that needs to be treated as is impotence in men. Women who have accepted their sexual function as a normal aspect of adult life are at least as capable as men of enjoying intercourse and reaching orgasm, and often more capable; this has been clearly demonstrated by direct observation by Masters and Johnson (1966, 1970); they have also shown that the distinction between a so-called 'clitoral' and 'vaginal' orgasm is physiologically incorrect, the clitoris being the main source of sexual excitement leading to orgasm whether it is stimulated by external manual manipulation or by the penis during penetration of the vagina.

Apart from these general psychosocial considerations and misconceptions there are a number of individual factors that can make a woman frigid. Thus, the partner may be the wrong one for her physically or emotionally, or the circumstances may be unfavourable to allow her fully to relax during intercourse. Moreover, the female usually needs to be sexually aroused by her partner to reach a sufficient state of excitement. Hence, if the male's sexual technique and his awareness of his partner's needs are defective this state will not be reached and orgasm will not occur. When this happens repeatedly and the woman remains disappointed and frustrated this may lead to more persistent frigidity.

More basic psychodynamic factors causing frigidity are:

1 Ignorance or erroneous ideas about intercourse, e.g. fear of being damaged by the penis or inadequate contraceptive measures with fear of pregnancy.

2 Guilt about sexuality.

3 Fear of losing control during intercourse.

4 The belief that intercourse is a dirty or aggressive act.

5 Unconscious fixation on the father or a brother.

6 Rejection of her feminine role and envy of the male ('penis envy'), often associated with conscious or unconscious homosexuality.

Treatment

This is similar to that for males.

1 In mild cases, or if frigidity is only a temporary phenomenon, discussions leading to better understanding and sex education may be all that is required. This may also include the male partner if his attitude and technique are unsatisfactory.

2 In more severe or persistent cases formal psychotherapy or psychoanalysis may be needed.

3 As in impotence Masters and Johnson's (1970) method may be used, both partners being seen together; the male partner is helped to understand the woman's physical needs and sensitive areas, and learns how to arouse her physically in whatever manner is desired by her, until ultimately she is able to respond and achieve orgasm.

4 If severe mental illness is present this will require separate treatment.

UNCONSUMMATED MARRIAGE

Non-consummation means that there has been no, or only very shallow, penetration by the penis into the vagina. This state, if not associated with obvious organic pathology in either partner, is a psychosexual problem and may go on for months or years. The wife develops adductor spasm of the thighs and spasm of the vagina as soon as penetration is attempted, so-called vaginismus. The husband is frequently passive, and does not 'bother his wife' sexually. The wife's psychosexual problems may take several forms, e.g.:

1 She is emotionally immature, frightened of sexuality and is convinced that penetration is painful and impossible, wanting only to be held and caressed like a child.

2 She is over-aggressive either openly or covertly towards her husband and resents the feminine role.

3 She wants a baby, but without intercourse.

Treatment consists of physical examination and demonstration to the wife that her vagina can admit one or more examining fingers without pain. This is followed by psychotherapy of the wife, and usually of the husband as well. Both may be treated together as in the Masters and Johnson technique (1970) (see p. 109). This has proved of value, but clearly depends on considerable patience and co-operation on both sides; it is likely to be successful only where sexual inadequacy is the major symptom in an otherwise compatible partnership, and to fail — even if it could be attempted — in pairs whose sexual difficulties are simply the focus for other underlying conflicts (see p. 256).

TRANSVESTISM AND TRANS-SEXUALISM

Transvestism is the desire to cross-dress; this may lead to guilt and anxiety in the patient, or to unhappiness in the sexual partner; it is sometimes, though not necessarily, associated with homosexuality. Many transvestites are content with their condition and do not ask for treatment, or refuse it if offered.

Trans-sexualism is the desire to change sex, the person being convinced that his anatomical make-up is contrary to his gender role. He may, therefore, ask for hormone treatment or an operation. It is often difficult to decide whether the patient will be better off if either request is granted or will get severely depressed instead. In latter years surgical intervention is being carried out more often than in the past, and some satisfactory adjustments have been made as a result. Psychotherapy, other than supportive, is usually ineffective.

FETISHISM

Occasionally a male may require the presence of a specific article, e.g. a particular scent or piece of clothing, to be worn by the woman before he can achieve sexual intercourse. It becomes the pathological condition of fetishism when the sexual excitement is entirely dependent on this article.

EXHIBITIONISM AND SCOPOPHILIA (VOYEURISM)

These conditions are the counterpart of one another. Scopophilia is the state of sexual excitement and pleasure derived from viewing sexual activity. Exhibitionism, or 'indecent exposure', is the state of sexual excitement and pleasure in displaying the genitals to a member of the opposite sex. It is almost completely a masculine activity, and often leads to discovery and prosecution.

SADISM AND MASOCHISM

These are another pair of polar opposites. In sadism (named after de Sade), the sexual excitement is found in the inflicting of pain upon another person, e.g. whipping, caning; in masochism (named after Masoch), the excitement is derived from having pain inflicted on oneself. One can observe sadistic tendencies in people who have an extreme need for self-aggrandisement and lust for power over others, and masochistic tendencies in those who are excessively humble and submissive.

In both these sets of polar opposites it is common to find evidence of both traits, with one particularly predominating, e.g. the voyeur with some exhibitionist tendencies.

BESTIALITY

Intercourse with animals, usually by male adults, but occasionally by females, is most common in rural areas, and where custom permits it; it is more likely in some defectives and psychopaths.

TREATMENT

In general, psychotherapy is the treatment of choice; much depends on the patient's and his partner's readiness to cooperate. Psychotherapy may be helpful in exhibitionism, sadism, masochism, fetishism and transvestism; fetishism may also respond to aversion therapy. Most transsexuals are resistant to treatment but occasionally benefit from surgery.

FURTHER READING

Comfort, A. (1972). *The Joy of Sex*. Quartet Books, London.
Deutsch, H. (1945). *Psychology of Women*. Grune and Stratton.
Ellison, C. (1968). 'Psychosomatic factors in the unconsummated marriage'. *J. Psychosom. Res.*, 12, 61.
Freud, S. (1905). *Three Essays in Sexuality*. Standard edition, Hogarth, London, vol. 7.
Friedman, L. J. (1962). *Virgin Wives: a study of unconsummated marriages*. Tavistock Publications, London.
Katchadourian, H. A. and Lunde, D.T. (1972). *Fundamentals of Human Sexuality*. Holt, Rinehart and Winston, New York.
Masters, W. H. and Johnson, V. E. (1966). *Human Sexual Response*. Churchill, London.
Master, W. H. and Johnson, V. E. (1970). *Human Sexual Inadequacy*. Churchill, London.
Michael, R. P. (ed.) (1968). *Endocrinology and Human Behaviour*. OUP.
Randell, J. (1970). 'Transvestism and trans-sexualism'. *Brit. J. Hosp. Med.*, 3, 211.
Rosen, I. (ed.) (1964). *Pathology and Treatment of Sexual Deviations*. OUP, London.

20 *The schizophrenias*

Schizophrenia is almost certainly not a single disease entity but comprises a number of severe mental disorders, with a variety of symptoms and of different aetiologies. They have in common the fact that the patient has, to a greater or lesser extent, lost touch with reality. He lives in a fantasy world of his own which feels real to him; i.e. he lacks insight, and it is often difficult to make emotional contact with him; his thought processes are disordered, his affect is disturbed in a variety of ways; his volition may be impaired and his behaviour is abnormal, governed, as it is, by his fantasy life rather than by outer reality. One essential feature is that these disorders occur in the absence of coarse brain disease.

It used to be stressed that the manifestations of the schizophrenias are not psychologically understandable but this applies only if the observer restricts himself to the rational common-sense aspects of human behaviour. The more sensitive sophisticated observer, aware of unconscious mental processes ('primary process thinking') can get in touch with the patient's inner world and understand the psychological meaning of some of the patient's communications and behaviour, especially as he is getting to know him better.

It also used to be thought that schizophrenia, which is characterized by a tendency to remissions and relapses, and may become chronic, would inevitably lead to gradual deterioration of mental and social functioning. This is, however, not necessarily so; some patients may only have one acute schizophrenic episode, and others who suffer from relapses do not necessarily become chronically disabled. This is especially so if given modern treatment (see below) and if they are not subjected to severe stresses.

In view of the uncertainty of what constitutes a schizophrenic illness and on account of the many variations with which it may present, psychiatrists differ in their readiness to attach the label of schizophrenia to a particular patient. For example, patients are more often diagnosed as schizophrenic in the United States than in Britain where more rigid criteria tend to be used for making the diagnosis (see p. 48).

INCIDENCE

The incidence of schizophrenia in the general population is about 0.85%. Its various forms, acute and chronic, are still responsible for a high proportion of patients in mental hospitals. Although attempts have been made to reduce the number of psychiatric beds by improved methods of rehabilitation and early discharge, this has not been very successful because of the lack of facilities to look after them in the community. Thus about 40% of all hospital beds in Great Britain are still in mental hospitals and smaller psychiatric units in general hospitals; almost half of these are occupied by schizophrenic patients. Early discharge of acute schizophrenics often leads to re-admission within a year, either because the strain of looking after a disturbed schizophrenic patient at home poses too great a strain on the rest of the family and he himself deteriorates or relapses, or because of the lack of hostel accommodation for chronic and elderly patients.

SYMPTOMATOLOGY AND MENTAL STATE

This can be considered under several headings but in any one schizophrenic patient not all the following manifestations are necessarily present; the diagnosis should not be made on the basis of one or two isolated symptoms but only on the total picture the patient presents.

1 *Withdrawal from reality into fantasy*

With varying degrees of lack of insight; although patients often maintain a remarkable and sometimes heightened awareness for the events in the environment, including the attitude and behaviour of the observer. Their reaction to his and other people's behaviour is, however, likely to be determined by their fantasy life and therefore, often seems exaggerated or inappropriate to the observer. Contact may, therefore, be difficult to establish and the observer needs to make a special effort to do so, if possible (see p. 120).

2 *Thought disorder*

This is a characteristic feature of schizophrenia but may only develop gradually as the disease progresses. For purposes of description it can be divided into the following groups.

(a) Disorder of the form and stream of thought

When present this is diagnostic of schizophrenia provided it occurs in the presence of clear consciousness and in the absence of organic brain disease. There may be impairment of the ability to think in abstract terms so that words are used and proverbs interpreted in a concrete fashion (*concrete thinking*). The sequence of thoughts may be determined by incidental associations (as in free association), such as sounds, alliterations, clang associations or rhyming (e.g. 'it is quarter to two; I must buckle my shoe, blue'). It is this lack of meaningful causal links which is the outstanding feature of formal thought disorder. There is an inability to maintain the boundaries of the problem and to focus on a particular thought (*overinclusive thinking*); e.g. a patient says 'I feel everybody is sort of related to everybody'. New words may be invented or two words may be condensed into one and given special meaning by the patient (*neologism*); e.g. the words cat and mouse are made into 'catamouse'. Words may get muddled up (word salad) so that sentences become incomprehensible. The train of thought may suddenly be changed so that a logical sequence of thought may go off at a tangent onto another sequence (*tangential thinking*); or the sequence of thoughts may jump slightly off course (*knight's move thinking*). Or the train of thought may suddenly be interrupted and after a brief pause a new, totally unconnected thought may take over (*thought blocking*); although characteristic of schizophrenia, this may also occur when people are over-anxious or physically exhausted. The thought process may be slowed down (*poverty of thought*) or speeded up (*pressure of thought*); however, the former also occurs in depression and the latter in manic states. The same word or idea may be repeated several times (*perseveration*) or a word used by another person may be repeated by the patient (*echolalia*).

(b) Disorders of the possession of thought

The patient may feel that his thoughts are not his own (*alienation of thought*) and have the sensation that his thoughts are taken away from him (*thought deprivation*), or that alien thoughts are being put into his mind (*thought insertion*). In *thought broadcasting* he has the feeling that other people know what he is thinking. Sometimes he may hear his own thoughts.

(c) *Disorder of the content of thought*

These are delusions, i.e. the patient holds a false, unshakeable belief, despite all evidence to the contrary, which is not in keeping with his educational, social and cultural background. The patient may suddenly attach special, delusional significance to some experience (e.g. a patient who saw an aeroplane fly overhead suddenly knew with absolute certainty that this meant he was the Messiah); these are referred to as *primary delusions* and occur especially at the onset of acute schizophrenia. Secondary delusions may be built around the primary delusion to justify and elaborate the primary one.

The commonest types of delusions are persecutory in nature (*paranoid delusions*) so that the patient believes he is being persecuted or accused by individuals, groups or organisations, e.g. Jews, Freemasons or communists. He may believe that events in his surroundings have a special significance for him (*ideas of self-reference*), e.g. seeing a car with a particular registration number may mean that the driver is following him. Another may have grandiose delusions so that he believes he is some important person such as Jesus, God, Napoleon or the Queen; or is connected with such important people. *Hypochondriacal delusions* are common in schizophrenics: the patient believes that his body is undergoing some bizarre change or that he has some dreadful illness like cancer or venereal disease. *Delusions of guilt*, though more common in psychotic depression, occur in schizophrenics, the patient believing that he has committed a terrible sin and is eternally doomed.

The following extract from a schizophrenic patient's letter to the psychiatrist serves as an example of schizophrenic thought disorder:

Apologise; and I might find some new fun, I.
NO PROMISES   MIND YOU.
WITH LOVE AND MORNINGTON CRESCENT.
    I find the going hard, will heart and mind and body please be sufficient for the intellectual on the found on the street

one. I met your secretary at the MORE House and did SOWE promised her help with a PROCALATION and then never saw her again to hear if she was in the left mind. Hope your RIVERS for a long time. Come and drink tea, sea and have a bite to eat on Thursday 6.30. And if you NEED to get rid of that painting now's the chance. I'll introduce you as the painter so as to enable you to put sickness out of your mind for at least ½ an hour.

Natalia (also Natalie)

3 *Disorders of perception*

These are *illusions* (misinterpretation of external stimuli), which of course occur in normal people, or *hallucinations* (perceptions in the absence of corresponding external stimuli). The commonest hallucinations in schizophrenics are auditory ones; but visual hallucinations may occur, and so may hallucinations of touch, taste or smell. The nature of the hallucinations and illusions is usally in keeping with any delusional beliefs the patient may have; e.g. a patient with paranoid delusions may hear voices talking to him or about him in derogatory, accusing terms.

4 *Disorders of affect*

Although often described as flat, or inappropriate to what the patient is talking about, his affect may be one of anxiety, e.g. if he feels and hears himself to be persecuted; elated if he has grandiose delusions, sometimes to the point of being ecstatic, e.g. if he has had a primary delusion of being God or Jesus; or depressed, e.g. if he is painfully aware of the fact that he is undergoing a serious change of his personality. He may also feel perplexed by what is happening to him. It is particularly in chronic schizophrenics that lack of emotion (flatness of affect) and incongruity of affect may be observed, but even here the apparent flatness and inappropriateness may cover up other emotions the patient is hiding from the observer.

5 *Disorders of behaviour*

The patient may show bizarre mannerisms, and repetitive or interrupted movements; or he may be immobile as in catatonic stupor, or prone to outbursts of violent, aggressive behaviour, e.g. if he is paranoid and feels himself threatened or attacked. Others may lack volition or feel that their motor behaviour is not under their own control but controlled from outside (passivity feelings).

6 *Relationship to the observer*

The attitude of the observer — doctor, nurse, social worker or psychologist — usually has a profound effect on the patient's feelings and behaviour. If the observer treats the patient as an object rather than as a person deeply disturbed by what he is experiencing, he will withdraw further, turn away from him or become aggressive, frightened or depressed. If, on the other hand, the observer makes a genuine attempt to understand the meaning of the patient's communications and behaviour, the patient may gradually feel more trusting and his behaviour may become less disturbed. It is sometimes possible to understand the nature of the patient's delusions, hallucinations and thought disorder in the context of his previous life experience, especially within his family (Laing 1960); as a result he may become less perplexed and frightened by what is happening to him and the more bizarre symptoms may diminish, at least temporarily during an interview. It must, however, be remembered that the patient may also feel threatened by an observer who tries to make close contact with him too quickly. A sensitive and cautious attempt at making meaningful contact with the patient is, therefore, essential to make him feel that he is being respected and treated as an individual.

Comments from recovered patients make it plain that this is often a turning point for them. On the other hand it is tragically possible that, in the past, failure to understand this interaction has led observers to push the incipient schizophrenic deeper into his illness.

7 Symptoms of chronic schizophrenia

In chronic cases there may be gradual deterioration of all mental functions, but this may be partly due to prolonged institutionalisation. Kraepelin's (1890) original term *dementia praecox* was replaced by the term schizophrenia by Bleuler in 1911 as dementia does not necessarily occur, nor does the condition always start, in young people. The term schizophrenia, which refers to a process of fragmentation of mental processes, not necessarily progressive, is therefore more appropriate.

MAIN CLINICAL GROUPS

It is only the predominating features of these groups which are given below. There are many mixed, atypical cases and in the course of time the same patient may show some of the features of several different types.

1 Hebephrenic

The condition usually occurs in the younger age group, from late adolescence to the mid-twenties, and starts insidiously or acutely. There is thought disorder and disturbance of affect which may be incongruous and blunted, or the patient may appear depressed, silly, giggling or abnormally cheerful, excited, irritable, anxious or perplexed. Hallucinations, changeable fantastic delusions, ideas of reference and depersonalisation develop gradually. His behaviour is often very disturbed, showing either lack of volition and initiative; bizarre, repetitive mannerisms; or outbursts of aggressive or anti-social behaviour.

2 Paranoid

The onset is somewhat later in life and may occur in the thirties or later. Suspicions, persecutory delusions and hallucinations are characteristic; as a result the patient may be fearful or depressed, and he may show aggressive outbursts or periods of withdrawal and isolation. Thought disorder may be absent or only develop as the illness progresses (see also paranoid states p. 128).

3 *Catatonic*

The commonest feature is some degree of rigidity and poverty of movement, sometimes amounting to *catatonic stupor*; negativism may occur which may consist of refusal to eat and to obey commands so that the patient may lie in bed, mute, immobile, soiling himself and failing to respond to the observer although he may respond after an interval, especially when left alone. He may maintain stereotyped postures the observer has placed him in (flexibilitas cerea). Hallucinations, delusions and thought disorder may become more obvious when he comes out of his stuporose state.

At other times there may be outbursts of extreme excitement, fear, rage, and destructive, violent behaviour (*catatonic excitement*).

4 *Simple*

This may be difficult to diagnose as the onset, usually in younger people, is insidious, and thought disorder, delusions and hallucinations may only develop as the condition progresses. The patient gradually loses interest, is unable to work, or shifts from job to job, and he may end up as a tramp, ineffective, solitary and apathetic, even though he may earlier on have been an active, intelligent person. The condition is slowly progressive and may lead to severe mental deterioration.

AETIOLOGY

The schizophrenias are probably multifactorial in origin and result from the interaction of psychological stresses, physical influences and a genetically determined constitution.

1 *Heredity*

The work of Shield and Slater and others has shown that the expectancy rate for schizophrenia in relatives of schizophrenic patients is greater than in the general population (general population 0.85%, parents 5-10%, siblings 5-15%). This could be due to the effect of a psychotic parent or child on the other family members but the importance of genetic factors is supported by studies of twins. Earlier claims suggested as high a concordance rate as 65% for schizophrenia in identical twins, even if brought up apart. More recent studies in Scandinavia and in Finland suggest a much lower concordance rate of 40% or less but even this is considerably higher than the expectancy rate of 15% in ordinary siblings. Genetic factors therefore play some part.

2 *Family environment*

Family studies have drawn attention to disturbed interaction in the families of schizophrenics, e.g. *double-binding*, parents giving the child contradictory messages by word or behaviour so that he can do nothing right, *invalidation*, the imposition of false or contradictory roles all of which lead to disturbed personality development; at the same time the presence of a psychotic member has a disrupting effect on the family, thus establishing a vicious circle. Claims have also been made, as the result of psychoanalytic treatment of schizophrenics, that a disturbed mother-child relationship at very early stages of infantile development may be of aetiological significance. The main difficulty in all these studies is that similar abnormalities in family interaction can also be observed in normal families and in families of patients suffering from psychiatric illnesses other than schizophrenia, but quantitive studies suggest that they are more common in the latter (Wynne 1967).

3 *Prepsychotic personality*

Not uncommonly schizophrenia develops in a particular type of person with a shy, seclusive, sensitive, day dreaming and introspective nature, the so-called schizoid personality. This may itself be the result of a disturbed family environment as described above. These facts have been used by Adolf Meyer in his concept of schizophrenia as a process of progressive maladaption of a person to his environment, and explain much of what is seen in schizophrenic thinking and behaviour. This takes into account the schizoid personality's steadily increasing propensity to evade or retreat from stresses and difficulties by the use of excessive fantasy, rather than by dealing with his troubles.

4 *Physical type*

Kretschmer (1936) and later Sheldon et al. (1940) have held the view that schizophrenic patients have certain statistically definable trends towards the so-called asthenic or ectomorphic bodily constitution but a schizophrenic illness is by no means limited to this type of physique.

5 *Biochemical changes*

Schizophrenic reactions can follow the administration of certain drugs, e.g. mescaline, amphetamine, which can cause a paranoid psychosis if taken over a long period and in large doses by amphetamine addicts, and LSD. Much work has been done in investigating the possible biochemical mechanisms involved and the view that abnormalities of adrenaline or of nitrogen metabolism might be responsible for schizophrenic illnesses has been put forward. However, so far there is no consistent evidence of any specific biochemical abnormality consistently associated with schizophrenia.

PROGNOSIS

This varies considerably with age, type and duration. Prognosis is worse in younger patients, in cases without marked precipitating stress, in insidious development, in cases with persistent hallucinations, and in hebephrenics. Spontaneous recovery may occur in 5% and some improvement in 35% of cases. Treatment has increased these figures from 30% to 60%. (These figures are rough since valid follow-up is difficult.) Prognosis also depends on the home atmosphere. Discharge to a disturbed family or intense emotional involvement with a close relative may provoke relapses; cautious and gradual rehabilitation in a stable, supportive environment may aid recovery and prevent relapses.

TREATMENT

Treatment may be considered as a series of steps, as follows:

1 *Admission*

Admission to hospital, compulsorily on occasion, offers the best chance of intensive treatment and is sometimes necessary for the protection of the patient and those around him. But it may lead to institutionalization in a hospital whose staff is inadequate. The pros and cons of admission must therefore be weighed at the start.

2 *Drugs and shock treatment*

Many of the acute and serious symptoms can nowadays quickly be brought under control with physical treatments. The phenothiazine derivatives are usually the first line of treatment, and if effective, the patient may have to stay on a maintenance dose for long periods up to a year or two. The following are especially useful:

Chlorpromazine (Largactil)	50-300 mg t.d.s.
Trifluoperazine (Stelazine)	5-15 mg t.d.s.
Perphenazine (Fentazin)	2-20 mg t.d.s.
Thioridazine (Melleril)	25-200 mg t.d.s.
Fluphenazine decanoate (Modecate) (intramuscularly)	25 mg fortnightly

It is usual to start with a smaller dose and to increase the dose gradually to obtain symptomatic relief. Close supervision is needed on account of such side effects as hypotension, Parkinsonism (which should be prevented by simultaneous administration of disipal, 50 mg t.d.s.), or toxic effects such as skin reactions, and occasionally jaundice or agranulocytosis. These drugs are potentiated by alcohol. Modecate constitutes a great advance, especially for patients who cannot be relied upon to take pills regularly.

In acute cases, especially for catatonic and depressive symptoms, and if drug treatment has failed, ECT may produce quick benefits, sometimes in combination with phenothiazines. Insulin coma, often used before the advent of phenothiazines, has now been discontinued.

3 *Psychotherapy*

Supportive psychotherapy is essential in order to establish a relationship with the patient and to provide sympathy, understanding and tolerance of disordered thought and behaviour, even if the patient appears to ignore it at first. Shortage of doctors makes it rarely possible to provide individual relationships, but by involving the nursing staff and by running wards and day hospitals along therapeutic community lines, similar results can be obtained.

Intensive analytical psychotherapy has been used. Here an intense transference relationship is allowed to develop and therapy may have to continue for several years. One of the aims is to overcome the patient's withdrawal and to help him understand the meaning of his fantasies and thought disorder but it is essential to emphasize contact with reality throughout. The outcome of such treatment is dubious and intense psychotherapy may be harmful. Modified psychotherapy can, however, be of considerable help to some patients, in combination with or following treatment with phenothiazines, which should not be delayed.

4 *Surgery*

For a few very disturbed patients who have failed to respond to all other methods a modified leucotomy has been used to allow the patient to live a quieter life but with blunted emotion: cingulectomy has proved successful in a few cases (see p. 342).

5 *Social rehabilitation*

The above methods may be considered as preparing the way for rehabilitation, a gradual re-introduction to ordinary life. It is directed mainly towards stimulating outgoing activities. Re-education may have to begin with the very fundamentals of life, such as feeding and personal hygiene. It will move on to taking part in social activities and responsibilities, part-time and later full-time work, in gradually increasing degrees and with support. A day hospital may be very useful for such rehabili-tation. After-care hostels are essential for those who have either no families to go back to or whose families have a disturbing effect on the patient.

Without these, early discharge — as recommended as official policy on many occasions — may do more harm than good to the patient; and his presence in a family or community which is not prepared to receive him may be too much for them and prevent them from trying again later.

FURTHER READING

Coppen, A., and Walk, A. (1967). 'Recent developments in schizophrenia', *Brit. J. Psychiat.*, Special publication No. 1.

Fish, F. J. (1962). *Schizophrenia.* Wright, Bristol.

Freeman, T. (1969). *Psychopathology of the Psychoses.* Tavistock Publications, London.

Kendell, R. E. (1972). 'Schizophrenia: the remedy for diagnostic confusion'. *Brit. J. Hosp. Med.*, 8, 383.

Kretschmer, E. (1936). *Physique and Character.* Routledge, London.

Leff, J. P. (1972). 'Maintenance therapy and schizophrenia'. *Brit. J. Hosp. Med.*, 8, 377.

Laing, R. D. (1960). *The Divided Self.* Tavistock Publications, London.

Mayer-Gross, W., Slater, E., and Roth, M. (1969). *Clinical Psychiatry*, Baillière, Tindall and Cassell, London, Chapter 5.

National Schizophrenia Fellowship (1974). *Living with Schizophrenia.* Surbiton.

Sheldon, W. H. et al. (1940). *The Varieties of Human Physique.* Harper, London.

Wing, J. K. (1972). 'Epidemiology of schizophrenia'. *Brit. J. Hosp. Med.*, 8, 364.

Wynne, L. C. (1967). In *The Transmission of Schizophrenia*, edited by D. Rosenthal and S. S. Ketz, Pergamon, New York.
Besides these, there are two books which enable the reader to feel what schizophrenics may experience.
Barnes, M. and Berk, J. (1971). *Mary Barnes: Two Accounts of a Journey Through Madness*. Penguin.
Green, H. (1964). *I Never Promised You a Rose Garden*. Pan, London.

21 Paranoid states

DEFINITION

The term paranoia antedates Hippocrates but in his writings appears to have been used as the equivalent of 'insanity' today. The term reappeared in the eighteenth century as a name for delusional and delirious disorders. In Kraepelin's work on a system of mental disorders published in the 1880s it was more narrowly defined as a rare diagnostic entity.

In current usage the term paranoid indicates the presence of feelings of persecution of varying degrees, from a defensive suspicious attitude in a patient with a personality disorder, to a psychosis in which there are firmly held systematized delusions of persecution; grandiose ideas or delusions may accompany these; ideas of reference, i.e. a tendency to regard outside events as referring to oneself, a marked form of ego-centricity, are a part of the persecutory grandiose range of reaction. Patients are often very secretive about their suspicions and delusions and it may be difficult to establish their nature even if the patients' behaviour suggests they are acting on the basis of such ideas.

In psychodynamic terms the paranoiac uses the psychological mechanisms of denial and projection. These mechanisms are normal components of everyone's defensive system used in dealing with psychological conflict, but the paranoid person uses them to a greater degree and more persistently. An example of the simplest form of dynamic formulation would be that the patient cannot accept his hostile feelings for a particular person, denies them, projects them on to that person and then feels the latter to be hostile to himself.

INCIDENCE AND SYMPTOMS

Paranoid reactions occur in many different conditions. They are an essential feature in the paranoid psychoses, and an occasional symptom in almost the entire range of psychiatric diagnoses. They may appear in normal people under the influence of adverse circumstances, such as isolation by deafness or other physical disability, or, in refugees among people whose language or customs they don't understand. They may be produced by drugs e.g. hashish, LSD, amphetamine.

1 *Paranoid psychoses*

This heading comprises a continuum ranging from the condition described by Kraepelin as paranoia, in which there are persecutory and grandiose delusions with an otherwise normal personality and without hallucinations, through paraphrenia, in which there are some schizophrenic symptoms, to a schizophrenic illness with paranoid features. In fact most patients with paranoid delusions do develop schizophrenic symptoms and there can be no clear distinction between the three groups.

The term 'paranoia' may be usefully kept to describe an insidiously developing system of delusions arising in middle age in a preserved personality; any stressful event, and later the whole of his environment may be incorporated into his system. This leads to increasing antagonism with his neighbours, and isolation. A feature of the condition is that some patients may appear to be able to lead relatively normal lives, but direct questioning will reveal an intact delusional system, which may also come to light if the patient is under stress. In paranoid schizophrenia (see p. 121) there is little systematisation of delusions, but quick changes of ideas and moods and more abnormal behaviour, and gradual deterioration may occur. Suicide is a risk in severely persecuted patients, and some patients will attack their supposed persecutors' life or property; these risks must be assessed in the management of the patient.

2 *Affective disorders*

In severe depression there is sometimes a paranoid element with the patient fluctuating between a feeling that his misery is a just punishment for his wickedness, and a feeling that it is due to persecution he hasn't deserved. (But paranoid psychoses sometimes present as depressive illnesses.)

Manic and hypomanic patients may show paranoid reactions only partly understandable as due to opposition to their conceit and overactivity; treatment is more difficult.

3 *Personality disorders*

Some people are abnormally suspicious, sensitive to criticism (real or imagined) and find it very difficult to trust or understand other people. They are often hostile in attitude and liable to experience considerable difficulties in interpersonal relations, with increasing personal isolation. This represents a life-long personality pattern, with no deterioration, but such a condition may be pre-psychotic.

4 *Organic psychoses*

Paranoid reactions are relatively common in the psychiatric complications of organic disease (see p. 148). There may be difficulty in the differential diagnosis of paranoid features accompanying senile dementia and paraphrenia of late onset. In some epileptics there are personality changes which may include a general paranoid attitude. A schizophrenia-like illness, usually with paranoid features, may be associated with temporal lobe epilepsy and other local cerebral lesions.

5 *Drugs*

Paranoid reactions are common in the psychiatric disorders associated with alcoholism. The latter, if chronic, is usually detectable, but *alcoholic hallucinosis* may be difficult to distinguish from paranoid schizophrenia. This and the psychosis associated with cocaine addiction usually produce vivid and terrifying paranoid delusions and hallucinations. In *amphetamine psychoses* the clinical features are indistinguishable from paranoid schizophrenia, except that the condition shows rapid remission when amphetamine is withdrawn, which will usually be the case when the patient is admitted to hospital. Urine tests will reveal the presence of amphetamine, but need to be done during the initial period of admission to establish the diagnosis.

TREATMENT

General management

Paranoid patients tend to arouse anxiety and hostility in others, which, if expressed, will aggravate the patient's suspiciousness, tendency to blame others and isolation. On the other hand the paranoid patient is liable to attribute to his doctors motives and actions hostile to himself. Often the most difficult part of the management of the paranoid patient is to get him into a treatment situation. In-patient treatment is not always required, and by steering a middle-course between impatience with the patient's distortions of reality and arousing his suspicions by trying to establish a closer emotional relationship than he can tolerate, the general practitioner may be able to provide enough support to enable the patient to keep his symptoms under control, to avoid intolerable emotional isolation and to continue his usual occupation. Compulsory powers under the Mental Health Act may be necessary to detain a patient in hospital if in-patient treatment is required. Once in hospital the general approach is the same. The relatives will need support and explanation of the patient's behaviour, from the GP or PSW.

Drugs

The phenothiazines, especially trifluoperazine (stelazine), have proved useful in the symptomatic treatment of paranoid illnesses, reducing tension and anxiety and interrupting the vicious circle liable to develop as the hostile patient provokes hostile reactions which in turn make him more hostile.

FURTHER READING

Fish, F. J. (1962). *Schizophrenia.* Wright, Bristol.
Rolfe, Fr. (1963). *Hadrian the Seventh.* Penguin. (A fascinating auto-
biographical account of paranoid fantasy by an author who happens to
write well; see also the play *Hadrian VII*, and Symons, A. J. A., *The
Quest for Corvo*, Penguin.)

22 Alcoholism

PUBLIC OPINION AND PREVALENCE

Alcoholism in UK is at present far less prevalent than in the
days of Dickens or Hogarth, and it is less common than in
certain other countries, such as USA or France. However, it still
constitutes an extremely important problem, not only numeric-
ally but also through its effects on the individual, his family and
the community. In 1951 WHO published Jellinek's estimate of
86,000 'chronic alcoholics' (i.e. those with definite mental and
physical complications) and a total of 350,000 alcoholics in
England and Wales; there are a number of indirect signs pointing
to an increase since that time. As on an average the alcoholic's
behaviour closely involves the lives of three or four other
members of his family it is evident that even today far more
than a million people in this country are directly or indirectly
affected by this illness. Unfortunately there is still a considerable stigma attached to it, so that both the alcoholic himself
and his family are deterred from seeking advice early on from
fear of not being understood or of being criticized by the
doctor. But the idea is gaining ground that the alcoholic is a sick
man in need of the doctor's help. The medical student should
realize that early diagnosis is all important; such complications
as cirrhosis of the liver and dementia are fortunately rare and
occur at a late stage of the illness so that diagnosis must not be
delayed until such complications supervene.

DEFINITION

There is no completely satisfactory definition but the one most widely quoted has been proposed by WHO in 1952: 'Alcoholics are those excessive drinkers whose dependence upon alcohol has attained such a degree that it shows a noticeable mental disturbance or an interference with their bodily and mental health, their inter-personal relations, and their smooth social and economic functioning; or who show the prodromal signs of such developments. They therefore require treatment.'

SYMPTOMATOLOGY

Alcoholism may be (1) acute, or (2) chronic.

1 *Acute intoxication.* Two uncommon varieties include acute hallucinosis and mania a potu, both often resulting from single heavy doses.
2 *Chronic alcoholism.* Symptoms rarely bring the patient to the doctor because of his lack of co-operation and insight; he is usually brought by his relatives, e.g. under threat of divorce or of losing his job. Early symptoms include poor concentration, poor memory, quick changes in mood to depression, euphoria, or aggressiveness in response to small stimuli, inability ever to refuse a drink, increasing self-centredness, diminution of higher ethical standards, plausibility and facile inventiveness.

The progress from initial social drinking to fully established alcoholism in most cases takes many years, often 10 to 15, and has been divided by Jellinek into four 'phases':
1 The 'pre-alcoholic' phase (relief drinking and tolerance increase).
2 The 'prodromal' phase (ushered in by 'blackouts', i.e. amnesias for events that happened whilst he was drinking without being drunk).
3 The 'crucial' phase (starting with 'loss of control').
4 The final 'chronic' phase, characterized by prolonged alcoholic bouts. It is in this 'chronic phase' with too little food that physical symptoms may arise from damage either to the

liver (fatty infiltration being a much more common occurrence than the relatively rare cirrhosis), or to the stomach, or cerebral or peripheral neurones.

Korsakov's syndrome. Here peripheral neuritis and opthalmo-plegia are associated with invention of fantastic stories told very plausibly to meet gaps in the patient's recent memory (confabulation).

Delirium tremens. An acute attack of terror and restlessness associated with vivid and usually frightening visual hallucinations in which often all types of strange animals (but hardly ever 'pink elephants') may be sighted. This may result from sudden withdrawal; so may *epileptiform fits*.

'Dipsomania' or Jellinek's 'epsilon alcoholism' consists of periods of compulsion to drink to excess, usually with periods of complete sobriety (or more rarely moderate drinking) in between.

AETIOLOGY

As in drug dependence in general, the exact causation is still obscure; the person's mental and physical make-up ('host'), the environment and the pharmacological nature of alcohol as a physical dependence-producing 'agent', all play a part in interaction with each other. Mental make-up is clearly one of the most important factors: thus inadequate neurotics, people with strong emotional needs, low frustration tolerance, anxiety or depression may more often be tempted to use alcohol. Small amounts alleviate tension initially, but gradually increasing amounts are needed. Alcoholism may then become a learned habit. Associated inadequate diet may result in the physical and mental complications of deficiency syndromes.

Some alcoholics are psychopaths, but the great majority are not. Other people may become alcoholics, if frequently exposed to heavy drinking as a consequence of their job.

Prognosis depends largely on the underlying personality and on environmental factors such as support by the family.

PREVENTION

Intensive campaigns for prevention are being waged in various European countries where alcoholism is far more prevalent than here; they are said to be hindered by local vested interests in wine producing countries such as France, by climatic conditions such as Finland and Sweden, and by local customs, such as distilling one's own plum brandy in Yugoslavia. In this country much has been achieved by restrictive, rather than by prohibitive, legislation, as for instance by cutting down opening hours in pubs, by heavy taxes on alcoholic drinks, by diluting beer, and so on; but important steps remain to be taken in convincing the sufferer that if he seeks early treatment he will get it without moralizing condemnation, and in ensuring this by adequate training and education of medical students and other professional groups. Thus education of the professions as well as of the lay public, research, early treatment and legislative measures are all important in the task of prevention.

THE GP's ROLE

The GP's functions in the first instance are:
1 to avoid a critical, rejecting, condemning attitude.
2 to provide sympathy, hope, understanding and some explanation of what treatment (including psychotherapy) can achieve; and to reassure the relatives as well as the patient. No treatment of an alcoholic is complete without involving his family in the therapeutic programme. Alcoholism must be accepted as an illness, not as a crime; but this does *not* mean that the patient can do nothing to help himself; while learning that to a large extent recovery is up to him he also has to learn to accept help from others in the process of helping himself.
3 to arrange any more specialized physical and psychological treatment.

TREATMENT

This can be sometimes as an outpatient but frequently admission is necessary to a specialized unit provided by the

NHS (e.g. St. Bernard's Hospital, Middlesex, and Warlingham Park Hospital, Surrey) or in a few private nursing homes.

Physical treatment

Alcohol is usually withdrawn suddenly and completely; tranquillizers, non-barbiturate hypnotics, intensive vitamin medication, restoration of metabolism and of fluid and electrolyte balance are all required during this initial phase. The risk of withdrawal convulsions in very heavy drinkers may necessitate prophylactic use of anti-convulsant drugs. If treatment at home is all that is possible, massive vitamin B1, e.g. in the form of injections of 'Parentrovite', and adequate sedation must be given and supervision will be needed; possibly in the acute stages, when treated at home, tapering of alcohol may be the safer method in very heavy drinkers.

Acute detoxication must always be followed by long-term treatment, including psychotherapy.

Psychotherapy

Although alcoholism may finally assume the importance of an 'illness' in its own right, it very commonly starts for some underlying psychological reason. Some form of psychotherapy, especially group therapy, is often needed to give the patient a measure of insight and motivation. The alcoholic usually hopes to be able to learn to drink in moderation, but during treatment he will have to learn that this is no longer possible for him and that in order to lead a normal and useful life he will have to avoid drink altogether. He must also give up any other drugs such as barbiturates, to which some alcoholics may be addicted as well. The difficulty in accepting the fact that he is unable to control his drinking is the most serious hurdle in the treatment of alcoholics. Rather than admit this inability alcoholics habitually resort to defence mechanisms such as outright denial, repression, rationalization and projection, and they need to acquire some insight into these while in treatment.

Anti-alcoholic drugs

Certain drugs are best regarded as adjuncts to psychotherapy, but not as replacements for it. There are two different types:

1 Drugs sensitizing the body to alcohol, i.e. 'antabuse' (disulfiram) and 'abstem' (CCC). These are given daily. They inhibit the enzyme which carries the alcohol breakdown beyond the acetaldehyde stage, so that if alcohol is taken the acetaldehyde level rises in the blood; this may produce very unpleasant and sometimes dangerous symptoms, such as hypotension, vasodilation (flushing), tachycardia, nausea and terror. The patient must thoroughly understand the mechanism involved and must be strongly warned of the possible dangerous consequences entailed if he is foolish enough to risk drinking on top of these drugs. He may also be given a preliminary alcohol-antabuse or abstem test while in hospital. Of course, he may often prefer to give up these tablets rather than his drinking, and in such cases this form of treatment fails. But in suitably motivated patients this method may provide a very useful adjunct. On no account must these tablets be given unbeknown to the patient (e.g. by putting them into his tea). These tablets act as conscious deterrents; they are not usually used as aversion treatment.

2 Aversion therapy with apomorphine or emetine. These drugs when injected over a short period repeatedly with alcoholic drinks will cause vomiting and a conditioned reflex will be established, so that later on vomiting may follow alcohol without the emetic.

Social therapy

Major help is given by AA (Alcoholics Anonymous) (HQ telephone: 01-352 9669) a fellowship of recovered alcoholics and of those wanting to recover. They have branches in all parts of the British Isles and are very anxious to help if the alcoholic asks for it. AA have been of considerable assistance to many thousands of alcoholics; AA provides a feeling of belonging and AA members are always ready to answer telephone calls made by the sufferer, asking for help at times of crises, anxiety, depression and threatened or actual relapses of drinking.

Incidentally, suicidal attempts — often with fatal outcome — are quite common in alcoholics and so are accidents due to an overdose of sleeping tablets. AA can be of great assistance to the doctor, probation officer, social worker, etc., in their efforts to help the alcoholic. The treatment of alcoholism requires integrated teamwork.

Aftercare is the most important phase in treating the alcoholic. Halfway houses to assist the homeless or single alcoholic after discharge from hospital, or from prison, or the down-and-out alcoholic may provide very valuable service. Support after his return to the community by social workers, by AA, by his GP, or by his priest may all be very helpful.

There are now a number of voluntary organizations helping the alcoholic, e.g. the Reginald Carter Foundation (34 Seymour Street, W1, 01-262 6689), which is a free clinic, and a number of special NHS out-patient clinics.

Spelthorne St Mary (Harpenden, Herts.) is an Anglican Nursing Home for female alcoholics and addicts.

The Society for the Study of Addiction (London) is a scientific society interested in all aspects of dependence on alcohol and other drugs. It meets at least 4 times a year in London; visitors are welcome. Official journal: *British Journal of Addiction*.

The Medical Council on Alcoholism is a medical organization active in educating doctors in the problem of alcoholism and in encouraging research.

FURTHER READING

Edwards, G. (1968). 'Patients with drinking problems'. *Brit. Med. J.*, 2435.
Glatt, M. M. (1972). *The Alcoholic and the Help he Needs*. London.
Jellinek, E. M. (1960). *The Disease Concept of Alcoholism*. Hillhouse Press, Newhaven.
Kessel, N. and Walton, H. (1965). *Alcoholism*. Penguin.

23 Drug dependence

DEFINITION

Drug dependence — as defined by the WHO subcommittee — is a state arising from repeated administration of a drug on a periodic or continuous basis. Its characteristics vary with the agent involved so that one can speak of drug dependence of amphetamine type, of cannabis, or morphine, cocaine, LSD (lysergic acid diethylamide) or of barbiturate type. These are all at present encountered in this country.

PREVALENCE

Although barbiturate dependence and, to a lesser extent, amphetamine dependence among the middle aged, especially women, have been common in this country for over 15 years, public and professional interest and concern have been attracted to the problems of drug abuse and dependence only over the past ten years or so since young people began to abuse amphetamines, cannabis (marihuana and hashish), heroin and cocaine. No exact figures are available but, as very rough estimates, there may be 3,000 to 5,000 methadone and heroin addicts, a hundred thousand or more regular cannabis users (as cannabis is not used therapeutically and its use and possession is legally prohibited, all smokers of cannabis reefers are legally 'abusers'), possibly 150,000 to 200,000 barbiturate abusers and 'addicts', 150,000 or so amphetamine ('pep pill') abusers and 'addicts' and perhaps 1,000 to 3,000 LSD 'trippers'. But the situation changes rapidly, and all these figures are no more than very rough guesses and may be too low. Alcholism with an estimated figure of 300,000 to 500,000 victims still constitutes the most important form of drug dependence in this country.

AETIOLOGY

The exact causation of the condition is not yet clear, but the original mental and physical make-up, the social environment and the pharmacological effect of the drug may all play a part. For example, psychopathic and highly neurotic individuals run a greater risk of becoming drug abusers and psychologically dependent than the average individual, if drugs are available. On the other hand, where a society accepts drug taking as the 'done thing' and regards the drugs (e.g. cannabis) as harmless even people without marked emotional disturbance may start taking drugs, e.g. for 'kicks' in the case of pep pills, or for expansion of consciousness in the case of LSD. As in the USA, so also in this country there exist special sub-cultures among some sections of the young — with special attitudes and ideas and their own slang — where drug taking may be a custom. Overprescribing by a handful of London doctors has been named by the second Brain Committee (1965) as the main reason for the heroin-cocaine epidemic among the young.

CHARACTERISTICS OF DRUG DEPENDENCE

1 A strong desire (or craving) to continue taking the drugs in later stages of certain types of dependence, often at any price, possibly leading to asocial or antisocial behaviour.
2 A state of tolerance so that the user has to take increased doses to obtain the desired effects. The degree of tolerance varies from drug to drug, e.g. young addicts may take 100 mg or more of heroin or methadone per day, the normal therapeutic dose being 10 mg.
3 The appearance of a withdrawal syndrome when the drug is discontinued or sharply reduced. Such withdrawal symptoms may be only psychological, i.e. with those drugs which produce emotional (psychological) dependence only, or both psychological and physical. In order to avoid confusion and verbal or semantic arguments WHO recommended recently that the terms 'habituation' (roughly meaning psychological dependence), and 'addiction' (roughly meaning physical dependence) should be replaced by the more inclusive term 'dependence'.

CLASSIFICATION OF DEPENDENCE PRODUCING DRUGS

Various classifications have been used, and are confusing. It is common to speak of soft and hard drugs; the 'soft' are amphetamines, cannabis, LSD, barbiturates, and the 'hard' opiates and their synthetic equivalents, and cocaine. It must, however, not be thought that 'soft' drugs are relatively harmless, e.g. amphetamines, barbiturates and LSD (which is the best known major 'hallucinogenic' drug) can produce states of psychosis, quite apart from the risk of dependence.

Some drugs produce 'psychological' (emotional) dependence only: viz. cannabis, cocaine, LSD. (Amphetamines are also generally included in this group though there is some EEG evidence that they can sometimes produce physical dependence.) The withdrawal symptoms with such drugs are psychological in nature (e.g. anxiety, tension, irritability, depression). On the other hand, there are drugs which also produce physical dependence, e.g. barbiturates and alcohol, which on sudden discontinuation may lead to epileptiform convulsions and delirium tremens; and the opiates.

Heroin and cocaine are often mentioned in the same breath but are functionally quite different drugs, heroin being a narcotic, cocaine a stimulant. They were often taken at the same time by addicts in an attempt to counterbalance each other's unpleasant extreme effects. Others took heroin and methedrine, or more recently methadone and methylphenidate (Ritalin). The great majority of drug misusers at present take any kind of addictive drug they can get hold of.

SYMPTOMATOLOGY

Symptoms of drug dependence obviously vary with the type of agent. The harm may be to the individual only, or to society, too. Intoxication may be acute or chronic. In the case of chronic barbiturate intoxication, the picture may closely resemble long-standing alcoholism, e.g. ataxia, slurred speech, confusion (see p. 133). Symptoms of chronic amphetamine intoxication include loss of appetite and weight, insomnia at night with drowsiness by day, irritability, tension, and sometimes a picture simulating paranoid schizophrenia; amphetamine withdrawal may give rise to severe depression. Cocaine abuse may lead to a paranoid state and to hallucinations (which are characteristic, being tactile, or 'haptic'), but neither amphetamine nor cocaine leads to a physical abstinence syndrome. Withdrawal of the opiates, on the other hand, does so and produces very characteristic and often very painful features including yawning, sweating, running eyes and nose, dilation of pupils, diarrhoea, goose flesh, severe aches in limbs and abdominal cramps. Thus the withdrawal symptoms are often the opposite to symptoms of intoxication.

In general, people who become dependent on drugs show a progressive mental, physical and moral deterioration and an addict may commit acts quite foreign to his original personality. The latter cannot therefore be discovered by simply observing his behaviour.

Symptoms vary of course also according to the manner the 'addict' takes his drugs. Thus 'sniffing' cocaine intranasally is less harmful than the methods more usual in this country of injection intramuscularly ('skin-popping') and intravenously ('mainlining'). Young people involved in this country's present-day epidemic of drug taking unfortunately tend to progress from oral drug taking to 'skin-popping' and 'mainlining', and the intravenous injection of heroin and methamphetamine is a very popular and extremely dangerous form of drug abuse. Injection using unsterile, 'communal' syringes and needles carries the additional hazards of septicaemia and hepatitis. Because of these and also of malnutrition, lowered resistance to intercurrent infections, accidental and intentional overdose, and accidents, the average addict's life expectation is very much reduced.

The addict tends to be interested mainly in his next dose: in severe cases he will steal, lie, beg or (occasionally) use force to get it: he develops some skill in 'confidence tricks' (conning) which become a pleasure in themselves.

TREATMENT

Treatment of the *acute phase* is no more than the start of a long-drawn-out programme of long-term treatment and rehabilitation with a well mapped out after-care programme. This unfortunately is only an ideal as yet and has not been attained in practice. In the case of drugs producing psychological dependence only (e.g. the stimulants, cannabis, LSD) the drug can be withdrawn suddenly and completely; resulting depression must be watched for and treated. But those drugs which produce also physical dependence must not be withdrawn suddenly without providing adequate substitutes; thus barbiturates should be 'tapered' off slowly; whereas heroin can sometimes be replaced by the synthetic drug methadone ('physeptone') which can then itself be withdrawn within 10 days or so, but methadone itself can cause addiction. Tranquillizers and antidepressants will often be helpful; attention to the physical state of health, nutrition etc, are essential.

In hospital, drug withdrawal is usually not a very difficult task if the patient is prepared to collaborate. But the addict's co-operation is obtained only when he is regarded and approached as a sick man and not as a criminal.

Because of the over-prescribing by a few doctors the Government has accepted the second Brain Committee's recommendation to take the prescribing of heroin and cocaine to addicts out of the GP's hands and limit it to the staff of the newly established 'treatment centres'. Although maintenance on heroin is legally permitted, the staff of treatment centres will always try to motivate the addict towards giving up his drug taking although that is not always possible and is often resisted strongly and vociferously by the drug taker.

REHABILITATION AND AFTER CARE

Long-term treatment is much more difficult. Some form of psychotherapy and long-continued social support are necessary to help the addict to learn to live contentedly and usefully without recourse to drugs. But addicts are often immature, inadequate individuals with a low frustration tolerance and their dependence has probably lost them their job and isolated them from earlier friends and family; they therefore often return to their old haunts and to their circle of addicts, and relapses are common; in fact drug dependence (including alcoholism) must be regarded as essentially a relapsing illness. Long continued support is vital.

As the young drug abuser is often uneducated and vocationally unskilled, help with education, vocational guidance, and learning a trade will often be necessary. Social support for a time is essential.

PROGNOSIS

By and large the outlook for the established drug addict is not good; even patients who seem to do well in hospital may soon return to drug abuse when returning to the outside world. The better the underlying basic personality the better the prognosis; thus the average 'professional' addict (doctor, nurse, pharmacist, etc., for whom easy availability often plays an important role in drug taking) or 'therapeutic' middle-age addict (i.e. the one originally introduced to the drug by his doctor for a genuine medical indication) can be expected to do better than the young, little motivated, self-indulgent addict who started his drug taking career for 'kicks' or 'thrills'. The degree of social support, the possibility of keeping away from his former drug taking friends, the possibility of finding adequate substitute satisfaction are important factors. So is the type of drug with the intensity of (psychological) dependence. Cannabis does not often produce a strong psychological dependence but majority opinion among experts would strongly disagree with the view often put forward that it is harmless enough to be legalized. Heroin, cocaine and the amphetamines may lead to an intense degree of psychic dependence.

PREVENTION AND RESEARCH

Neither the punitive American approach (regarding the 'dope fiend' as a criminal) nor the formerly over-permissive 'British system' have been able to prevent the emergence of a widespread drug dependence problem. Fortunately the extent of the narcotic problem in Great Britain has remained much smaller than in the USA. Certainly seeing the addict as a sick person and not as a criminal is still foremost in the current approach in Great Britain, as exemplified in the official Outpatient Treatment Centres, and the principle of treating him in this way should encourage him to come forward for treatment at an earlier phase. Education of the professional and the lay public, research, and early diagnosis, treatment and legislative measures will all have to play their part in the task of preventing drug dependence, a task made the more important as treatment of the established state is so often difficult and disappointing. Medical students, social workers and probation officers need to know more about the problem than in the past; and for the education of the lay public it is necessary to present information in a non-sensational, objective and factual manner and to avoid glamorizing the addict. The task of providing factual information in this field is often extremely difficult for the question of escalation from soft to hard drugs is un-answered; it is true, on the one hand, that the great majority of young heroin addicts in this country have used amphetamine and cannabis; but it is equally true that the great majority of amphetamine and cannabis users in this country do not go on to heroin. In fact, escalation to LSD is more probable. This problem of escalation is only one of many examples which illustrate the vital need for research in this important modern medico-social problem.

Drug dependence is a complex problem of multifactorial causation requiring both in treatment and research a multi-disciplinary and interdisciplinary approach and teamwork. Future research will clarify to what extent methods such as the 'therapeutic community', group therapy, halfway houses, support by social workers and probation officers, groups formed by recovered addicts, chemotherapy etc., have their respective parts to play in a comprehensive approach. In the fields of research and chemotherapy, for example, an intriguing, promising method is currently being looked into in the USA, viz. the use of cyclazocine, a long-acting, orally effective, narcotic antagonist given in an attempt to block the euphoric action of heroin.

FURTHER READING

Edwards, G. (1969). 'The British approach to the treatment of heroin addiction'. *Lancet*, i, 768.

Glatt, M. M. (1974). *Drugs, Society and Man: A Guide to Addiction and its Treatment*. Medical and Technical Publishing, Lancaster.

Tylden, E. (1974). 'The clinical features of cannabis use'. *Practioner*, 212, 810.

Willis, J. (1973). *Addicts: Drugs and Alcohol Re-examined*. London.

24 Organic syndromes (organic psychoses)

These are the result of disturbed cerebral function, caused by structural disease or physiological dysfunction due to organic conditions.

They can be grouped as acute, subacute and chronic. A patient may pass easily from one form to another, and there is no dividing line. For example, a patient with an acute encephalitis may have an acute confusion; he may improve gradually, but be left with a chronic disability. Or a patient with a chronic cerebrovascular condition, and its psychiatric results, may suddenly develop an acute confusional state from a vascular accident.

INCIDENCE

Such cases are much commoner than is often realized. In 1954, for instance, a review was made of patients with physical disease who had been admitted to the psychiatric wing at UCH during five years (Stokes, Nabarro, Rosenheim and Dunkley, 1955). There were 8,480 of these; 329 of them had died, from senile or arterisclerotic dementia, or organic psychosis; and 109 of the latter had been admitted in a state of toxic confusion, many having been, unjustifiably, transferred from elsewhere. There were 208 other patients, who needed medical care in wards, for physical conditions.

AETIOLOGY

The common causes of these states are:
1 Infections:
    pneumonia
    peritonitis
    septicaemia
    typhoid
    malaria
    brucellosis
2 Metabolic:
    uraemia (often extra-renal)
    electrolyte disturbances, alkalosis, hyper- and hypo-calcaemia
    liver failure
    porta-caval encephalopathy
    porphyria
3 Endocrine:
    myxoedema
    hyperthyroidism
    Cushing's syndrome
    acute Addisonian state after steroids
    spontaneous or insulin-induced hypoglycaemia
4 Cerebral:
    minor strokes, arteriosclerotic cerebrovascular disease
    cerebral tumour — primary or secondary (e.g. to bronchus)
    cerebral abscess
    GPI
    encephalitis
    epileptiform equivalents
    trauma, including subdural haematoma
    degeneration, e.g. senile and pre-senile dementia, Huntington's chorea
5 Vitamin deficiencies: thiamine, nicotinic acid, B12
6 Cor pulmonale and chronic respiratory disease
7 Pernicious anaemia
8 Cachexia from malignant disease and malnutrition
9 Intoxication by drugs: bromides, amphetamines, CO, lead, mercury; alcohol, addictive drugs (see pp. 132, 139).

GENERAL SYMPTOMATOLOGY

The fundamental changes of organic psychotic states are:

1 Intellectual defects in orientation in space and time (resulting in confusion), memory change (including loss of recent memory and false recollection, comprehension and attention).
2 Emotional instability, and lability and absence of normal emotional response.
3 Changes in behaviour, e.g. self-neglect, incontinence, indecent behaviour and other antisocial conduct.

The *acute* organic psychosis is usually characterized by confusion and disorientation, often by hallucinations and by clouding of consciousness. The *chronic* organic psychosis may be characterised by dementia, i.e. irreversible changes in the CNS accompanied by intellectual deterioration — confusion (sometimes), disorientation, memory failure, lowering of personal and moral standards. Sometimes a chronic organic state may show itself almost entirely in the field of personality change with a decline in personal standards, but with negligible intellectual changes, e.g. in some patients with the 'post-encephalitic state'. A good example of the acute organic psychosis is delirium tremens; of the chronic organic state, the later stage of General Paralysis of the Insane (GPI).

The organic psychosis may present as an apparent endogenous or functional psychosis, e.g. GPI presenting as a manic-depressive illness or as a schizophrenic illness; a chronic alcoholic psychosis presenting as a paranoid illness. A cerebral tumour may present with *any* type of psychiatric picture. These examples serve to show the importance of a complete physical examination in all psychiatric patients. Patients regarded as 'neurotic' or 'nuisances' may have fatal organic disease, or may develop it.

SPECIAL SYNDROMES

Delirium

This is the most acute form of organic reaction. It usually starts with fever, apprehension and tremulousness; clouding of consciousness and disorientation appear later and are often accompanied by terrifying auditory and visual hallucinations. The symptoms are usually worse at night than by day.

Confusional state

This term is used to describe an illness which is a less acute reaction than delirium. A confusional state may be a brief acute reaction or an insidiously developing chronic illness, or it may start as an acute illness, fail to resolve and pass through a subacute into a chronic state.

Some of the causes of confusion present with certain patterns, e.g. the combination of confusion, hallucinations and bewilderment of the chronic alcoholic psychotic; the unconcerned deteriorating patient with GPI (it is a fallacy that GPI presents only with grandiose delusions — they account for only a small proportion of cases of this condition); the picture of mild or intermittent confusion with varying levels of consciousness seen in subdural haematoma; the paranoid hallucinatory state of amphetamine intoxication. But these are the common clinical pictures and they do not cover all cases of the particular illness concerned, e.g. GPI may present in early life in its congenital form as an apparent example of subnormality; early in adult life it may present as an apparent psychogenic illness, e.g. schizophrenia; in middle life it may present as the typical organic psychotic reaction; and in old age it may resemble a senile idiopathic dementia.

Porphyria has been much talked about since the suggestion that it was the cause of the recurrent insanity of George III, and so possibly a factor in the separation of the American Colonies from Britain. It is caused by an autosomal dominant gene, but does not produce symptoms in all affected. There are periodic attacks of confusion, with noisy outbursts and hallucinations, and accompanied by hypotension, abdominal pain and vomiting, polyuria and motor neuropathy. Barbiturates may precipitate an attack, or make one fatal from respiratory failure.

Sometimes schizophrenia, especially with an acute onset and in puerperal women, may for a short time resemble an acute confusional state though the correct diagnosis usually becomes obvious as the illness develops.

Chronic forms of organic psychosis are most prone to display personality changes, e.g. post-encephalitic state, chronic drug addiction.

Eventually, if the disease is progressive, all these differences become blotted out in the near complete erosion of all higher mental faculties in profound dementia.

DIAGNOSIS

In general the onset of psychotic or neurotic symptoms in a previously well-balanced subject should arouse suspicion. So should psychiatric states that are atypical. There is no need to emphasize the necessity for full clinical examination in all patients. If diagnosis is in doubt, however, the following are essential: haemoglobin, sedimentation rate, blood urea and electrolytes, W.R., chest X-ray and perhaps lumbar puncture, skull X-ray, B12 estimation, tests of thyroid function.

It is possible that some conditions that are now considered to be psychogenic may, in the future, be recognized to have an organic basis. It is known that severe depression may be produced by drugs such as reserpine or by jaundice, and such depression may improve with physical treatment. The full details of some underlying metabolic cause may ultimately be discovered. The same may hold for some schizophrenic reactions.

It is evident that there is in this field a great scope for collaborative research by psychiatrist, physician, biochemist and pharmacologist.

TREATMENT OF ACUTE SYNDROMES

Physical

First, this demands the energetic investigation and treatment of the underlying physical illness. The importance of this cannot be overstressed. There may seem to be little encouragement to pursue full clinical investigation in a restless, confused and even resistive patient; yet the patient's chance of survival may depend on these investigations being carried through. There is about a fortnight in which to work, because after that time the chances of a complete psychological recovery fall away quite rapidly.

An acute confusional psychosis may occur in association with a chronic medical condition. For example while the psychosis of myxoedema usually develops insidiously, it may first be brought to the notice of the physician when an acute psychotic episode has developed. Patients with acute confusion are often dehydrated, especially if they refuse food; so fluids in plenty should be given unless there is medical contra-indication. Vitamin or other specific factor deficiency is a primary defect in delirium tremens and may be an accessory factor in other confusional states, e.g. confusion of old age, malabsorption states; so injections of 'Parentrovite' may help in dealing with an acute confusional illness. The electrolyte balance must be controlled.

It is vital that in his delirium or confusion the patient's condition should not be made worse by retention of urine (maybe with overflow) or by impacted faecal masses in the rectum (maybe with spurious diarrhoea). It is important to get the patient out of bed as early as possible, especially if elderly. Confusional states are a special problem in the aged, and details of their management are separately discussed (see p. 000). If an acute episode occurs while a patient is in hospital, it is better for him to be kept where he is, but the staff will need support in nursing him.

Psychiatric

Although it may not be ideal to move a confused patient to strange surroundings, the multiple investigations necessary and the heavy nursing demands often make it imperative to nurse such patients in hospital.

The patient should be nursed in a cubicle or side room, both for his own welfare and also because he may be a distressing sight to others. Some patients may be so restless and disturbed or so terrified, e.g. in delirium tremens, that they should be cared for in a psychiatric rather than in a general ward. But to move them from one to the other, to strange staff and surroundings, may lead to confusion, and should be avoided if possible.

The relatives of such a patient should be encouraged to stay with him in turn. Where his hold on reality is blotted out by failure of recent memory, confusion and hallucinations, the presence of near relatives often has a reassuring, calming influence on him. His recognition of them often increases his tenuous hold on reality. It is particularly important that they should, if possible, be there at the critical times when he goes off to sleep and wakes up. So, if they are co-operative, they should not go away just because he has gone to sleep; their presence in a couple of hours may be most valuable. Of course he may be so seriously disturbed as to fail to recognize them and need continuous sedation throughout for a few days.

Another help for the patient is the wearing of name badges by the staff; and for the staff to refer to each other by name. It is no surprise if the patient is muddled when any one of half a dozen white-clad people arriving at his bedside answers to the name of 'Nurse'. Similarly, the patient should always be referred to by his proper name and not as 'Pop', 'Grandad' or 'old chap'. In the rush of admission to hospital he may have left behind his false teeth, his spectacles or his hearing aid; the absence of any or all of these may prevent effective communication between him and the staff.

Sedation

This is a difficult question and it is impossible to lay down hard and fast rules. In an acute short-lived psychosis like delirium tremens accompanied by frightening hallucinations, it is better for the patient to sleep through his illness, so that it is wise to give sedatives by day and by night. In confusion associated with cerebral anoxia, one has to steer a difficult path between giving so much sedation that the cerebral anoxia is increased and not giving enough so that the patient in his restlessness exhausts himself.

Again in a patient suspected of having a subdural haematoma one must watch for the development of neurological signs including changes in the level of consciousness, so that one needs to be sparing and cautious in giving sedatives. Nevertheless, in general, sedation takes the edge off a patient's confusion and restlessness and so makes it easier to administer the necessary medical treatment.

As a routine sedative, chlorpromazine by tablets, syrup or intramuscular injection (100-150 mgm) is probably the best. It is a reasonably safe sedative but:

1 It potentiates the effect of barbiturates and alcohol.

2 It occasionally causes hypotensive attacks.

3 It may cause liver damage or other toxic manifestations though these are uncommon where it is used for short periods.

Promazine and perphenazine are thought to be safer than chlorpromazine but are almost certainly less effective in acute disturbance. Diazepan (valium), 20-40 mg. intravenously is very useful in acute confusional states, especially in delirium tremens.

The short-acting barbiturates are often useful in the less severely disturbed patients. In geriatric patients or patients with severe renal disease they may be harmful and may easily produce the condition of barbiturate intoxication. There is no place for the long acting barbiturate, e.g. phenobarbitone, in the treatment of the acute or subacute organic psychosis.

Paraldehyde has limited uses, but is often of special value in delirium tremens and in a small minority of elderly patients. There is only one indication for giving this drug intramuscularly (8-14 mls): namely when the patient refuses a drug by mouth *and* when because of severe liver damage the uses of morphia, phenothiazines and barbiturates are all contra-indicated. Paraldehyde is still given intramuscularly far too often when another sedative would have worked as well or better. It is exquisitely painful when injected; and not infrequently leads to massive necrosis and sloughing at the site of injection.

Morphia (16-32 mgm) and hyoscine (0.3-0.6 mgm) combined is a very useful sedative in an acute emergency and where all other sedatives have failed. It is then justifiable to use it even in delirium tremens or cardiac failure, but it should only be used for two or three days while other longer-term sedatives are being considered.

TREATMENT OF CHRONIC SYNDROMES

In the milder cases it is often possible for the patient to live at home, particularly if his family are able and willing to give him the necessary psychological support. If possible, he should be encouraged to be active to the limit of his talents: the sheltered workshops for the disabled provide a most helpful, morale-sustaining service.

For the more severely demented or disturbed chronic psychotic, mental hospital care becomes essential. Often one is fighting a losing battle against a progressive dementing process. The basis of treatment is the preservation of the individuality, morale and personality of the patient for as long as possible. This is helped by meaningful activity, i.e. occupational therapy, social therapy and toilet training. Rarely the patient with severe personality changes following organic disease of the nervous system, e.g. post encephalitic syndrome, may need to be confined in some security institution.

There is no specific drug therapy in severe dementia. A programme of ordered activity is the best treatment for the patient but as the dementia progresses and the patient's social conduct and behaviour deteriorate his mode of life can often be rendered less trying to his immediate neighbours by the judicious use of tranquillizers, e.g. chlorpromazine, promazine, perphenazine, diazepam. These must be used with discretion so that the patient is not left in a state of drug-induced stupor.

REFERENCES

Barton, R. (1959). *Institutional Neurosis.* Wright, Bristol.

Gooddy, W., Gautier-Smith, P. C., and Dunkley, E. W. (1960). 'Neurological practice in a mental observation unit'. *Lancet*, ii, 1290.

Mayer-Gross, W., Slater, E., and Roth, M. (1969). *Clinical Psychiatry.* Chapters 7 to 10. Baillière, Tindall and Cassell, London.

Stokes, J. F., Nabarro, J. D. N., Rosenheim, M. L., and Dunkley, E. W. (1954). 'Physical disease in a mental observation unit'. *Lancet*, ii, 862.

Waldenström, J. and Haegen-Aronsen, B. (1963). 'Different patterns of human porphyria'. *Brit. Med. J.*, 2, 805.

25 Epilepsy

Epilepsy is a sudden discharge of grey matter of the brain. Alternatively, it may be described as a spontaneous self-sustained hyper-synchronous excessive discharge of cerebral neurones. Probably all epileptic attacks begin in a particular area of the brain that is locally hyper-excitable. This hyper-excitability usually arises from an area of acquired damage, such as tumour, vascular lesion or congenital deformity, but some epilepsies (particularly the very common febrile convulsions of early childhood) appear to arise from an inborn sensitivity of the brain that manifests itself at the younger ages only. The site of the focus, the pathways of spread of the abnormal discharge from the focus and the effects of the transitory post-ictal paralysis, are the main determinants of the clinical fit-pattern seen. The major seizure or grand mal attack may be the end result of discharge beginning in any part of the brain. It is the form of seizure that can occur in brains that are otherwise not susceptible to epilepsy, as is seen, for example, in ECT. It is of the utmost importance to get an accurate chronological description of patients' seizures in order to understand their evolution. A scheme of examination is given below.

The classification on pp. 162-3 has now been elaborated by an international committee. Certain terms are still in common use, such as petit mal, which may refer to several types of seizure, physiologically distinct and aetiologically different. In general, the fit-pattern enables one to determine the site of origin of the attack; the history of the length of attacks and accompanying signs and symptoms usually indicate the nature of the underlying lesion. Idiopathic epilepsy should not be used as a diagnosis, since it means only 'epilepsy of unknown origin'. All epilepsy is symptomatic, but the underlying cause may be unknown even after exhaustive investigation.

A logical classification of the psychological disturbances seen in association with epilepsy relates them as far as possible to actual epileptic attacks as observed in clinical fits or in the specific EEG discharges.

(a) *Pre-ictal disturbances.* Some chronic patients show increasing irritability and anxiety, and seem to be 'working up to a fit'. The physiological mechanism is unknown, and it is doubtful whether the behaviour is cause or effect of epileptic attacks (the precipitation of attacks by psychological events is common; the triggers are occasionally very specific, e.g. so-called musicogenic epilepsy).

(b) *Ictal disturbances.* These are almost solely confined to disturbances of consciousness which may be profound and total, as in major seizures, or transitory and in the nature of dreamy states, as often occurs in temporal lobe attacks, of which the patient may remember fragments of dream-like experiences as well as the actual happenings around him at the time of the attack.

(c) *Post-ictal disturbances.* After many forms of attack many patients have a temporary disturbance of consciousness in which they may act in all sorts of psychologically determined ways. This is particularly marked after major seizures and some temporal lobe attacks. The so-called epileptic furors usually occur at this stage, but criminal behaviour and dangerous violence is uncommon in epileptics at any time.

(d) *Psychological disturbances not related to attacks.* Psychological disorders apparently unrelated to ictal discharges are the most common forms of disturbance. For their assessment, a full psychiatric investigation is as essential as diagnosing the 'neurological' aspects of the epilepsy. Some patients with mental subnormality may also suffer from epilepsy, though only a small proportion of epileptics as a whole are subnormal. The more subnormal the patient, the more likely is epilepsy to occur. The subnormality and the epilepsy are both symptoms of underlying brain damage.

As regards behaviour disorders, patients with temporal lobe epilepsy appear to suffer from more severe disturbances than those with other forms of epilepsy, perhaps because of the special position of the temporal lobe in relation to emotional behaviour. A few adult patients show a paranoid hallucinatory psychosis that at times may be indistinguishable from schizophrenia. This often occurs after patients have been epileptic for some years and when the attacks are beginning to diminish.

However, the most common reactions are ordinary neurotic depressive disturbances. The epileptic personality is a long described and well recognized clinical entity with slowness, stickiness, paranoid tendencies and circumstantiality. It is probably a special case of the combined effects of temporal lobe epilepsy and adverse social circumstances. In epileptic children, a wide variety of disturbances is seen, but hyperkinesis and irritability are particularly common at the youngest ages.

The following factors in order of importance are to be taken into account in assessing psychological changes in all epileptics:

1 The pre-existing genetic inheritance.
2 The brain damage of whatever cause that is responsible for the epilepsy.
3 The possible physiological effects of the fits themselves; in practice only fits causing anoxia (i.e. status or severe major seizures) result in further psychological changes.
4 The effects of family attitude and social problems (epilepsy is still a dread disease in folklore; many patients suffer unnecessary restrictions as regards education, employment and recreation).
5 The anticonvulsant drugs in large doses may have a slight sedative effect but these effects are often exaggerated.

THE DIFFERENTIAL DIAGNOSIS OF 'ATTACKS'

The word attack is meant to cover in the broadest sense episodic disturbances of consciousness and/or behaviour that usually last seconds or minutes rather than hours or days and are often stereotyped in form. There are four main groups of causes: epileptic, vascular, biochemical and psychogenic. By far the most important information comes from a minute account of what actually happens in the attacks, preferably from observers as well as from the sufferer. An exact description of one particular attack seen from the very beginning is more helpful than an impressionistic summary of many. Words such as epileptiform, hysterical and so on, should not be used. The following points may be noted though not all of them are usually necessary in every case:

1 The circumstances of the attack: What time of day or night was it? What was the patient doing at the time? Was he tired or hungry or emotionally upset?

2 Note the first thing seen by an observer and/or whether the patient had a warning (aura) of which he speaks, or which (in children, for example) can be inferred from his actions (for example, holding the abdomen as if in pain).

3 As far as possible in chronological order, note the pattern of movements — jerking, or writhing, etc., whether they begin symmetrically or on one side and affect arm before leg, or vice versa. Note if the movements are alternate, as in bicycling, or simultaneous.

4 Look for evidence of autonomic change — flushing, pallor, sweating, drooling of saliva, state of pupils.

5 If the patient can still speak, ask him for any subjective changes in sensation in the body, or changes in the appearances of noises or objects seen. If he is speechless or unconscious, ask these questions as soon as he comes round and can reply.

6 Observe roughly how long the attack takes and what the state of the patient is afterwards. Sleep or drowsiness is common. Note whether the course of the attack seems to be affected by the circumstances surrounding the patient, for example, whether movements are more violent if restraint is attempted. If attacks of more than one form occur, obtain separate descriptions of the commonest types.

Epileptic

Epileptic attacks characteristically last seconds rather than minutes, and attacks without any disturbance of consciousness are rare. The pattern of the major seizure, or grand mal attack, is the most stereotyped of all, and details of it are less important than the details of minor attacks and of the exact way in which the generalized convulsion began. There are several common patterns of minor seizure and patients may suffer from more than one form, e.g. petit mal (or absence), myoclonic jerks (focal or generalized), focal motor attacks with or without auras. These should, if necessary, be imitated to the examiner by the observer attempting to describe the attack seen. Such mimicry is much more accurate than verbal description. Attacks often occur in sleep, or when the patient is alone. Injuries are possible as a result of falling in the attacks when they occur without warning.

There are three common groups of symptoms of particular diagnostic difficulty. In young children, under the age of 2 years, when typical epileptic attacks are common, there are also breath-holding spells. These are psychogenic in origin and are the reaction to frustration of children who are otherwise fairly normal though possibly rather bad-tempered. The children after some minutes of normal crying in rage take a deep breath and hold it until unconsciousness may supervene for a few seconds with a few jerkings of the limbs (jactitations). The second common group of diagnostic difficulties concerns adults who may have a variety of turns consisting mostly of subjective experiences, panic states, epigastric sensations, giddiness, fullness in the head, and so on. Their time course may be variable and it is difficult to sort out whether they are epileptic or purely psychogenic. The two, of course, often co-exist in the patient with temporal lobe epilepsy. This is the commonest form of epilepsy causing such attacks on an epileptic basis, and it is usually associated with psychological disturbances. In old age there is the problem of the differential diagnosis of senile falls, that is to say, the apparent sudden losses of posture in old people with or without a transient loss of consciousness. These may be epileptic, cerebro-vascular or cardio-vascular in origin.

Vascular

Attacks on a vascular basis involving loss of consciousness usually result from an impairment of the function of the heart or of the major vessels of the brain. By far the commonest form, especially in young people, is the faint due to a temporary failure of sufficient blood supply to the brain. It usually occurs with the subject standing, sometimes sitting, but never lying down unless he has serious heart disease. There is usually a sensation of 'going off' which, combined with the pallor, slow small pulse and sweating, usually make the diagnosis. A few jerks of the body from the cerebral anoxia or rarely, more definite epileptic phenomena, are sometimes seen, particularly when the circulation is beginning to be restored.

Such attacks are common in young people, in starvation, in situations of stress and anxiety and in women rather than men.

Several serious forms of heart disease can produce sudden unconsciousness from failure of the circulation, for example Stokes-Adams. In such cases there is always other evidence of pre-existing heart disease.

Cerebro-vascular disorders are very varied in form, depending on which blood vessel of the brain is involved. The basilar artery region supplying the brain stem and mid-brain produces the widest variety of atypical turns, with transient paralyses, disturbances of speech and consciousness. These usually last minutes or hours rather than seconds. In older people transient losses of speech or weakness of limbs are very common, and it is sometimes difficult to sort out whether they are epileptic or vascular, particularly since an old vascular lesion can certainly become epileptogenic.

Under the vascular heading may be included, for convenience, attacks of labyrinthine origin, so-called Menières, in which the patient has sudden paroxysmal giddiness that may cause loss of posture. Headaches, particularly of the migrainous variety, probably also have a basis in vascular spasm. Their symptomatology may resemble epileptic attacks but is of longer duration.

Biochemical disorders

Two simple and transitory forms of attack, where the symptoms are biochemical in origin though the initial cause of the attack is psychogenic, are the breath-holding spells in infancy already mentioned and the tetany, numbness and tingling following hyperventilation that occur in some neurotic adults.

Several metabolic diseases can produce sufficient interference with cerebral function to produce unconsciousness. Hypoglycaemia is the commonest one, but failure of function of liver (cholemia), kidney (uraemia), can also produce periods of unconsciousness. These usually last hours or days rather than minutes. The differential diagnosis depends on specialized medical knowledge and confirmatory laboratory investigations.

Under this heading may be included the effects of drugs, of

which by far the most common and important are the barbiturates and alcohol. The latter, after some years of addiction, is often associated with transitory losses of consciousness or posture that may simulate vascular disease and/or epilepsy. Any patient who has periods of drowsiness or amnesic episodes where it is difficult to obtain supporting evidence from observers should be suspected of drug addiction and/or alcohol. The nystagmus sometimes found in barbiturate intoxication is often absent in chronic addicts.

Psychogenic disorders

This general term is preferable to hysterical as disturbances of behaviour can occur in a variety of psychiatric conditions. For example, catatonic schizophrenics may have sudden periods of mutism or immobility or sudden outbursts of violence. The tantrums and rage attacks of behaviour problems in children can also hardly be regarded as purely hysterical without this word losing all specificity. The malingerer is also a different psychological problem, but one rarely seen in civilian practice.

The commonest forms of psychogenic attack are 'hysterical' in the sense that they occur in neurotic personalities with other evidence of emotional disturbance. The forms of seizure are very variable and no typical patterns can be described. The seizures normally occur when the subject is not alone and the attention paid to the attack by others usually results in an increase in the violence of the movements or noises made. The patient's behaviour may be altered by the attention of others even when seemingly unconscious and without any subsequent memory of the attack.

Both epileptic and hysterical attacks may occur in the same patient at different times, but apparently hysterical episodes can also occur during the post-ictal confusional phase following a short epileptic attack, the movements of which may be forgotten by observers in the light of subsequent excitement.

STATUS EPILEPTICUS

The patient may fail to recover consciousness between a series

TABLE II: *Proposed international classification of epileptic seizures*

Clinical seizure type	Electroencephalographic expression	
	Ictal	Interictal
I. Partial seizures	Discharge more or less localized over one or, sometimes, both hemispheres	Local discharges, generally over one hemisphere only
A. 1. With motor symptoms 2. With special sensory or somatosensory symptoms 3. With autonomic symptoms 4. Compound forms	Local contralateral discharge	Local contralateral discharges
B. With complex symptomatology (which may sometimes begin with elementary symptomatology) 1. With impaired consciousness alone 2. With intellectual symptomatology 3. With affective symptomatology 4. With 'psychosensory' symptomatology (illusions, hallucinations) 5. With 'psychomotor' symptomatology (automatisms) 6. Compound forms	Unilateral or bilateral discharge, diffuse, or focal in temporal or fronto-temporal regions	Unilateral or bilateral, generally asynchronous, focus; usually in the temporal regions)
C. Secondarily generalized	Above discharge becomes secondarily and rapidly generalized	
II. Generalized seizures	Bilateral, essentially synchronous and symmetrical discharge from the start	Bilateral, essentially synchronous and usually symmetrical discharges
A. Non-convulsive seizures 1. With impairment of consciousness only (a) Brief duration (beginning and ending abruptly) (b) Long duration ('absence status') 2. With other phenomena associated with impairment of consciousness		
B. Convulsive seizures 1. Myoclonic jerks 2. Clonic seizures 3. Tonic seizures 4. Tonic-clonic seizures		
III. Unilateral or predominantly unilateral seizures in children Characterized by clonic, tonic or tonic-clonic convulsions, with or without an impairment of consciousness, expressed only or predominantly on one side. Such seizures sometimes shift from one side to the other but usually do not become symmetrical	Partial discharge very rapidly spreading over only one hemisphere Or discharges generalized from the start but considerably predominant over one hemisphere	Focal contralateral discharges Bilateral and synchronous symmetrical or asymmetrical discharges
IV. Erratic seizures in new-born With variable tonic and/or clonic convulsions, generally unilateral, sometimes alternating or generalized	Various patterns, often localized but variable from time to time and from area to area	Variable

(Gastaut Classification, from Epilepsia 1964, 297, 306, simplified)

Anatomical substrate	Aetiology	Age
Various cortical and/or sub-cortical regions Usually in the cortical region of one hemisphere Usually cortical and/or sub-cortical, temporal or fronto-temporal regions (including rhinencephalic structures), unilateral or bilateral	Usually related to a wide variety of local brain lesions (cause known, suspected or unknown). Constitutional factors may be important	Possible at all ages but more frequent with increasing age
Unlocalized (? meso-diencephalon)	No cause found, or diffuse or bilateral lesions, or toxic and/or metabolic disturbances (constitutional factors may be important) B3: organic aetiology is usual	All ages A1a: especially in children B2, 3: especially in children B4: all ages except infancy
Cortical and/or sub-cortical Region in one hemisphere un-localized (? meso-diencephalon)	Wide variety of focal, unilateral brain (constitutional factor may be important) no cause found, or diffuse or multiple bilateral lesions, or toxic metabolic perturbations, generally in immature brain (constitutional factors may be important)	Almost exclusively in very young children
Cortical and/or subcortical region in one or both hemispheres, or unlocalized	Focal or diffuse lesions of diverse aetiology or metabolic and/or toxic. Constitutional factors and cerebral immaturity are important	Limited virtually to the new-born

of fits. Death from exhaustion may occur. Admission to hospital is recommended, but intravenous anaesthetics may be required at once: e.g. phenobarbitone 200 mg, or sod. amytal 500 mg. Diazepan 10 mg. intravenously, the dose to be increased if necessary, has been found to be very effective. Paraldehyde 5-8 ml. intramuscularly is still useful occasionally.

TREATMENT OF EPILEPSY

Acute

Treatment of a fit consists of the 'first-aid' measures of keeping the air-way clear, and preventing injury. The fit is horrifying for others, in particular relatives, to watch and re-assurance is required.

Treatment of *status epilepticus* has been described above.

Long-term

The long-term treatment by the GP depends on finding the correct drugs for the individual, on which specialist help may be desirable, and on helping the patient and family treat the illness with as little prejudice and fear as possible.

The drug treatment of epilepsy may take some time to establish. A change of drugs is often needed in adolescence, as the child gets bigger, and also the fit patterns often change. In general, there is no need to start anti-convulsant therapy with the patient's first attack as many people have one or two attacks in their lives that do not need treatment. But if fits recur and drugs are required, phenobarbitone, 30 mg, and phenytoin, 90 mg b.d. should be given, and increased gradually, if necessary to the limit of tolerance as shown by the appearance of blurred vision or ataxia. Tridione 300-1800 mg daily may be used to control petit mal attacks, but may cause skin rashes, and there is a risk of aplastic anaemia.

The parents of children with fits always require careful handling with an explanation of the nature of the child's disability, the need for a regular régime of treatment, and, as far as possible, normal outlets for exercise and social development. Special schooling is needed only for those who have the additional handicaps of mental backwardness or behaviour disorders, or associated physical disabilities, for example, spastic hemiplegia. Every child with continuing fits needs a careful social and psychological examination. There are particular problems at the school leaving age as suitable sheltered employment may be difficult to find. Behaviour disorders are as likely to occur from the patient's resentment of society's attitude to him as from an 'epileptic temperament'.

Inevitably there are disabilities which the patient has to accept; restrictions on employment, on sport undertaken, on driving, and on marriage. Each depends on individual assessment of the risks: and the GP, supported by a specialist, can often allow the patient to accept reasonable ones, though employers and licensing authorities are cautious.

Surgery is discussed below (see p. 342).

FURTHER READING

Falconer, M. A. (1974). 'Mesial temporal sclerosis as a common cause of epilepsy'. *Lancet*, 2, 767.

Hill, J. D. N. (1972). 'Treatment of the epilepsies'. In Sargant, W., and Slater, E., *Physical Methods of Treatment in Psychiatry*, Livingstone, Edinburgh, Chapter 9.

Scott, D. F., (1969). *About Epilepsy.* Duckworth, London.

The February 1973 issue of The British Journal of Hospital Medicine contains several articles on epilepsy including one on its surgical treatment.

26 Psychiatric illness in old age

A person with chronic psychiatric illness or subnormality may simply live on into old age, e.g. the organic psychotic, the chronic neurotic, the psychotic; i.e. the person who is already handicapped and isolated, becomes more deeply so. Besides these, the following syndromes occur in old people.

DEPRESSION

This may occur in one of the three following forms:

1 As part of a cycle of recurrent depressive attacks.
2 As agitated depression, with marked guilt feelings and unworthiness, considerable somatic preoccupation, e.g. 'Inside stopped up' — 'Bowels rotting away'.
3 As simple reactive depression.

All are important, because, if they are energetically treated, the prognosis is good: and because the risk of suicide in depression rises quite rapidly after 60 — until it falls again in extreme old age when physically impossible.

Treatment

Treatment has been described above (see p. 80); but in old age, special questions arise with ECT. Sometimes an elderly patient presents with a mixed picture of deterioration and depression. Some people do not do well on ECT, which accentuates the confusion and seems to speed the dementing process. Similarly if an elderly patient remains confused for more than 24 hours after an application of ECT it should be abandoned. On the other hand, severe depression can be even more unpleasant than dementia, and may respond to ECT, which is then worth a short trial.

PARANOID ILLNESS

This is not uncommon in old age — particularly among the deaf and the isolated. The persecutory and delusional system, often with auditory hallucinations, is often local and limited, i.e. it refers to events in the patient's own room or house or immediate surroundings but would not be cured by a move. The condition may closely resemble paranoid schizophrenia as seen in earlier age groups (Kay 1972).

Treatment

Phenothiazine drugs often help the patient, or may enable him to live with his delusions and to be less disturbed by them. Most important of all is the attitude of the patient to his doctor. If he feels that his doctor is one in whom he can confide without being ridiculed, then a most useful bond between the two has been forged and he will feel he has a friend in whom he can trust. The doctor must not buy peace by agreeing with the patient about his delusions, for this is to confirm him in his psychosis. But he should not oppose him, or he may simply provoke reiteration and antagonism. He should make it clear that while he understands that the patient genuinely believes this, he (the doctor) cannot share his belief, but that he does appreciate how real and unpleasant it is for the patient and that he is ready to hear anything that he has to say about himself and his illness. It is surprising how many elderly paranoid patients can on these terms accept their doctor as a person to whom they can unburden themselves, so that they can stay in the outside world. Hospitalization should be avoided, wherever possible, but just occasionally the patient's conduct becomes so anti-social as to make this step necessary.

The alleviation of isolation is essential where possible. Relatives must be encouraged to keep in touch, and to avoid antagonising him.

ACUTE CONFUSIONAL STATES

These have already been described (p. 148). No GP will go long without meeting with one of these illnesses. There are three points to consider:

1 The fact that physical illness or deterioration may cause confusional states.
2 The need for investigation.
3 The problems of admitting the elderly to hospital.

1 *Physical illnesses*

These are legion, and have already been discussed (p. 147).

Severe physical pain also seems a potent factor in the development of confusional states. This may be due to retention of urine with overflow; impacted rectal masses, with or without spurious diarrhoea; impending or actual gangrene of limb; or glaucoma.

Relief of any of these underlying conditions may effect a miraculous improvement in the patient's psychological state. His restlessness should be controlled by tranquillizers or sedatives and energetic treatment of the primary physical condition pursued.

2 *Investigation*

With the ever increasing biochemical and technical advances, the investigation and treatment of disease imposes greatly increased demands on the patience and co-operation of our patients which a number of elderly patients find too great. As a general principle, if old people can be investigated as outpatients, this should be done, even if it means that the diagnosis is reached rather more slowly. It is no profit to the patient (or the NHS) if after extensive treatment or high-powered investigation you are left with a permanently confused patient who will need long-term psychiatric care. Nevertheless, many old people require admission either because their illness is acute — the medical or surgical emergency — or because the investigations cannot be done outside.

3 *Admission to hospital*

We may first consider the attitude of the old person to hospital. For such a person death is not far off in time — it is an ugly fact which he cannot escape. To him hospital is often a place where you go to die and this adds to his fears.

Investigations and operations which make demands on him should be postponed (unless essential) until he is thoroughly settled into the ward, and has lost any confusion he had. An operation should be postponed, if possible, until any depression has lifted: or the patient may simply die from it.

The hospital inevitably demands a greater or less degree of

conformity among its patients, but for the elderly it may mean a prohibition of a life-long habit, or idiosyncrasy, when he already feels himself severely threatened. The ward which can tolerate the minor eccentricities of the elderly will get better results and fewer cases of confusion.

Another disturbing feature for the patient is that he feels himself at the mercy of doctors and nurses young enough to be his grandchildren. This handing over of oneself to the 'very young' can be a frightening and humiliating experience for the elderly.

A potent factor in precipitating disorientation and confusion is the impaired sight and hearing of the elderly. This is particularly so at nights when confusion so often first manifests itself. In the darkened ward in strange surroundings, the patient finds orientation and interpretation of strange sights and sounds difficult. Often misinterpretation (illusion) leads to a failure of orientation and this to confusion with hallucinosis. Once this state has been established it is difficult to reverse the process.

GENERAL PRINCIPLES OF TREATMENT

There are certain principles which will help the elderly patient, and minimize any psychiatric disabilities.

1 Admission to hospital (general or psychiatric) should be only when necessary.
2 Single cubicles should be provided to which the patient can be admitted and nursed while he is becoming oriented to his new surroundings. He needs the light until he is firmly asleep and a regular sedative (see below) over his first few nights, so that he does not lie awake wondering where he is. He will not become a drug addict and may well avoid becoming a psychiatric casualty. Four or five days spent in this way produce a more co-operative patient more willing to fight for his life. Abolishing this period may produce a perfect medical or surgical result but a demented patient.
3 The patient should be nursed, later, in small rooms rather than large wards, so that he is able to form relationships with a small group of patients, rather than no relationships with a large ward full of 'other' patients.

4 Staff should wear name labels, so that the patient can know to whom he is talking.

5 A patient is often helped by the presence of a near relative or friend sitting by his bedside, and this kind of visiting should be encouraged: it is as important as in a children's ward.

6 The patient should be got out of bed at the earliest opportunity.

7 Sedatives: Every doctor and every nurse and many a patient has his or her favourite sedative. For the elderly simple measures, the hot sweet milk drink, a hot toddy are not to be despised. If this is what the patient has been used to, it is stopped at his risk (and the doctor's).

Useful simple sedatives are Welldorm, Promazine and Chlorpromazine. Paraldehyde is occasionally useful (only by mouth, never by injection in the elderly).

8 Analgesics: Pain often produces a restless confused patient, and pain-relieving drugs in adequate doses are indicated, including Pethidine or Morphia if the pain is severe. Addiction hardly ever develops after the age of 60.

FURTHER READING

Kay, D. W. K. (1972). 'Schizophrenia and schizophrenia-like states in the elderly'. *Brit. J. Hosp. Med.*, 8, 369.

Post, F. (1965). *The Clinical Psychiatry of Late Life*. Pergamon, Oxford.

27 Dementia

Dementia can arise from various causes, and its age of onset varies greatly.

It has been usual to describe two main types:

1 *Senile dementia* with a slow steady march to increasing dementia.

2 *Arteriosclerotic dementia*, an illness whose general progress is downhill punctuated by cerebrovascular episodes with exacer-

bation of confusion, transient paralysis or aphasia. Emotional lability is common.

There are also the *presenile dementias*, known as *Pick's disease* and *Alzheimer's disease*. Each has symptoms of focal cerebral degeneration, as well as dementia. The onset is usually between 40 and 60; the aetiology is obscure and possibly genetic. *Huntington's chorea* consists of an insidious deterioration of various parts of the brain especially the corpus striatum due to a simple Mendelian dominant. Jerky movements occur early; complete dementia is gradual but certain.

The normal changes of old age become steadily more marked. Confusion and disorientation appear; often these appear first only at night but sooner or later become present throughout the twenty-four hours. There is a falling off of personal standards and incontinence frequently occurs.

The patient, because of the contraction of his span of attention and failure of recent memory, may become a danger to himself, e.g. he wants to light a gas ring or stove, he turns on the gas but before he can apply a light he has forgotten what he set out to do and so the gas remains unlit; later he may be found dead in a gas filled room. Or he sets out to cross the road, but he cannot hold in his attention simultaneously the desire to reach the far side pavement and the necessity to look both ways before crossing, so that he steps out in front of an oncoming vehicle.

Another distressing feature is that many patients are very restless by night, and rise in the small hours of the morning and insist that they must get up and go to work. Such behaviour can make care of the elderly at home impossible and can be a great nuisance in a hospital ward.

Sometimes the first sign of dementia is shown in a deterioration of social behaviour and the patient may find himself charged in court, e.g. with some sexual offence, often against young children, or with shoplifting. When an elderly patient, previously of good character, finds himself in this position it is the urgent duty of the patient's doctor to make sure that the offence has not been committed as the result of dementia. Not every elderly accused person has dementia but the occasion does demand urgent psychiatric investigation, including psychometric tresting and clectro-encephalography.

DIAGNOSIS AND MANAGEMENT

Because there is no treatment for dementia the doctor has a heavy responsibility not to accept the diagnosis without excluding every other possible cause, and without an accurate history; if the history is short, some systemic physical cause which is reversible may be operating (see p. 147); even if the history is a long one, the condition may possibly be due to a slowly growing tumour or subdural haematoma.

But for dementia itself treatment is impossible. In the early stages much can be done to prevent or minimise its effects and avoid suffering and isolation by a full understanding of the psychological stresses in old age, as discussed in detail later (see p. 299). Other points on the handling of psychiatric symptoms in elderly people have already been described (see p. 169).

The management of the severely demented patient (Arie 1973) demands a great deal of care and supervision in a safe but stimulating environment. The strain of providing this at home may ultimately become too great for the relatives; in such cases, and if the patient has no family to care for him, admission to a residential home or other institution may become essential.

FURTHER READING

Arie, T. (1973). 'Dementia in the elderly: management'. *Brit. Med. J.*, 2, 602.

Corsellis, J. A. N. (1969). 'The pathology of dementia'. *Brit. J. Hosp. Med.*, March, 65.

Roth, M. and Myers, D. H. (1969). 'The diagnosis of dementia'. *Brit. J. Hosp. Med.*, March, 765.

Slater, E. and Roth, M. (ed.) (1969) 'Ageing and the mental diseases of the aged'. In Mayer-Gross, Slater and Roth, *Clinical Psychiatry*, Baillière, Tindall and Cassell, London.

28 The psychosomatic approach to illness

DEFINITION

The term 'psychosomatic' is used in different ways (Wolff 1971). By 'psychosomatic disorders' are meant certain specific illnesses with definite organic pathology in the origin of which psychological factors, usually prolonged emotional stress, are thought to play a major role. These include ulcerative colitis, duodenal ulcer, some cases of asthma (allergy and infection being important alternative or additional causes), migraine, some types of dermatitis and urticaria, and possibly some cases of essential hypertension.

However, whether these disorders are regarded as psychosomatic or not, and whether others, like coronary disease, rheumatoid arthritis and some endocrine disorders like hyperthyroidism are added to the list, does in our present state of incomplete knowledge depend a great deal on the orientation of the physician, i.e. on whether he favours a purely organic approach or whether he believes in the importance of psychological factors.

It is often more useful to speak of a 'psychosomatic approach' to illness in order to draw attention to the fact that in many illnesses psychological factors related to the patient's life situation may play some part in determining the onset and progress of the condition even though physical factors may be of equal or major importance. The following are a few examples. The onset of pulmonary tuberculosis often coincides with a period of emotional stress; thyrotoxicosis may develop during an acute crisis in the patient's life; the progress of diabetes is often influenced by the patient's personality, which affects his ability to co-operate in treatment, and stress may aggravate the condition. Similarly, and in an even wider sense the expression 'psychosomatic medicine' or 'whole person medicine' is used to describe an approach to all illnesses, structural or functional, in which, where aetiology and treatment are concerned, the patient is considered as a whole, equal attention being paid to physical, psychological, inter-personal and social aspects and to their interaction.

INCIDENCE OF STRESS DISORDERS

That there is a high incidence of stress disorders or emotionally determined illness in the population has been shown by several studies, and especially by Halliday (1949). He (1946, 1949) has pointed out that social factors may be partly responsible for the changing incidence of various stress disorders, from time to time and from culture to culture; thus the incidence of hysterical symptoms has decreased and that of psychosomatic disorders has increased since World War I. Rosenbaum (1954) has suggested that the fact that the incidence of peptic ulcers in men has increased and that of women decreased since the turn of the century, might be related to the change in the social status of women; this allows the latter a greater degree of freedom in giving expression to aggressive feelings, and also to their drives for either dependency or independency according to their needs, while men have less opportunity of expressing their aggressive drives and also find themselves in a more dependent position at home. Whether this is in fact the case and whether it relates to ulcer formation is unproven. Statistical studies by Hopkins (1956), Shepherd et al. (1966) and the College of Practitioners (Watts 1962) have already been quoted (see above, p. 49).

'STRESS' AND ORGANIC ILLNESS

It is widely accepted that stress plays a major part in the causation of psychiatric illness but the exact relationship between stress and organic illness is less clear.

The word 'stress' is here used to refer to the internal emotional stress set up in the patient and not to the external stressful situation which causes it. To give one example to illustrate this distinction: if a weak and dependent wife feels angry at her husband's aggressive behaviour she may be unable to show her anger because of a conflict between her desire to do so and her fear of the consequences. This conflict or internal stress, if maintained over a long period, may lead to the development of a psychosomatic illness. Another more confident and independent woman may react to the same external, stressful situation by standing up for herself so that she has less internal conflict and does not fall ill. In other words, the stress which is responsible for the illness is the internal emotional stress due to conflict which prevents open expression of feelings and not to the external stressful situation itself.

Knowledge is gradually accumulating on the neurological and endocrine mechanisms through which such internal stress can lead to physiological and hence, perhaps, to pathological changes (see p. 45). Much research in psychosomatic medicine is concerned with elucidating the physiological mechanisms involved (Levi 1972). Thus, stress is known to influence the secretion of the anti-diuretic hormone by the posterior pituitary, to increase the production of nor-adrenaline by the adrenal medulla and of corticosteroids by the adrenal cortex and to increase thyroid activity. It affects the autonomic nervous system causing, for example, vasco-constriction and a rise of systolic and diastolic blood pressure and changes in gastric secretion and motility (see p. 183). In all these and similar physiological reactions the hypothalamus, the reticular formation and limbic system play a prominent part. For example, peptic ulcers can be produced in monkeys by electrical stimulation of the hypothalamus. It is thus easy to understand that emotional stress can cause physical symptoms through physiological dysfunction and possibly more lasting pathological changes in various peripheral organs.

PERSONALITY

While experimental work in man is mainly concerned with physiological responses to stress rather than with the production of actual organic illness, evidence is accumulating gradually that there is some correlation between such illnesses and the patient's personality and his life situation. This is derived from two main sources.

First, attempts have been made, mainly by means of questionnaires, to correlate certain types of personality with certain specific psychosomatic disorders. Thus, patients with ulcerative colitis tend to have rigid, obsessional, dependent types of personality and to be people who have difficulty in expressing their feelings. However, it is very doubtful whether there is in fact one specific type of personality for each psychosomatic disease.

The other, probably more fruitful source is the detailed investigation of individual patients in the course of psychotherapy and their close observation over long periods. These studies throw light on the manner in which conscious and unconscious conflicts related to the patient's life situation and inter-personal relationships are correlated with the development and disappearance of psychosomatic manifestations, several of which, such as asthma, migraine and colitis, may even be seen in the same patient, either at the same or at different times. Moreover, a psychosomatic illness may be replaced by a psychoneurotic or even a psychotic illness, either spontaneously or during psychotherapy. Constitutional and other physical factors, and the patient's past personality development and present-day stresses, all play their part in determining whether a patient under stress develops a neurotic, psychotic or psychosomatic — and more particularly *which* psychosomatic — symptom or disorder.

DIAGNOSIS

In addition to the usual medical procedures, a psychosomatic assessment should include a detailed enquiry into the patient's life history from childhood onwards, his present life situation and his personality make-up. It is usually not possible, or even desirable, to attempt this in a single session. A series of interviews, preferably not conducted along formal psychiatric lines, is usually required before anything like a complete picture can be drawn. The general practitioner is sometimes in a particularly good position to do so, partly because he has an opportunity of getting to know his patient over a long period, and partly because he is already familiar with the family background which plays such an important part in the development of psychosomatic illness. In hospital practice close collaboration between physicians and psychiatrists experienced in the psychosomatic approach is often essential (Lipowski 1967; Wolff 1970). The following points are of particular importance:

1 What was happening in the patient's life around the time of onset of his illness?

2 Are there are circumstances in the patient's family or work situation which expose him to persistent stress?

3 How does the patient handle his emotional reactions, e.g. can he release his feelings or does he tend to 'bottle them up'?

4 In particular, how does he deal with feelings of anger and with his sexual wishes?

5 Is there a history of previous stress disorders, psychosomatic or psychoneurotic, and what was the patient's life situation when they occurred?

6 Are there any indications from the patient's early history that insecurity, excessive anxiety on the part of the parents, frequent illness or other factors in childhood might have laid down a pattern which predisposed to the development of stress disorders; or that he was taught to 'bottle up' his feelings?

In eliciting this and other relevant information it is usually best to encourage the patient to talk freely, and to listen rather than to ask too many direct questions. It is often helpful first of all to explain in simple terms, perhaps by means of a few examples, that emotional upsets can have an effect on the body and that this is the reason why we should like to know more about the patient's life history and present circumstances. Patients with psychosomatic disorders tend to be particularly reluctant to admit that they have serious psychological problems, and too premature a suggestion that they might be suffering from an underlying emotional disturbance may increase their defences and make it more difficult, if not impossible, to elicit the necessary information. It should also be remembered that a patient's physical symptoms are often made worse if distressing and painful topics are discussed too soon. Thus, an asthmatic patient may develop an acute attack of asthma if he is handled too forcefully in a diagnostic interview. A patient and understanding approach is essential if the right kind of information is to be obtained without aggravating the patient's symptoms.

TREATMENT

Both the physical and psychological aspects must be considered.

1 Any medical or surgical treatment indicated by organic lesions and accompanying symptoms should be given.

2 To reduce stress in an acutely ill patient the doctor's attitude is fundamental. If he is sympathetic, prepared to listen, and reassuring, the patient's emotional tension and physical symptoms may both improve considerably. Such improvement is largely due to the establishment of a good doctor-patient relationship. The manner in which patient and doctor relate to each other and how this affects the patient's management has been described in detail by Balint (1964). At this stage one should avoid stirring up the patient's conflicts by premature discussion of painful topics. External stressful situations may have to be dealt with when possible, for example by influencing the patient's relatives. Sometimes removal from home to hospital or elsewhere may be necessary if the family situation is intolerable. For example, asthmatic children sometimes improve temporarily when they are separated for a while from an over-possessive mother, but other patients are made worse when they are separated from their relatives, and each situation must be judged on its merits.

3 Sedatives, tranquillizers and anti-depressant drugs have on the whole proved of relatively little benefit in psychosomatic illnesses but may be helpful for brief periods and during acute exacerbations. Hypnosis or narco-analysis is occasionally of use, e.g. in the treatment of asthma and dermatitis.

4 In patients who are not acutely ill and who are suffering from chronic or relapsing psychosomatic disorders the question should be considered whether they would benefit from formal psychotherapy in combination with, or instead of physical treatment. In general these patients are often more resistant to psychotherapy than psychoneurotic patients. HoweveIy, some of them benefit from brief psychotherapy and others from long-term analytically oriented psychotherapy but the treatment needs to be conducted with particular care in order to

avoid exacerbations of the organic illness. Whether or not formal psychotherapy is indicated and what form it should take should be determined by the nature of the underlying psychological disturbance and the patient's defences and personality structure, the indications for or against the different types of treatment being similar to those which apply to psychoneurotic patients (see pp. 307 and 347).

5 The fundamental principle in the treatment of all these patients is to treat not only 'the illness' but the whole person which means that attention must be paid to physical as well as psychological aspects, including his personality make-up, his internal conflicts and feelings and his inter-personal relationships and life situation.

FURTHER READING

Balint, M. (1964). *The Doctor, his Patient and the Illness*. Pitman, London.

Beaumont, W. (1833). *Experiments and Observations on the Gastric Juice and the Physiology of Digestion*. Allen, Plattsburgh.

Engel, G. L. (1964). *Psychological Development in Health and Disease*. Saunders, London.

Halliday, J. L. (1946). 'Epidemiology of psychosomatic affections'. *Lancet*, 2, 185.

Halliday, J. L. (1949). *Psychosocial Medicine*. Heinemann, London.

Hill, O. W. (ed.) (1970). *Modern Trends in Psychosomatic Medicine* 2. Butterworth, London.

Hopkins, P., and Wolff, H. H. (1965). *Principles of Treatments of Psychosomatic Disorders*. Pergamon, Oxford.

Levi, L. (1972). *Stress and Distress in Response to Psychosocial Stimuli*. Pergamon, Oxford.

Lipowski, Z. J. (1967). 'Review of consultation psychiatry and psychosomatic medicine'. *Psychosom. Med.*, 29, 153.

Rosenbaum, M. (1954). 'Psychosomatic aspects of patients with peptic ulcers'. In Wittkower, E. D. and Cleghorn, R. A. (eds.), *Recent Developments in Psychosomatic Medicine*. Pitman, London.

Shepherd, M., Cooper, B., Brown, A. C., and Kalton, G. W. (1966). *Psychiatric Illness in General Practice*. OUP, London.

Wolf, S. G., and Wolff, H. G. (1943). *Human Gastric Function*. OUP, London.

Wolff, H. H. (1970). 'Practice and teaching of pyschosomatic medicine in general hospitals'. In Hill O. W. (ed.), *Modern Trends in Psychosomatic Medicine* 2. Butterworth, London.

Wolff, H. H. (1971). 'Basic pyschosomatic concepts'. *Postgrad. Med. J.*, 47, 525.

29 Various psychosomatic disorders

This and the next sections describe the commoner psycho-somatic disorders, i.e. conditions with structural lesions in which emotional factors play a major aetiological role. For the sake of completeness some conditions have also been included in which there is abnormality of physiological function of psychological origin. Although they are listed according to the different systems of the body involved, in practice several of these psychosomatic disorders may be present at the same time or occur at different times in the same patient's life.

CARDIOVASCULAR SYSTEM

Essential hypertension

It is, of course, widely recognized that acute emotional disturbances such as anger and fear give rise to a temporary increase of blood pressure; this has been demonstrated in normals and in hypertensive patients in interview situations. It is thought that in some patients with a genetic predisposition to hypertension prolonged emotional stress may lead to a maintained increase of blood pressure and ultimately to persistent hypertension.

This has been shown to be so in patients whose parents rejected them as soon as they began to show aggression; they came 'to live in fear not to be accepted . . . then become very angry, but then . . . ashamed' (Van der Valk 1964). Constitutional or other physical factors must be of importance as well, as similar observations have also been made in patients with other psychosomatic disorders, and in normal people.

Psychotherapy directed at releasing aggression has had some success in reducing hypertension (Hambling 1952). Malignant hypertension has been improved by leucotomy, presumably because it enabled the patient to benefit from psychotherapy and to tolerate conflict situations better than before (Groen et al. 1964).

Effort syndrome

This condition is also known as da Costa's syndrome, Soldier's heart, or disordered action of the heart (DAH). It was described as prevalent in the American Civil War, and both World Wars. At present it is rarely seen.

It consists of dyspnoea, precordial pain and palpitation on exertion: and is accompanied by anxiety focussed on the heart's function. No physical abnormality is to be found: except that the condition may be grafted on to an existing, but symptomless, minor cardiac abnormality, for example an innocent murmur, if the patient has been told about it.

The anxiety may be due to genuine fear of a cardiac lesion, and its effects, or to some other cause, e.g. fear of death or of cowardice, and be focussed on the cardiac symptoms.

Treatment must follow a complete physical examination, and must consist in tackling the basic anxiety. Graduated rehabilitation may be necessary to restore confidence.

Coronary artery disease

Although several factors undoubtedly contribute to the development of coronary disease the actual onset of a coronary thrombosis may be precipitated by emotional stress. In such cases psychological factors are of obvious aetiological importance but it is uncertain to what extent they also contribute to the development of the arterial changes in the coronary vessels over longer periods.

After a coronary, anxiety is likely for a few days, and depression some days later; both are usually temporary and respond to simple reassurance. Tricyclic antidepressants are to be avoided, as they may produce further cardiac damage (Baxter 1974). In some patients, long-term rehabilitation will be required.

Nixon (1970) has described the typical personality of a coronary patient as obviously proud, with intense underlying aggression and the symptoms of irrational insecurity, competitiveness, and inability to relax, which he displays as the attack threatens; these are accompanied by changes in the fourth heart sound. Treatment consists in taking the patient off work without the stigma of a psychiatric diagnosis, getting him to express his feelings, often physically, and graded mental and physical rehabilitation.

Paroxysmal tachycardia

Excitement may bring on such attacks in a predisposed individual.

Cerebro-vascular accidents

Again the onset of a stroke often coincides with an emotional crisis, e.g. sudden anger and loss of temper, which may have provoked a sudden rise in blood pressure.

Raynaud's disease

The peripheral vasoconstriction due to increased sympathetic activity is frequently increased by emotional stress and may diminish when this is relieved.

GASTRO-INTESTINAL SYSTEM

Gastro-intestinal symptoms are among the commonest psychosomatic reactions and may affect any part of the gastrointestinal tract. Anorexia, difficulty in swallowing (globus hystericus), nausea, vomiting, abdominal pain, constipation and diarrhoea are common symptoms due to disturbance of function which may be clearly correlated with periods of stress. The following disorders with actual structural lesions are of particular importance.

Peptic ulcer

The emotional state has a profound effect on gastric function. The classical observations by William Beaumont (1833), of changes in the gastric mucosa and secretions seen through the gastric fistula of his patient Alexis St. Martin when the latter was fearful or angry, offered firm objective evidence. In the equally famous study by Wolf and Wolff (1943) of their patient Tom it was found that anxiety, resentment and hostility were associated with changes in gastric vascularity, secretion and motility. Later work suggests that the way in which gastric motility, secretion and vascularity are affected by such emotions as anger, fear, frustration and conflict varies according to the patient's personality and the particular conscious and unconscious factors involved (Rosenbaum 1954), and more recent studies on an infant called Monica, with a gastric fistula, by Engel et al. (1956) showed that when she related actively to others her gastric secretion increased; when she withdrew it diminished. Mirsky (1950) has demonstrated that people who develop peptic ulcers have a higher pepsinogen secretion than normals and that pepsinogen production is increased by emotional stress.

There can be no doubt that in clinical practice peptic ulcers often develop and relapses occur at periods in the patient's life situation during which he is exposed to severe or persistent stress. Disturbed interaction in the family or excessive pressure or conflict at work are common precipitating factors. There is also some evidence that patients with peptic ulcers have certain personality characteristics in common. They are often dependent people who over-compensate for their dependent needs by becoming ambitious, hard working and successful; others reveal their dependency more openly. However, such characteristics can be found in many other psychosomatic and also psychoneurotic disorders so that the exact significance of these observations is still uncertain. Physical and constitutional factors may determine whether patients with such conflicts and personality structures will develop a peptic ulcer or some other psychosomatic disorder.

In treatment, equal attention must be paid to the physical and psychological aspects. Once an ulcer has developed and especially if complications such as pyloric stenosis have arisen, physical treatment must have priority. But full understanding of the psychological factors involved will make it possible for the doctor to plan the patient's management in such a way that the emotional aspects are taken into account. Thus a good doctor/patient relationship and frank discussion of emotional problems may be more effective than excessive preoccupation with dietary measures. Formal psychotherapy is hardly ever indicated on account of the ulcer alone but may, in selected cases, be valuable if the patient is aware of unresolved psychological conflicts and wants to resolve these in psycho-therapy. Discussion with relatives may be helpful if inter-personal conflict is an important factor and working conditions may have to be reviewed and changed if necessary.

Irritable bowel syndrome

Attacks of abdominal pain and diarrhoea or constipation are commonly the result of spasm or increased activity of the colon in over-controlled patients who are in emotional conflict and are unable to express their feelings, especially those of aggression and sexuality.

Ulcerative colitis, anorexia nervosa and obesity

These are important enough to be dealt with separately (see pp. 201 and 196).

GENITO-URINARY SYSTEM

Frequency of micturition is a common symptom due to anxiety. Retention of urine in the absence of an organic cause is seen occasionally as a hysterical symptom. Bedwetting in children is usually due to an emotional disturbance (see p. 235). The various abnormalities associated with sexual and reproductive function, such as impotence, frigidity, disturbances of menstrual function and pregnancy are all dealt with elsewhere.

MUSCULO-SKELETAL SYSTEM

Muscular and skeletal pains, unless due to definite organic disease, are often of psychological origin related to emotional tension. Common examples are headaches, stiffness and pain in the neck, shoulders, limbs and back — so-called fibrositis or muscular rheumatism. A minor local physical abnormality sometimes focuses the patient's attention on a particular part of his body and after that he reacts to emotional stress by developing symptoms in the same area or, conversely, muscular spasm resulting from his painful area may lead to further pain, disability, irritability and depression, and generalised tension increases. Pain in the face is another similar condition and may be difficult to distinguish from dental conditions. The patient usually becomes increasingly pre-occupied with these various painful conditions and this leads to secondary anxiety and depression. Sometimes the particular symptom may indicate the nature of the underlying psychological problem in so-called body language, e.g. having pain in the neck may be a way of saying that somebody else 'is a pain in the neck'.

Torticollis, involuntary spasmodic pulling of the head to one side (Meares, 1973; Tibbets, 1971) and occupational cramps, e.g. writer's cramp and musician's cramp (Moldofsky, 1971) are special examples of localised muscular contraction. In torticollis, in particular, there may be organic changes, i.e. spasm and hypertrophy of the sternomastoids. Psychological factors in the shape of personal stress and conflict, e.g. in a marital relationship undoubtedly play an important part but, once established, physical factors contribute to maintaining the condition. The same applies to occupational cramps. Tics, brief irregular purposeless repeated movements, for example of the face, commonly start in childhood. The Gilles de la Tourette syndrome is a rare condition in which tics and more widespread involuntary movements are associated with the compulsive utterance of swear words and obscenities. In these various functional motor disorders physical and psychological factors usually co-exist.

Treatment is often difficult. Physiotherapy and pain-relieving drugs may prove ineffective. These patients are often very reluctant to consider that their physical symptom could be partly of emotional origin. Careful exploration and discussion is necessary to help them accept this. Psychotherapy may then prove helpful in some cases. Sometimes there may be an underlying depression and the symptom may respond to an anti-depressant drug combined with psychotherapy.

Rheumatoid arthritis

To what extent this has a psychosomatic basis is undecided but attacks are often precipitated by stressful events in a patient's life, and long-standing personality problems often associated with repressed aggression are found in many of these patients. Ludwig (1954) believes that regression occurs when their defences are broken down by severe stress or frustration. Therapy, though mainly physical, must include support and sympathy from the GP: some patients may need formal psychotherapy. The relations of psychological stress to this and other auto-immune disease is fully discussed by Solomon (1970) and Moldofsky (1970).

CENTRAL NERVOUS SYSTEM

Migraine

There is usually a familial predisposition but emotional conflicts are of considerable importance. These patients are often ambitious, outwardly calm but beneath this there may be a great deal of anxiety and conflict. During formal psychotherapy such patients are often found to have strong aggressive fantasies and they conceal basic feelings of dependency. It is doubtful whether any of these findings can be regarded as specific for migrainous subjects but in treatment the importance of psychological factors must be taken into account. A few benefit from analytical psychotherapy.

ENDOCRINE FUNCTIONS AND DISORDERS

This is of particular importance in the consideration of psychosomatic disorders for two reasons: emotional stress is known to affect the function of several endocrine glands, and conversely endocrine disorders affect the mental state and human behaviour.

Stress and the adrenal cortex

Adreno-cortical activity, as measured by the plasma cortisol or 11-OHCS level, or by the 24-hour urinary excretion of cortisol metabolites has been shown to be increased by a number of stressful situations (Gibbons, 1968); it is raised in students about to take an examination, in members of boat crews before the start of a race, in patients anticipating an operation; and also over more prolonged periods in some, though not all, parents of children with leukaemia who were distressed by their child's illness, and who were the subjects of a special investigation. In the latter and similar studies it is of interest to note that the degree to which adreno-cortical activity is affected in individual patients depends partly on the degree to which they are able to defend themselves by denial against feeling too distressed in which case the cortisol levels are lower than in those whose defence mechanisms are less effective. Nabarro (1969) has also shown that the psychological stress associated with acute medical illness causes an increase in adreno-cortical activity as shown by an increase in Plasma 11-OHCS levels and an increase in the concentration of ACTH in the plasma. In psychiatric patients, too, adrenocortical activity is increased in most, though not all depressed patients and it falls to normal levels after recovery. All these changes in response to stress are presumably transmitted via the hypothalamic-pituitary-adrenal axis.

Cushing's syndrome

When the steroid level is raised as in Cushing's disease (or as the result of the administration of steroids), changes in the mental state are common; mood changes, depression or elation, may occur and so may psychotic states. It is often difficult to decide whether these psychiatric sequelae are the direct result of the increased steroid level or the indirect effect of the psychological stress associated with such bodily changes as hirsuties, obesity and the moon faced appearance, especially in women. Both effects may co-exist.

Adreno-genital syndrome

Here the increased androgen production, usually the result of bilateral adrenal hyperplasia or tumours, leads to the development of male characteristics in girls, often present at birth: female pseudo-hermaphroditism; in boys it leads to precocious puberty. The associated psychiatric problems are largely due to the indirect effect of the resultant difficulties in sexual adjustment; for example, if a girl is mistakenly regarded as, and therefore brought up as, a boy the resultant uncertainty about her sexual identity will cause serious psychological difficulties and sometimes extreme self-consciousness and social withdrawal. Such patients and their parents need careful handling from the beginning both from the physical and psychological angle (see p. 105).

Adrenal medulla

Selye (1950) drew attention to what he called the 'alarm reaction', a hormonal response to stress with certain adaptive and homeostatic functions in which the adrenal medulla as well as the adrenal cortex play an important role. Recent experimental work (Levi 1968) has shown that the catecholamine excretion levels, reflecting the secretion of adrenaline by the adrenal medulla, are profoundly affected by stressful emotional stimuli. Interestingly enough, pleasant stimuli causing amusement were in some individuals as effective in increasing adrenaline production as stressful and unpleasant stimuli. As in the case of steroid secretion, the personality of the individual plays an important part in determining the response.

Conversely, spontaneous excessive secretion of adrenaline as in patients with a phaeochromocytoma is known to produce periodic attacks of acute anxiety; this needs to be considered in the differential diagnosis of an anxiety state but the periodicity and the associated rise in blood pressure should assist in the diagnosis.

Diabetes

Here genetic and other primary physical causes are of major importance but diabetes is occasionally brought on by acute stress; and compulsive overeating of psychological origin leading to obesity may be another factor in predisposing to diabetes. That emotional stress can affect the blood sugar and insulin requirements of an established diabetic patient, and the fact that the blood level of ketones is raised by stress, sometimes leading to the onset of ketosis and diabetic coma, are well known. Conversely, the psychological effects of being diabetic and of needing insulin or to have to adhere to a diet are important factors to be considered in the management of all diabetics, especially in children. Hypoglycaemic attacks occurring in the course of treatment often present themselves with psychological symptoms, such as confusion and inability to think or concentrate, and may lead to abnormal behaviour. Rarely psychological symptoms of similar kind may occur as the result of spontaneous hypoglycaemia, as in patients with pancreatic islet cell tumours.

Obesity

Metabolic, endocrine and psychological factors are all of considerable importance. For many people eating may from childhood onwards continue to provide comfort and relieve anxiety or depression at times of stress, especially after painful losses and separations. Compulsive over-eating thus may complicate depression; it may also occur in the course of anorexia nervosa (see p. 198). The resulting obesity may cause psychological distress and depression, as well as physical trouble. The pattern of over-eating is notoriously difficult to treat and dieting may unmask depression; patients are rarely motivated to undertake psychotherapy, which anyhow is unsuccessful unless basic changes in the patient's personality and life situation are brought about. Joining a group like Weight Watchers can help to change eating habits.

REFERENCES

Beaumont, W. (1833). *Experiments and Observations on the Gastric Juice and the Physiology of Digestion.* Allen, Plattsburgh.

Bruch, H. (1957). *The Importance of Overweight*. Norton, New York.

Engel, G. L., Reichsman, F. and Segal, H. L. (1956). 'A study of an infant with a gastric fistula'. *Psychosom. Med.*, 18, 374.'

Gibbons, J. L. (1968). 'The adrenal cortex and psychological distress'. In Michael, R. P. (ed.). *Endocrinology and Human Behaviour*. OUP.

Groen, J. J., Van der Valk, J. M., and Bastiaans, J. (1964). 'A case of malignant hypertension, treated with prefrontal leucotomy and psychotherapy'. In Groen, J. J. (ed.), *Psychosomatic Research*. Pergamon, Oxford.

Hambling, J. (1952). 'Psychosomatic aspects of arterial hypertension'. *Brit. J. Med. Psychol.*, 25, 39.

Hill, O. W. (1970). 'Functional vomiting, abdominal pain and diarrhoea'. In *Modern Trends in Psychosomatic Medicine*, 2. Butterworth, London.

Levi, L. (1968). 'Sympatho-adrenomedullary and related biochemical reactions during experimentally induced emotional stress'. In Michael, R. P. (ed.), *Endocrinology and Human Behaviour*. OUP, London.

Ludwig, A. O. (1954). 'Rheumatoid arthritis'. In Wittkower, E. D. and Cleghorn, R. A. (eds.), *Recent Developments in Psychosomatic Medicine*. Pitman, London.

Meares, R. (1973). 'Spasmodic torticollis'. *Brit. J. Hosp. Med.*, Feb., 135.

Mirsky, I. A., Kaplan, S., and Broh-Kahn, R. H. (1950). 'Pepsinogen secretion (uropepsin) as an index of influence of various life situations on gastric secretion'. *Proc. Assoc. Res. nerv. ment. Dis.*, 29, 629.

Moldofsky, H. (1970). 'The significance of emotions in the course of rheumatoid arthritis'. In Hill, O. W. (ed.), *Modern Trends in Psychosomatic Medicine* 2. Butterworth, London.

Moldofsky, H. (1971). 'Occupational cramp'. *J. Psychosom. Res.*, 15, 439.

Nabarro, J. D. N. (1969). 'The metabolic and endocrine response to acute medical stress'. *Proc. Roy. Soc. Med.*, 62, 351.

Nixon, P. G. F. (1972). 'Rehabilitation of the coronary patient'. *Physiotherapy*, 58, 336.

O'Neill, D. (1955). *Modern Trends in Psychosomatic Medicine*. Butterworth, London.

Reiser, M. F., and Bakst, H. (1959). 'Psychology of cardiovascular disorders'. In Arieti, S. (ed.), *American Handbook of Psychiatry* vol. 1, Basic Books, New York.

Rosenbaum, M. (1954). 'Psychosomatic aspects of patients with peptic ulcer'. In Wittkower, E. D. and Cleghorn, R. A. (eds.), *Recent Developments in Psychosomatic Medicine*. Pitman, London.

Selye, H. (1950). *Stress*. Montreal.

Solomon, G. F. (1970). 'Psychophysiological aspects of rheumatoid arthritis and auto-immune disease'. In Hill, O. W. (ed.), *Modern Trends in Psychosomatic Medicine*, 2. Butterworth, London.

Tibbets, R. W. (1971). 'Spasmodic torticollis'. *J. Psychosom. Res.*, 15, 461.

Van der Valk, J. M. (1964). 'Blood pressure changes under emotional influences in patients with essential hypertension and control subjects'. In Groen, J. J. (ed.), *Psychosomatic Research*. Pergamon, Oxford.

Wolf, S. G. and Wolff, H. G. (1943). *Human Gastric Function*. OUP.

30 Respiratory disorders

BRONCHIAL ASTHMA

Aetiology and incidence

Asthma occurs in at least 1% of the population of England and Wales. The age of onset may be from infancy to old age but is most common under the age of 5 years and in boys at an earlier age than girls. A family history is present in 40% of all asthmatic patients. Recently the death rate has been rising, from 2 per 100,000 persons in 1959 to 3.7 in 1966 (Speizer, Doll and Heaf, 1968).

Asthmatic attacks are almost always caused by a combination and interaction of several factors. There are three main groups of these: allergic, psychological and infective. Commonly all three of these factors may operate together, but one or other of them is almost always dominant. It is often difficult to decide which factor is the most important and in particular whether psychological methods of treatment should be used in addition to physical methods. If the importance of psychological factors is overlooked, appropriate methods of dealing with them may be delayed until it is too late for them to have much effect.

There have been several surveys on this subject carried out in the last 10 years, especially by Rees (1964). It has been shown that the relative importance of the different factors varies with age:

1 In patients presenting in childhood the most common dominant factor is psychological.

2 In patients presenting from puberty to 35 years of age the most common dominant factor is allergic.

3 In patients presenting over the age of 35 the most common dominant factor is infection.

Allergic factors

These provoke constriction of the bronchi, swelling of the mucous membrane of the respiratory tract and hypersecretion of mucous membrane. The basic reaction which occurs is a cellular anaphylaxis due to the interaction of antigen and tissue fixed antibodies (reagins).

Reagins are gamma globulins present in sensitized (allergic) subjects and recently identified as IgE. It is reagins which are responsible for positive allergic skin tests. They can be passively transferred to non-atopic subjects (Prausnitz-Kuestner reaction) in whom their effect is only temporary.

The antigens which most commonly cause human allergic asthma are: house dust (a decomposition product of animal and vegetable dust from furnishings); pollens; airborne mould; house mites, and animal danders. Some show seasonal variation. In asthma due to inhalants, associated rhinitis and conjunctivitis are often seen. Experimental asthmatic attacks can be provoked by inhalations of antigens in allergic subjects. The results of desensitization treatment are good in patients with pollen allergy. Allergic factors in food are difficult to demonstrate as skin tests tend to be negative except in very severe and obvious cases. Allergy to food is common in young children. It must be remembered that allergic responses themselves can be affected by the patient's mental state and by hypnosis (Black, 1963), and that a prolonged search for allergic causes and unnecessary dietary and other restrictions may be harmful if it means that important psychological factors are being overlooked, and the patient becomes more preoccupied with his physical condition.

Psychological factors

Neurotic personalities are common and an unhappy home life and faulty parental attitudes are frequently found in parents of asthmatic patients. Attacks are often precipitated by stressful situations and symptoms may improve if a patient is removed from a stressful environment, e.g. to hospital, or in response to psychotherapy.

A considerable amount of research has been done on this subject, especially by authors working in the field of psychosomatic medicine, such as Groen and Bastiaans (1964) and their psychosomatic research team in Amsterdam, by Linford Rees (1964) and by McNichol and his colleagues (1973).

Although there is not one clear-cut personality type specific for all asthmatics, certain characteristics are commonly found in these patients.

A history of emotional insecurity in childhood is very common. Asthmatic children have a great need for affection, especially from their mothers, but if the parents are too authoritarian, rejecting, possessive, or manipulative, and are unable to tolerate expressions of anger, the child feels obliged to submit and to suppress any feelings of aggression out of fear of losing the parents' love; and some become perfectionist. This conflict persists throughout life, so that in any situation, as children or adults, in which the patients come up against others who are too demanding, possessive or authoritarian, they feel oppressed and smothered and their anger will be aroused; but instead of releasing it they tend to bottle it up, and develop an asthmatic attack. Their suppressed demandingness and aggression makes them egocentric and difficult to live with; they are prone to impulsive behaviour and jealous in their human relationships; but they are unable to verbalize their conflicts or to express their feelings. If they can be made to talk, they can often see that attacks are brought on by stressful situations similar to those they experienced in relation to their parents or siblings in childhood.

Conditioning has also been implicated in the production of asthmatic attacks. Thus, Decker, Pelser and Groen (1964) have shown that in two patients with allergic asthma whose attacks could be regularly precipitated in the laboratory by the inhalation of pollen and house dust respectively, attacks could later be produced by the identical procedure, though, unbeknown to the patient, no allergen was being inhaled. It must be stressed that such conditioning is only effective in a small proportion of patients and anxiety associated with the test procedure may be more important than conditioning proper. Conversely, asthmatic attacks can sometimes be relieved by suggestion or hypnosis, and prevented by de-conditioning.

Turnbull (1962) claims that asthmatic breathing may be learned at an early age as a result of frustration and that it may be reinforced by securing a satisfying response from an over-anxious mother.

Infective factors

These are of considerable importance in the very young and the elderly. Initial upper respiratory tract infections proceed to a secondary chest infection with asthma associated with productive cough and tenacious sputum. It is thought by some workers that bacterial allergy occurs in these patients but this has not been conclusively demonstrated.

Treatment

One must consider both physical and psychological approaches. Often both should be combined. A full review of the standard physical treatment is given by Nicholson (1965) For psychological treatment the following should be noted.

In childhood it is often essential to correct parental attitudes by dealing with the parents (Pinkerton and Weaver 1970). Occasionally, if the family situation is too disturbed the child may benefit from being temporarily removed from home to stay with friends, or at boarding school, or by admission to hospital. If it is possible to influence the parents to modify their attitudes and to become less anxious and over-protective, one may not only relieve the child's asthma at that stage, but one may also hope to prevent the tendecy to asthmatic attacks in years to come. A few children may benefit from more intensive psychotherapy.

When dealing with adult patients, except in clear-cut cases of allergy, the past and present life situation should be explored in detail for possible psychogenic factors. If these are found, detailed and patient explanation will usually be needed to convince the patient of their importance; and psychotherapy may be of benefit. Often a few interviews at a relatively superficial level in which a patient is allowed to release his feelings, for example to show anger or to weep, may be helpful provided the patient knows that he can always return for further interviews if he encounters stressful situations in the future or if his asthma recurs. Hypnosis has been found helpful in some cases (Maher-Loughnan et al. 1962).

In some patients, especially those who are young, flexible, intelligent and aware of their emotional problems, more intensive psychotherapy, either individually or in groups, may be indicated to deal with the underlying personality disturbance.

Whatever form of psychotherapy is used, it is most important to adopt a permissive, tolerant and understanding attitude as asthmatic patients respond badly to a critical, rejecting or authoritarian approach, which, by repeating the original conflict situation, may precipitate severe attacks of asthma. It should be stressed that it is essential to employ the usual symptomatic treatment with drugs while psychotherapy is being used. However, if psychotherapy is successful, it may be possible gradually to reduce whatever drugs are being used and sometimes to discontinue their use altogether.

It is clear, therefore, that close collaboration between physician and psychiatrist is essential unless one doctor is prepared to undertake both lines of treatment. Besides, the patient can get much help from the sympathetic support of his relatives, and they themselves may need information and help from the doctor to overcome their anxiety and sometimes to modify their behaviour and attitude towards the patient. This is especially important for the parents of young asthmatics and for the husbands or wives of patients.

VASOMOTOR RHINITIS AND HAY-FEVER

Although allergy plays an important part, these acute attacks of nasal congestion can often be correlated with periods of emotional stress in the patient's life situation. In general, anxiety and emotional tension increase the intensity of allergic responses under experimental conditions and Black (1963) has shown that allergic responses can be inhibited by direct suggestion under hypnosis.

HYPERVENTILATION

This is a common symptom in anxiety states, to be distinguished from physically-based dyspnoea: it often leads to tetany.

REFERENCES

Bastianns, J., and Groen, J. J. (1955). 'Psychogenesis and psychotherapy of bronchial asthma' in O'Neill, D. (ed.), *Modern Trends in Psychosomatic Medicine*. Butterworth, London.

Black, S. (1963). 'Inhibition of the immediate type hypersensitivity response by direct suggestion under hypnosis'. *Brit. Med. J.*, 1, 925.

British Tuberculosis Association (1968). 'Hypnosis for asthma'. *Brit. Med. J.*, 2, 71.

Decker, E., Pelser, H. E. and Groen, J. J. (1964). 'Conditioning as a cause of asthmatic attacks'. In Groen, J. J. (ed.), *Psychosomatic Research*. Pergamon, Oxford.

Groen, J. J., and Bastiaans, J. (1964). 'The psychosomatic approach to bronchial asthma'. In Groen, J. J. (ed.), *Psychosomatic Research*. Pergamon, Oxford.

Humphrey, J. H. and White, R. G. (1970). *Immunology for Students of Medicine*. Blackwell.

Maher-Loughnan, G. P. et al. (1962). 'Controlled trial of hypnosis in symptomatic treatment of asthma'. *Brit. Med. J.*, 2, 371.

McNichol, K. N., Williams, H. E., Allen, J. and McAndrew, I. (1973). 'Spectrum of asthma in children. III: Psychological and social components'. *Brit. Med. J.*, 4, 16.

Nicholson, H. (1965). 'The management of asthma'. *Practitioner*, 195, 742.

Pinkerton, P. and Weaver, C.M. (1970). 'Childhood asthma'. In Hill, O. (ed.), *Modern Trends in Psychosomatic Medicine* 2. Butterworth.

Rees, W. L. (1964). 'The importance of psychological, allergic and infective factors in childhood asthma'. *J. Psychosom. Res.*, 7. 253.

Speizer, F. E., Doll, R. and Heaf, P. (1968). 'Observations on recent increase in mortality from asthma'. *Brit. Med. J.*, i, 335.

Turk, J. L. (1972). *Immunology in Clinical Medicine*. Heinemann.

Turnbull, J. W. (1962). 'Asthma conceived as a learned response'. *J. Psychosom. Res.*, 6, 59.

31 *Anorexia nervosa*

HISTORY

Clear descriptions of cases of anorexia nervosa (nervous consumption or mental anorexia) have been given since Richard Morton's account in 1689, although, curiously, neither Hippocrates nor Galen mention it. In the literature, it has often been confused with Simmonds' Disease, which is a syndrome of dysfunction of many endocrines due to failure of the anterior pituitary, but in Simmonds' Disease the wasting is only terminal; and there is no evidence that anorexia nervosa is due to pituitary deficiency, although the latter (and hence thyroidal and gonadal hypofunction) may be secondary to the malnutrition.

The criteria for the use of the term vary considerably. While most psychiatrists agree in regarding anorexia nervosa as due to underlying psychological causes, for a long time surprisingly little was written about the syndrome in standard textbooks on psychiatry and psychotherapy, although in *Physical Methods of Treatment* Sargant and Slater give an optimistic account of the results of treatment with drugs.

There is an excellent monograph by Bliss and Branch (1960), who survey the literature in considerable detail and describe their own series of cases. Crisp (1965, 1967) has written a comprehensive survey.

INCIDENCE

Anorexia nervosa occurs overwhelmingly in emotionally disturbed adolescent girls, but has been recorded in older women, and, very rarely, in males. Twin studies have shown no evidence of a genetic basis (Crisp, 1967). The condition is commoner in higher socio-economic classes.

SYMPTOMS

Anorexia nervosa is better regarded as a symptom, or set of symptoms, than as a clinical entity. It can be part of a hysterical, obsessional, depressive or schizophrenic syndrome. It is therefore vital to consider the psychological and physical needs of each case afresh, if treatment is to succeed. Nonetheless, certain generalizations can be made.

The cardinal symptom is fear of gaining weight, which leads to dieting and hence to insidious wasting; three stone or more may be lost and the weight reach as low as 3½ or 4 stone. Dieting often starts in the teenage girl because she wants to slim, but after a while she cannot stop dieting, either because she feels full and uncomfortable as soon as she starts eating or because she develops such a fear of getting fat that she does not eat even when hungry. Carbohydrate foods in particular are avoided. Some girls pretend to eat and do not; some eat and then either purge themselves, or make themselves vomit; a few even concealing their vomit by various tricks. There may be brief periods when she eats excessively and then feels very guilty and again becomes anorexic. Her body image is usually distorted and unrealistic.

Energy is often maintained surprisingly long, but a collapse due to extreme emaciation may suddenly occur, and death has been recorded from intercurrent infection or emaciation.

Amenorrhoea is an early symptom, and even in successfully treated cases may be the last to go.

Naturally, such behaviour and the girl's appearance of extreme emaciation cause intense anxiety and frustration in those around, especially her mother, who responds by pressing her to eat and providing special meals to tempt her. This provokes more refusal and guilt, and increases the preoccupation of both with food; antagonism becomes chronic, and a reluctant patient is eventually brought to the doctor by an anxious and angry mother.

MENTAL STATE

The patient is extremely preoccupied with food, either with the difficulty in swallowing it, or with the horror of eating too much, from fear of getting too fat. She is generally withdrawn, resistant to advice or help and her symptoms produce around her an atmosphere of anxiety, irritation or despair, which makes her worse. She may mislead nurses by frank lies and denial, or by concealing food she pretends to have eaten.

Deeper investigations may reveal hostility to her parents, especially her mother, rivalry with a brother or sister (often a sister who is more outgoing, and so more attractive to her parents); guilt over aggression and sexual wishes; denial of femininity; and ideas of self-punishment. The patient often experiences her mother as domineering and over-controlling, feels herself to lack an identity of her own and wants at all costs to avoid becoming a grown-up woman like her mother. The physical manifestations described above are the results of these emotional conflicts.

The symptoms are nearly always accompanied by depression, and the patient obstinately clings to her pattern of behaviour and opposes efforts of help.

TREATMENT

An enormous range of physical and psychological treatment has been tried; every method has had its successes (which appear related to the therapist's confidence) but also its failures. Comparison of different treatments is difficult, owing to lack of controls and the inability to measure the effect of the doctor's consciously and unconsciously determined attitude.

There are two questions to be asked about every patient:

1 What is required to check further weight loss, and to prevent her death from emaciation?

Admission to hospital may be needed; chlorpromazine (50-100 mg, t.d.s. or more) and insulin (10 units t.d.s.) sometimes restore appetite quickly; tube feeding is now hardly ever needed since chlorpromazine has been introduced. Removal of pressure to eat and of tension at home may itself restore appetite; but in severe cases, strict supervision in hospital and high calorie diet are needed. When sufficient weight has been put on, they can be reduced, but a careful and regular check must be kept on the patient's weight.

2 What is the psychological background of the symptoms?

On this depends the type of psychotherapy to be given: but the first step must be for the therapist to establish a close rapport with the patient. He may have to dissociate himself from critical influences of the past, which have provoked guilt, resistance and further preoccupation with food. He must allow her to ventilate emotions long repressed and to rebuild lost relationships, e.g. with parents. The latter's collaboration in this may need re-education, if not therapy by PSW or psychiatrist. The patient often gets more depressed when she sees that her weight is increasing, as she fears fatness and adulthood. Prolonged psychotherapy is therefore essential.

In extreme depression, anti-depressant drugs may help.

Although one therapist must have overall responsibility, team work is essential between him, his immediate deputy (to cover his absences), a PSW to cope with relations and all the nursing staff involved. Any one may well feel helpless and angry at the patient's symptoms and frequent relapses, just as her parents have; the therapist must prevent this, e.g. by group discussion with them; family therapy may help in some cases. All must be prepared for progress to be slow, and for the stress and disappointment involved. Opinions differ as to how flexible the regime should be; every patient must be judged according to her need.

Since some anorexics resist treatment, the only line open may be supportive psychotherapy which may help the patient to a happier and more useful life, and cope with the occasional relapse. Although it is essential that an established case should receive full and comprehensive treatment, there are many girls who temporarily diet in order to slim, and who pass through this phase unharmed, and more quickly so if their parents resist the temptation to make an issue of it, and merely keep an unobtrusive eye on them.

PROGNOSIS

In spite of all treatment, some patients die; of Kay and Leigh's (1954) follow-up of twenty-five, six died, seven were still anorexic, and four others had other psychiatric symptoms. But more recently, treatment has been more successful, and a recovery rate of two patients in three has been reported by Crisp (1965) and Dally and Sargant (1966). In some patients the condition becomes chronic and a few ultimately commit suicide. Even those who have made a good physical recovery may be left with emotional and psychosexual problems requiring further psychotherapy. Others later overeat and become obese.

REFERENCES

Bliss, E. L., and Branch, C. H. H. (1960). *Anorexia Nervosa* (contains an extensive bibliography). Hoeber, New York.

Crisp, A. H. (1965). 'Clinical and therapeutic aspects of anorexia nervosa'. *J. Psychosom. Res.*, 9, 67.

Crisp, A. H. (1967). 'Anorexia nervosa'. *Hospital Medicine*, 1, 713.

Crisp, A. H. (1970). 'Psychological aspects of some disorders of weight'. In Hill, O. W. (ed.), *Modern Trends in Psychosomatic Medicine 2*. Butterworth, London.

Dally, P. (1969). *Anorexia Nervosa*. Heinemann, London.

Dally, P. J. and Sargant, W. (1966). 'Treatment and outcome of anorexia nervosa'. *Brit. Med. J.*, ii, 793.

Kay, D. W. K. and Leigh, D. (1954). 'The natural history, treatment and prognosis of anorexia nervosa'. *J. Ment. Sci.*, 100, 411.

Robertson, R. F. and Proudfoot, A. T. (ed.) (1973) *Symposium on Anorexia Nervosa and Obesity*. Royal College of Physicians, Edinburgh.

Sargant, W. and Slater, E. (1972). *Physical Methods of Treatment*, 5th ed. Livingstone, Edinburgh.

32 Ulcerative colitis: psychological aspects

INTRODUCTION

The view that psychological factors play a major role in the aetiology and course of ulcerative colitis was first put forward by Murray (1930) while he was still a medical student. Nowadays it is widely held that constitutional and physical factors, possibly the presence of antibodies in the colonic mucosa or other allergic and bacterial causes, may be of importance in causing the condition, but that stress factors often precipitate the onset of the illness and of relapses. It is equally important to remember that the symptoms of ulcerative colitis are themselves very distressing so that a vicious circle is easily set up.

The psychological aspects thus include:

1 The patient's personality make-up.
2 His reactions to recent stresses.
3 His attitude to his illness.

PERSONALITY

Many patients with ulcerative colitis are said to have characteristic personality traits. They tend to be somewhat obsessional, fastidious, over-conscientious, dependent and excessively vulnerable to humiliating events; they find it difficult to express anger and they bottle up their feelings. These characteristics are mainly acquired as ∵ result of childhood experiences, though heredity may play its part. They may be aggravated by the patient's reaction to the illness which makes him regress and increases his dependency and vulnerability. Groen and Van der Valk (1964) stress his passivity and his craving for affection, sympathy and admiration, although this may be covered up by a facade of apparent independence and conceit.

These traits are, of course, not unique to patients with ulcerative colitis, nor are they present in every case, but the frequency with which they occur suggests that they may play a part in determining the patient's reactions to stress and hence in affecting the onset and course of the illness.

Reaction to stress

A history of recent stress and conflict in relationships can be elicited in the majority of cases, provided they are allowed gradually to talk freely; if they are asked outright on this subject, they often deny any trouble, or any connection with their symptoms. The precipitating stress which usually precedes the onset of an acute attack by a few days or a week or two is often an injury to their security, because they have been deprived of affection on which they relied, or to their self-esteem (especially in the presence of others). Bereavements, rejections and criticism are especially important. As they cannot express their hurt feelings, their reaction becomes one of inward resentment at a real or imagined affront; though they are unable to admit this, or their ineffectiveness, even to themselves.

Attitude to the illness

The persistent and distressing symptoms of diarrhoea with

blood and mucus in the stools and fear of relapses, and the possibility that they may one day need surgical treatment make them anxious and depressed and often interfere with their social life and personal relationships. Fear of smelling, urgency and sometimes incontinence are particularly troublesome. If they require an ileostomy they may develop further anxieties, e.g. that they will become unacceptable as sexual partners and hence may either never get married and have children, or be rejected by their friends, husband or wife. They may not voice these anxieties unless specifically asked by an understanding doctor, and open discussion to prepare them for surgery is essential (see below). In fact, many patients greatly improve psychologically after surgery, and talking to other patients who have, say, had an ileostomy done and who lead a satisfactory life may help them to accept an operation.

PSYCHO-PHYSIOLOGICAL OBSERVATIONS

Physiological studies, e.g. direct observation of the colonic mucosa in patients with a colonic fistula, have shown that anger or anxiety evoked by discussing stressful topics are accompanied by colonic over-activity and mucus secretion, and ultimately, if it persists, hyperaemia and bleeding. On the other hand relaxation of the colon can be obtained by getting the patient to speak of his achievements or to talk on neutral topics.

DIAGNOSIS

Ulcerative colitis is not difficult to diagnose, but the possibility of carcinoma of the colon, either at the start or developing later, must always be remembered.

It is more difficult to decide on the extent to which psychological and physical causes are each responsible. It is likely, from the nature of the patient's symptoms and personality, that psychological factors are often missed, and psychotherapy neglected.

TREATMENT

1 Medical and surgical treatment and their indications are not described here; but they must always be provided, whether in conjunction with psychotherapy or not. In every case a good personal relationship must be established with the patient, usually at first by the GP or physician, and the patient must be encouraged to talk freely about any recent stresses and conflicts in his life. If necessary a psychiatrist should be called in at this stage. As the condition is potentially fatal, psychotherapy must never be relied upon exclusively. In advanced cases treatment with steroids or surgical intervention must not be too long delayed. Surgery must also be considered in chronic patients with extensive disease, in view of the risk of a carcinoma developing.

2 In an acute case, the provision of intensive support, avoidance of frustrations and the acceptance of the patient's dependence by the medical and nursing staff may reduce the physical symptoms, as well as the emotional crisis. To avoid relapses long term supportive psychotherapy may be helpful. This is usually best done by the patient's physician or GP to whom the patient must have easy access, so that he can rely on him at once if new problems or stresses arise.

3 Formal psychotherapy may be helpful in selected cases to deal with any underlying personality disorder. This applies particularly to young, flexible and intelligent patients who are aware of their personal problems, who are willing to accept intensive psychotherapy and in whom the organic changes are less acute and not too far advanced. It must however, be remembered that such treatment must be conducted with great care, since breaking down the patient's defences prematurely or the development of a negative transference may lead to an acute and potentially fatal relapse or, alternatively, to a psychotic breakdown. Schizophrenic breakdowns have also been described in patients with colitis not undergoing psychotherapy (O'Connor 1970). Careful assessment by a psychotherapist is therefore needed to decide whether or not a patient is suitable for formal psychotherpay, following the ordinary supportive psychotherapeutic methods which should have been made available.

There are some studies which suggest that psychotherapy combined with physical treatment is more effective than physical treatment alone (O'Connor et al. 1964). But no large series of comparable cases, subjected to controlled observations and treatment is yet available. Meanwhile it seems logical to suppose that the disease has several possible causes, some psychological, some physical; and that whichever is the prime cause, a psychophysical vicious cycle may develop, which needs treatment on all fronts; how much of each must be determined by the details of each case. Cooperation between all members of the treatment team is essential to avoid confusing the patient by contradictory opinions.

REFERENCES

Groen, J. J. and van der Valk, J. M. (1964). 'Psychosomatic aspects of ulcerative colitis'. In Groen, J. J. (ed.), *Psychosomatic Research*. Pergamon, Oxford.

Murray, C. D. (1930). 'Psychogenic factors in the aetiology of ulcerative and bloody diarrhoea'. *Amer. J. Med. Sci.*, 180, 239.

O'Connor, J. F. et al. (1964). 'Evaluation of the effectiveness of psychotherapy in the treatment of ulcerative colitis'. *Annals Int. Med.*, 60, 587.

O'Connor, J. F. (1970). 'A comprehensive approach to the treatment of ulcerative colitis'. In Hill, O. W. (ed.), *Modern Trends in Psychosomatic Medicine*, 2. Butterworth, London.

33 The thyroid gland and psychiatric illness

The thyroid gland and mental function are intimately related. The secretion of thyroid hormones is known to be under the control of the hypothalamus and there is increasing evidence that stressful environmental events, particularly those causing a psychological disturbance, may influence the output of these hormones via the release of TSH by the pituitary gland. Depending probably upon genetic factors such emotional stress may produce either an increase or a decrease in the circulating hormones (Hamburg and Lunde 1967). Further, the syndromes of hyperthyroidism and hypothyroidism once established are both associated with a disturbance of normal mental functioning (Whybrow et al. 1969).

HYPERTHYROIDISM AND ANXIETY

Whether or not hyperthyroidism may be precipitated by psychological stress has been debated since 1803 when Parry first described thyrotoxicosis and noted that the illness had been immediately preceded by a frightening experience. Although some physicians maintain that such an event is merely coincidental and that a careful history would usually reveal hyperthyroid symptoms developing prior to the trauma there is evidence that in some persons psycho-dynamic factors do play a contributing part in the pathogenesis of the disease.

The majority of the persons who develop thyrotoxicosis have a family history of the disturbance, suggesting a genetic predisposition. Psychiatrists familiar with the illness have also noted that hyperthyroid persons as a group frequently have strikingly similar personalities. One writer has colourfully characterized the way of life as that of 'inhibited martyrdom' (Wallerstein et al. 1965). A detailed history frequently reveals that because of family circumstances the individual was forced into an early independence of his parents, hence usually missing many of the usual gratifications of childhood. Probably as a compensation there is often a premature striving for self-sufficiency with the shouldering of family responsibilities at an early age and an excessive concern for the care of others. Such an adjustment is precarious and in later life the disruption or threat of disruption of a close emotional tie, such as the death of a near relative or the breakup of a marriage, will precipitate the clinical picture of thyrotoxicosis if there is a genetic predisposition to the illness.

Two studies in particular lend support to these observations. In one (Dongier et al. 1956) psychiatric patients without biochemical or clinical evidence of hyperthyroidism but with personality characteristics as just described were found to have a significantly more rapid turnover of radioactive iodine in the thyroid gland than did patients without such character traits. Another, more recent study has shown that one may predict individuals with 'thyroid hot-spots' by a knowledge of their personality constellation (Wallerstein et al. 1965).

Once the clinical syndrome of hyperthyroidism is developed there invariably occurs psychological disturbance secondary to the abnormal thyroid metabolism (Whybrow et al. 1969). One of these is anxiety which may predominate as a symptom and give rise to diagnostic confusion. Some of the symptoms of hyperthyroidism closely resemble those of an anxiety state and indeed may be produced by a similar physiological mechanism. Many of the physiological accompaniments of anxiety are mimicked by sympathetic stimulation and adrenaline secretion and it is established that hyperthyroidism increases the sensitivity of the tissues to both of these. Thus, some of the symptoms of hyperthyroidism such as tremor, tachycardia and sweating may be attributed to hypersensitivity to sympathetic stimulation and can be relieved to some extent by drugs such as propranolol and reserpine, which are known to reduce the quantity of noradrenaline available in the central nervous system.

Certain symptoms, however, are peculiar to hyperthyroidism and therefore of great value in differentiating it from anxiety states. Perhaps the most distinctive is the combination of weight loss with a good and indeed often excessive appetite. Anxious people may lose weight but if they do so it is usually because their appetites are poor. Hyperthyroid patients also often report an intolerance of heat and an increase in sweating. This may be obvious on shaking hands with the patient when the hot sweaty hand of hyperthyroidism contrasts markedly with the cold, clammy palm of the anxious person.

Palpitations, that is, abnormal awareness of the heart's action, are commonly felt by both hyperthyroid and anxious patients. What is significant about this symptom in the hyperthyroid subject is that it is most noticeable when the patient is resting quietly and, like the sensation of subjective anxiety also present in thyrotoxicosis, is usually unrelated to specific thought content.

Physical examination of the patient may reveal features characteristic of hyperthyroidism such as one or other of the peculiar eye signs or a firm enlarged thyroid with a vascular bruit. However, in the majority of hyperthyroid patients now referred to hospital these helpful features are absent and the diagnosis can only be firmly established by laboratory tests such as radio-iodine uptake, serum protein bound iodine (PBI) and the tri-iodothyronine uptake test.

Should the hyperthyroidism remain undiagnosed and untreated, psychiatric symptoms become more apparent and increasingly distressing to the patient as the level of circulating hormone rises. A mild delirium occurs with increasing irritability, difficulty in concentration and some impairment of recent memory. Difficulty is found with simple mental arithmetic and the patient becomes aware of a mild confusional state which may merge into perceptual distortion and even frank hallucination, when he usually presents to the psychiatrist with a picture of psychosis. There is nothing specific about the psychotic picture, the thought content of which is determined by the individual's previous personality, and life experience. Depressive symptoms, however, are notable for their absence. Although a sadness of mood may be present prior to the onset of the thyrotoxicosis, this is rarely seen during the illness itself despite considerable physical disability.

Treatment of the psychic disturbance secondary to the increased metabolism of hyperthyroidism lies, of course, in the successful treatment of the thyrotoxicosis itself. Essentially this can be achieved by the administration of antithyroid drugs, by surgical removal of part of the thyroid gland or by selective irradiation of the gland by means of radio-iodine. Although all of these are efficient means of reducing thyroid function to a normal level they do not do so immediately and thus symptomatic treatment of the anxiety or the psychotic symptoms secondary to the delirium may be necessary. Reserpine is of value here, as are the minor tranquillizers (such as Diazepam) for anxiety, and the phenothiazines may be used to reduce psychotic disturbance.

As the individual improves emotional support is important and indeed some persons may need formal psychotherapy to improve their previously fragile psychological adjustment to life circumstance.

HYPOTHYROIDISM AND DEPRESSION

It is not known whether emotional stress contributes to hypothyroidism in humans (Gibson 1962) although in certain animals physical stress may inhibit production of thyroid hormone, as will electrical stimulation of the posterior hypothalamic area (Reichlin 1964). That florid psychic disturbance may occur secondary to hypothyroidism is well known, however. Indeed, at times persons with 'myxoedematous madness' (Asher 1949) may be referred directly to a psychiatrist and because of the specific treatment available for this psychotic illness, recognition of the syndrome is very important.

Like those with hyperthyroidism persons with myxoedema invariably have a mental disturbance (Whybrow et al. 1969). This may be only a mild impairment of recent memory and difficulty in concentration reflecting an early delirious state. However, if left unchecked for a long period of time this will progress eventually to an irreversible dementia.

In contrast to hyperthyroidism where sadness during the actual illness is a rarity, persons with hypothyroidism frequently complain of a marked depression which at times may mimic the syndrome of melancholia. They become preoccupied with morbid thoughts, are tearful, guilty and have suicidal ideas. The physical symptoms of motor lethargy, diminished appetite and constipation may also suggest melancholia. Hence, in a person who is depressed *and* confused it is always important during the physical examination to look for other stigmata of hypothyroid illness as treatment of the psychiatric symptoms may then be largely one of replacement of thyroid hormone.

The difference in mood between hyperthyroidism and hypothyroidism is of considerable interest to the psychiatrist. It suggests that in some way an excess of thyroid hormone may 'protect' the individual against sad feelings. Some thyrotoxic people for example become depressed about the situation immediately preceding their illness only as they return to an euthyroid state. One implication is that thyroid hormones might be found helpful in the treatment of melancholia, and recent studies using tri-iodothyronine as an adjunct to antidepressant drugs suggest that indeed a much more rapid recovery from the depressive illness is obtained than when

210   Part V *Psychosomatic conditions*

treatment is with antidepressant drugs alone (Prange et al. 1969).

Myxoedema is a much commoner cause of psychosis than generally believed (Asher 1949). The symptoms are not specific but paranoid ideas are common and generally clear up quickly with thyroid treatment.

Besides this a condition of irritability, lassitude and being 'out of sorts' may well occur in a slightly hypothyroid patient, and puzzle his physician, though a second attack will at once be recognized by the patient for what it is.

REFERENCES

Asher, R. J. (1949). 'Myxoedematous madness'. *Brit. Med. J.*, ii, 555.

Dongier, M., Wittkower, E. D., Stephans-Newsham, L. and Hoffman, M. M. (1956). 'Psychophysiological studies in thyroid function'. *Psychosomatic Medicine*, 4, 310.

Gibson, J. G. (1962). 'Emotions and the thyroid gland: a critical appraisal'. *J. of Psychosomatic Research*, 6, 93.

Hamburg, D. A., and Lunde, D. T. (1967). 'Relation of behavioural, genetic and neuroendocrine factors to thyroid function in genetic diversity and human behaviour'. Edited by J. N. Spuhler. Aldine, Chicago.

Prange, A. J. et al. (1969). 'Enhancement of imipramine antidepressant activity by thyroid hormone'. *Amer. J. Psychiat.* 126, 457.

Reichlin, S. (1964). 'Function of the hypothalamus in regulation of pituitary-thyroid activity'. In *Brain-Thyroid Relationships*, CIBA Foundation Study Group No. 18. Little, Brown, Boston.

Wallerstein, R. S., Holzman, P. S., Voth, H. M. and Uhr, N. (1965). 'Thyroid "hot-spots", a psychophysiological study'. *Psychosomatic Medicine*, 27, 508.

Whybrow, P. C., Prange, A. J. and Treadway, C. R. (1969). 'Mental changes accompanying thyroid gland dysfunction. A reappraisal using objective psychological measurement'. *Arch. Gen. Psychiat.*, 20, 48.

Whybrow, P. C. and Ferrell, R. (1974). 'Thyroid state and human behaviour'. In Prange, A. J. (ed.), *The Thyroid Axis, Drugs and Behaviour*. New York.

34 Psychological aspects
of skin disease

For two reasons psychological aspects are of special importance in skin disorders. Firstly, emotional factors play an important part in the onset and maintenance of many common dermatological conditions; and secondly, having a skin disease often causes emotional disturbance to the patient, and sometimes also to people in his environment. There are several reasons for this: skin lesions are often visible and unsightly, thus making the patient self-conscious and embarrassed; they may arouse fears of having been infected or of infecting others, especially in cases of venereal disease or scabies but also when the condition is in fact not infectious; if there is itching the conflict between wanting to scratch at the expense of further damage to the skin, or abstaining from scratching leads to tension and anxiety, and after an attack of scratching the patient may feel guilty and depressed; itching also leads to mental irritation, insomnia and depression; some skin diseases tend to be chronic, and patients may get depressed as the result and project their feelings of frustration at not getting better on to their doctor. Whether or not, in an individual case, psychological factors may have played a part in originally causing the disorder, a vicious circle is often set up as these emotional reactions may in turn aggravate or prolong the illness.

PSYCHOSOMATIC SKIN DISEASES

Everyday experience shows that mood changes influence the function of the skin. Thus shame and embarrassment lead to vasodilatation making people blush, while anxiety and fear may lead to vaso-constriction causing pallor, and to increased sweating.

Experimentally it has been demonstrated by Graham and

Wolf (1950) that the state of the blood vessels in the skin can be altered by emotional stress; similarly the effect of stress on palmar sweating has been studied by MacKinnon (1964); the fact that emotional tension alters the electrical resistance of the skin (galvanic skin response) is secondary to altered function of the sweat glands. It has also been shown that the vascular component of the skin response to the local injection of tuberculin can be inhibited by hypnosis (Black 1963). Itching can also be reduced by relaxation or hypnosis and is increased by emotional stress.

There is thus a good deal of evidence that skin function can be affected by psychological factors but opinions still differ as to the relative importance of such factors in different skin conditions. It is likely that in the individual patient several factors, including constitutional, allergic, infective and psychological ones, often play a combined role but in the following conditions psychological aspects tend to be of special importance.

Pruritus. The itching may be generalized, or localized to the nape of the neck or to the genital region and the anus. Physical causes must, of course, be excluded but the majority of these cases are psychogenic; conflicts concerning sexuality and aggression are likely to exist and patient, prolonged psychiatric investigation may be needed to bring these factors to light.

Excessive blushing may accompany feelings of embarrassment and anger. It occurs more often in young women than in men, and may lead to further embarrassment.

Rosacea is characterised by prolonged and persistent redness of the middle of the face. It occurs most frequently in middle-aged women and may be connected with problems relating to guilt and embarrassment.

Hyperhidrosis. Excessive sweating, particularly of palms, soles and axillae, often starts in adolescence and is frequently due to psychological conflict.

Urticaria. Unless of definite allergic origin, attacks of urticaria are often brought on by acute emotional stress and conflict.

Neuro-dermatitis. Here long-standing psychological problems may be present and superimposed acute emotional stresses often precipitate or aggravate attacks. Conflict connected with suppressed aggression and sexual problems may be especially important. Itching is often intense and scratching may be associated with erotic sensations.

Infantile and atopic eczema and the asthma-eczema syndrome. Constitutional factors are of decisive importance here. Psychologically these conditions in children are found in a setting in which there is a disturbed relationship between mother and child. This may be slight or transitory or, in the early stages, easily corrected by discussion with the mother. If this is not so the relationship between mother and patient may deteriorate further. The mother begins to feel incompetent and she may seem to reject the child who, in turn, feels himself to be a nuisance and unwanted. These feelings are somatized into itching followed by scratching and deterioration of the eczema. A vicious circle of ambivalence with the eczema at its centre is established between mother and child. Emotional and intellectual development of the patient may increasingly be interfered with and retarded, and lead to a personality disorder which accompanies and outlasts the chronic eczema.

Alopecia areata or patchy hair loss may have acute emotional stress as a contributory aetiological factor.

Psoriasis is one of the most common chronic dermatoses of unknown aetiology. In some patients the signs and symptoms of their particular form of psoriasis, unsightly, scaly patches on exposed body surfaces or in the scalp, itching or shedding of scales in the bed, bathroom or wherever they go unclothed, or the reaction of people in their environment to them cause intense and sometimes severe emotional distress and disturbance in their personal and working life. In some patients the severity of the disease itself can be improved by psychotherapy.

Artefacts (dermatitis artefacta). Quite apart from the fact that in many skin diseases the patient may scratch and make his skin worse and produce excoriated lesions, psychiatrically ill patients may consciously or unconsciously damage their normal skin, e.g. by burning or cutting themselves, or by means of chemicals applied to or even injected under the skin, thus producing a variety of lesions. The patient may be unaware of what he is doing or conceal the truth. It is more important to discover the underlying reasons than to make him 'confess' — even if caught in the act; a punitive attitude will make it impossible to discover the underlying psychological conflict and merely result in a more antagonistic and miserable patient. A

personality disorder or depressive illness is often found to lie at
the root of this condition.

Trichotillomania. Compulsive pulling out of hair, which may
lead to a considerable degree of baldness. This is always the
result of a severe underlying psychiatric disturbance, often a
personality disorder.

PSYCHIATRIC DISORDERS FOCUSSED ON THE SKIN

The above conditions have been labelled as 'psychosomatic'
because psychological factors may, in varying degrees, play a
part in the causation of the diseases described. In addition
patients with psychiatric disorders may present themselves with
the fear of having something wrong with their skin without this
being the case, or they may become excessively concerned with
a minor abnormality of the skin while psychologically ill. Thus
a patient with an anxiety state may watch his skin for the
presence of blemishes which he or she would ordinarily ignore;
a depressed patient may become hypochondriacally pre-
occupied with the idea that he has got a skin disease;
occasionally a patient with a psychotic illness may develop the
delusion that he is infested with parasites, so-called acaro-
phobia.

TREATMENT

This clearly depends on the correct assessment of both physical
and psychological aspects of the disorder. Unless one is dealing
with a skin disorder of physical origin which is being treated
successfully and quickly by purely physical means, it is
important to get to know the patient well and to find out what
was happening in his life when the illness commenced or got
worse, and also how he is reacting to his illness. Patients often
benefit once they realize that the doctor recognizes that they
may have developed a skin disease in response to stress; and to
be able to talk about themselves and about their anxiety
concerning their skin condition may itself have a therapeutic
effect, in combination with whatever physical treatment is
required. This is specially important during periods of unavoid-

able stress which has precipitated or produced an exacerbation of a skin disorder.

In children, e.g. those with the eczema-asthma syndrome in which the mother-child relationship is of special importance, work with the mother may be as essential as the treatment of the child. Sometimes the child may have to be admitted to hospital or convalescent home. Such separation from the mother may occasionally be helpful but in other cases it may do further damage to the relationship between the child and his mother.

In adults with chronic or relapsing skin diseases, such as dermatitis and eczema, unless of proven allergic origin, more formal, long-term psychotherapy may be helpful. In patients who are beginning to be aware of underlying problems, often connected with sexual and aggressive conflicts, analytical psychotherapy may be of benefit. Occasionally hypnosis has proved useful in bringing a severe attack of dermatitis under control (see p. 325). Group therapy or common problem groups may bring about improvement in the skin condition itself or at least lighten the excessive burden which the patient has allowed the dermatosis to impose on him and enable him to lead a richer and more satisfying life.

FURTHER READING

Altschulova, H. J. (1958). 'Psychotherapy of the asthma-prurigo syndrome in children'. *A Crianca Portuguesa*, xvii, 683.

Altschulova, H. J. (1971). 'Psychiatric aspects of the asthma-eczema syndrome in children and young people with special reference to depression'. In *Depressive States in Childhood and Adolescence*, Stockholm.

Black, S. (1963). 'Inhibition of the immediate type hypersensitivity response by direct suggestion under hypnosis'. *Brit. Med. J.*, 1, 925.

Graham, D. T. and Wolf, S. (1950). 'Pathogenesis of urticaria. Experimental study of life situations, emotions and cutaneous vascular reactions'. *J.A.M.A.*, 143, 1396.

MacKinnon, P. C. B. (1964). 'Hormonal control of the reaction of the palmar sweat index to emotional stress'. *J. Psychosomatic Research*, 8, 193.

Musaph, H. (1964). *Itching and Scratching: Psychodynamics in Dermatology.* Karger, Basel.

Obermayer, M. F. (1955). *Psychocutaneous medicine.* Thomas, Springfield, Mass.

Wittkower, E. and Russell, B. (1953). *Emotional Factors in Skin Disease.* Hoeber, New York.

35 *Disorders of menstrual function*

THE NORMAL MENSTRUAL CYCLE: HORMONAL AND EMOTIONAL

Helene Deutsch (1945), whose work on the psychology of women remains unsurpassed, writes concerning menstruation: 'The first genital bleeding mobilizes psychic reactions so numerous and varied that we are justified in speaking of the psychology of menstruation as a specific problem ... The extent to which the organic and psychic influence each other is a matter for experimental investigation.' Benedek and Rubinstein (1939) correlated the emotional states of a series of patients under psychoanalytic treatment with their basal body temperatures and vaginal smears. They reported a correlation between each hormonal variation of the sexual cycle and the psychodynamic manifestations of the sexual drive; thus, parallel to the hormonal cycle, there is an emotional cycle. Both together constitute the sexual cycle, which has four stages:

1 *Oestrogenic phase.* Active interest in the sexual partner, with coitus as the aim.
2 *Ovulation.* Some emotional tension just before ovulation; such tension is usual during hormonal change.
3 *Progesterone phase.* The woman is emotionally more relaxed. Interest in the sexual partner is less direct and the woman is more concerned with her own body, so that she is more passively receptive to male sexual advances. She has phantasies of having a child or a positive wish for a child.
4 *Premenstrual phase.* As progesterone production diminishes the woman becomes less loving and mature. This is the phase where there may be pre-menstrual tension.

AMENORRHOEA

Primary functional amenorrhoea

This is simply a delayed onset of menstruation. The prognosis for normal sexual development and reproductive function is good; the use of endocrine preparations is inadvisable, for patients usually respond to reassurance, explanation and time. Deeper psychotherapy is indicated for long-standing immaturity and adolescent conflicts.

Secondary functional amenorrhoea

A. *Personality structure*
Two main types are seen:
1 Those who are basically hysterics, showing their major conflict in the area of feeling and attitudes to their feminine role.
2 Dependent clinging personalities, childlike emotionally, however gifted intellectually, who tend to think, 'Who will help me?' rather than, 'How can I cope?'

B. *Precipitating stress*
1 Separation from parents, e.g. when the patient leaves home for study or job, or separation from husband, e.g. in divorce. This tends to occur in the dependent type. Usually menstruation starts as the patient gets to know people again.
2 Transient amenorrhoea during times of emotional stress. For example, this was common during the bombing of London, or after a fright such as attempted rape.
3 Obesity. Treatment for obesity may succeed, but psychotherapy is often needed as well.
4 Pseudocyesis. A rare condition in which the woman is convinced she is pregnant when this is not so.
5 Amenorrhoea may be an early symptom of anorexia nervosa.
6 Amenorrhoea may be part of a tension syndrome.

C. *Amenorrhoea of organic origin* can cause insecurity and fear of reproductive incompetence and loss of femininity. In such an emotional environment any surgical or endocrine treatment may be hampered, or even thwarted at times, unless the meaning of menstruation to the woman concerned is explained and resolved.

THE PREMENSTRUAL SYNDROME

Definition and incidence

The premenstrual syndrome covers symptoms which recur regularly at the same phase of each menstrual cycle, usually occurring during the premenstruum, but occasionally at ovulation or the beginning of menstruation.

The syndrome is common among those who have previously suffered from toxaemia of pregnancy or puerperal depression, among hypertensives and sufferers from glaucoma. The incidence is increased with the approach of the menopause and with increasing parity.

Aetiology

Originally the syndrome was thought to be due to a high oestrogen/progesterone ratio, but more recent work suggests that it is due to the effect of the rapidly falling oestrogen/progesterone levels on the hypothalamic-pituitary-adrenal axis. Symptoms arise from selective temporary failure of adrenal functions; the mineralocorticoids causing water and sodium retention and potassium depletion, the glucocorticoids causing the transitory hypoglycaemia, and the failure of the cortico-steroids causing the allergic phenomena.

Symptoms and signs

The symptoms are of wide diversity and many occur together. The onset is usually gradual, rising to a crescendo at the premenstruum and then ending abruptly with the onset of the full menstrual flow. The commonest symptom is often referred to as 'premenstrual tension' and is manifested as a triad of lethargy, irritability and depression. Other symptoms include headache, backache, asthma, epilepsy, rhinitis, vertigo, nausea and urticaria.

Oedema, especially of the ankles, is common. Fluctuations of weight and blood pressure may be noted if frequent readings are taken. Facial pallor and puffiness and spontaneous bruising may occur during the premenstruum. Pain and swelling in the breasts are common.

Diagnosis

The only positive method of diagnosis available today is the simple and inexpensive method of recording the dates of menstruation and the symptoms. The menstrual chart will show the recurrence of symptoms always at the same phase of the menstrual cycle, usually during the premenstruum, and occasionally a short attack at the time of ovulation. Helpful diagnostic pointers obtained during history taking include:

1 *Normal painfree menstruation.* Indeed so natural is their menstruation that many sufferers are unable to relate menstruation to the relief of symptoms until it is revealed on a menstrual chart. If dysmenorrhoea occurs it is the congestive type with heavy, dragging, continuous lower abdominal pain, commencing during the premenstruum and increasing in severity until the onset of the full menstrual flow.

2 *Effect of pregnancy.* Patients conceive easily and most experience an exceptionally severe and prolonged attack of symptoms at the time of the first missed menstruation, but after the first trimester has passed the majority become free from symptoms and experience a feeling of well-being during later pregnancy. Those whose symptoms do not disappear during the middle trimester are likely to develop toxaemia of pregnancy. 78% of cases of toxaemia develop premenstrual symptoms later.

3 *Effect of childbirth.* There may be a recurrence of symptoms during the puerperium, and puerperal depression is common among those who felt exceptionally fit during pregnancy.

4 *Effect of oestrogens.* Oestrogens are often given for treatment of menstrual disorders or to suppress lactation. Patients with the premenstrual syndrome complain of nausea and

vomiting with even the smallest doses of oestrogen.

5 *Weight fluctuations.* Patients are apt to give their weight as 'within half a stone' or explain that 'it's never the same two days running'.

6 *Effect of prolonged standing.* The tendency to develop oedema of the ankles leads to difficulty when the patients are required to stand for long periods; patients often recognize this and avoid situations requiring prolonged standing.

7 *Effect of stress.* All symptoms are increased in severity and duration at times of stress.

Social significance

Mild cases of the premenstrual syndrome are of relatively little importance, bringing only minor discomforts to sufferers. In its advanced forms it is of considerable social importance, for the spontaneous, frequent and irrational outbursts of women during the premenstruum have shattered the happiness of the home, and led to divorce and suicide, serious accidents, crimes of violence and battered babies (Dalton 1964). Studies have shown that during the premenstruum and early menstruation of schoolgirls and women prisoners behaviour deteriorates, mental ability declines, and there are more failures in examinations and increased absenteeism from work. A decreased resistance to bacterial and viral infections, lowered pain tolerance, increased allergic reactions and frequency of pyrexia result in over half of all admissions to medical and surgical wards occurring during the premenstruum or early menstruation. No woman's medical history should be considered complete unless it also contains the date of the last menstrual period.

Treatment

Not all cases of the premenstrual syndrome require treatment; often recognition of the condition and simple explanation will suffice.

1 *Symptomatic treatment.* This is indicated in mild cases and while the diagnosis is being made on the menstrual chart. Drugs

of addiction must be avoided as treatment is likely to continue for years. In selecting a drug for symptomatic treatment care must be taken to select one in which the side effects will not aggravate any other symptoms that may also be present. Thus tranquillizers or sedatives may help the tension or irritability but they nearly always increase the mental and physical dullness and the accident-proneness. Anti-histamines for the relief of urticaria or rhinitis may serve only to increase the lethargy. Phenylbutazone for the relief of joint pains may increase oedema. Fluid restriction and salt limitation are helpful. Fluids are limited to one pint per day. Diuretics are valuable, especially where there is evidence of oedema, weight gain or abdominal bloatedness. When oral diuretics are used a potassium supplement is always indicated, for it is probable that there is already potassium depletion, as indicated by the almost universal lethargy which accompanies other symptoms.

2 *Hormone therapy.* This is indicated in severe premenstrual tension, especially in cases of premenstrual depression, epilepsy, asthma and migraine. *Progesterone* is the hormone of choice and can be administered as pessaries, suppositories, intramuscular injections or implants. Pessaries or suppositories in daily doses from 200 mg to 400 mg may be given initially from midcycle until the onset of menstruation. In subsequent cycles the dose is gradually adjusted to produce relief of symptoms with the shortest therapeutic course. Daily or alternate day injections of 10-100 mgs may also be given.

When a patient is symptom-free on progesterone she may be given a *progesterone implant* of ½ to 1 g implanted into the fat of the abdominal wall. This gives freedom from symptoms for 3-18 months. Progesterone should not be confused with synthetic progestogens, e.g. nor-ethisterone or hydroxyprogesterone caproate, which can be taken orally or by long-acting injections, and which lower the plasma progesterone level, thus causing an exacerbation of premenstrual symptoms.

3 *Psychotherapy.* This may also be required as a useful adjunct, but in a controlled series it was found of no value when used alone.

FUNCTIONAL DYSMENORRHOEA

Common symptoms are pain, nausea, vomiting, fainting.

Causation

It is important to emphasize that dysmenorrhoea is not yet fully understood. Moon (1950) said, and it still remains true, 'Although the importance of psychogenic factors in the evaluation and treatment of primary dysmenorrhoea is recognized, such factors are not a principal cause or even an essential feature of the condition. Severe and intractable dysmenorrhoea can be found among healthy and well-developed girls who are free from neurosis'. Nonetheless, both physical and emotional factors must be considered in every case.

1 *Ovulation*. Wilson and Kurzok (1938) state, 'the presence of menstrual cramps without organic disease means that ovulation has occurred. One cannot have functional dysmenorrhoea without prior ovulation.' This explains why the onset of dysmenorrhoea is usually from 6 to 24 months after the menarche, and the first periods are generally anovulatory, of the oestrogen withdrawal type. Dysmenorrhoea does not occur until the pituitary ovarian axis has matured sufficiently to achieve ovulation and the consequent production of progesterone.
2 *Emotional factors*. Intolerance of discomfort related to the flow, often associated with conflict over developing femininity, or to other stress has been described (O'Neill 1951).

Sturgis (1962) describes a typical personality as one who shows a marked dichotomy, being able, competent and effective between periods, but dependent and childlike with the dysmenorrhoea. This dichotomy reflects the conflict over wishes to stay as the mother's child, and wishes to grow into a mature woman and escape her domination. This conflict and some dysmenorrhoea are both common in adolescent girls and usually resolve with time when they leave home and become emotionally independent.

Wittkower and Wilson (1940) describe two main personality groups: (1) Masculine women rejecting the female role, and (2) women with small juvenile faces and fragile physique, who had shut-in personalities, and were over-attached to their parents.

O'Neill (1951) describes two clinical types of dysmenorrhoea: (1) Hysterical reactions to the period, and (2) dysmenorrhoea as a reaction to stress.

Less common, and more refractory to treatment, is a masochistic pleasure derived from the painful periods.

Treatment

From the above it follows that there are two valid approaches to treatment:
1 Suppression of ovulation.
2 Psychotherapy to help the patient to mature as a woman and be capable of adequate motherhood.

MENORRHAGIA

Blaikley (1949) who was not a psychiatrist but a practising gynaecologist wrote that 'the importance of recognizing an underlying emotional origin of menorrhagia lies first in the possibility of cure by appropriate advice, reassurance, or even formal psychotherapy, and secondly in the avoidance of unnecessary surgery — even such radical operations as hysterectomy may have been contemplated'. He also reports that 'when doing a hysterectomy on women whom I have thought to be a little over-emotional I have several times noted that the uterus flushes and blanches, and flushes again. The endometrium has appeared normal, and I believe I have done hysterectomies where the cause, or at least an important aggravating factor, has been emotional'. He comments on the relationship of fatigue to heavy periods. For example members of the WAAF engaged on night work plotting enemy aircraft during the war complained of menorrhagia, but improved with a change to day work and a less exacting job. Hopkins (1959) has described the management of psychogenic menorrhagia in general practice.

The *menopause* is described separately (see p. 299).

REFERENCES

Benedek, T. (1952). *Psychosexual Functions in Women.* Ronald, New York.
Benedek, T. and Rubenstein, B. B. (1942). *The Sexual Cycle in Women: the relation between ovarian function and psychodynamic processes.* Nat. Res. Council. Washington.
Blaikley, J. B. (1949). 'Menorrhagia of emotional origin'. *Lancet*, 2, 691.
Dalton, K. (1964). *The Premenstrual Syndrome.* Heinemann, London.
Deutsch, H. (1945). *The Psychology of Women.* Grune and Stratton, London.
Hamburg, D. A., Moos, R. H. and Yalom, I. D. (1968). 'Studies of distress in the menstrual cycle and the post-partum period'. In Michael, R. P. (ed.), *Endocrinology and Human Behaviour.*
Hopkins, P. (1959). 'Menorrhagia in general practice'. *Medical World*, 1.
Moon, A. A. (1950). 'Dysmenorrhoea and the climacteric; psychosomatic assessment and treatment'. *Med. J. Austral.*, 1, 174.
O'Neill, D. (1951). 'Incidence of the Atalanta syndrome'. *Postgrad. Med. J.*, 27, 468.
Rees, W. L. (1953). 'The premenstrual tension syndrome and its treatment'. *Brit. Med. J.*, i, 1014.
Sturgis, S. H. et al. (1962). *The Gynaecological Patient: a Psycho-Endocrine Study.*
Wilson, L. and Kurzok, R. (1938). 'Studies on motility of human uterus in vivo'. *Endocrinol.*, 23, 79.
Wittkower, E. D. and Wilson, A. T. M. (1940). 'Dysmenorrhoea and sterility, personality studies'. *Brit. Med. J.*, 2, 586.

36 Organic gynaecological conditions with associated psychological problems

Certain psychological characteristics arc sccn in patients suffering from gynaecological conditions. Each patient's fears and anxieties, the nature of her relationship to other people, as well as her social situation, may all influence her attitude to treatment, and her response to it, more particularly in gynaecology than other branches of medicine because her views of herself as a woman, wife and mother are intimately involved. Gynaecological operations in general are more often followed by psychological complications than other surgical procedures.

CONGENITAL ANOMALIES

May be discovered in adolescent girls or young women who need a minor corrective surgical operation on their genitals, or have defective or absent gonads.

On learning about the defect the patient may become introverted, asocial and depressed, or deny that she minds at all, saying she wants to forget about it; so before surgery or hormone therapy is contemplated some form of counselling may be needed. Whether she will be capable of a sexual relationship, or have children, will probably cause her grave anxieties and she may be too afraid to ask in a straightforward way.

If she becomes depressed, in accepting the physical limitations in herself as a woman, she will need support, so that she can later go on to find satisfaction in other fields where she can still feel valued.

The usual family tensions may be felt to be even less tolerable to a girl with this added handicap, so she may need treatment from a psychotherapist as well as sensitive counselling from her gynaecologist for her specific difficulties.

ENDOMETRIOSIS

Endometriosis seems to be found more among women of the high socio-economic groups. As such, it has been correlated with delayed or deferred motherhood. The personality type is mesomorphic but underweight, overanxious, intelligent, egocentric and perfectionist; these characteristics represent a personality pattern in which marriage and child-bearing are likely to be deferred and therefore predispose to prolonged periods of uninterrupted ovulation.

TRICHOMONIASIS

Evidence exists that recurrent attacks which do not respond readily to treatment may be correlated with emotional stress.

NEURODERMATITIS OF THE VULVA

This occurs predominantly in overactive, oversensitive persons, particularly those who suffer from psychosexual disorders; often severely disturbed women with marital friction, frigidity, dyspareunia, fear of pregnancy, who need, but respond only slowly to psychotherapy.

HYSTERECTOMY

Counselling is often required before hysterectomy because there are many common fears about this operation, e.g. that the patient or her husband will no longer be able to enjoy intercourse, that she will become hirsute, obese or insane. Women who have not reached the menopause, even if they do not want more children, get reassurance of their femininity from their periods.

A patient tends to rely for support on her gynaecologist. The psychiatrist must guard against weakening this relationship of trust by transferring her away from the surgeon in whose hands lies the decision for positive therapy. Only when the situation is made intolerable by neurosis should a psychiatrist intervene — of course with the gynaecologist's consent.

Patients who enjoyed masochistic pleasure from their dysmenorrhoea may substitute other symptoms after hysterectomy, such as headache, fatigue, insomnia.

Convalescence after hysterectomy is likely to be free of emotional trouble in those who are not in conflict over their femininity, either because they have accepted and enjoyed it fully, or because they have rejected it and enjoyed other satisfactions in careers, etc. There is seldom loss of libido after operation for cervical cancer, but the patient may need reassurance from her gynaecologist on this. But disturbed convalescence was found more often by Sturgis among those married women with children who were not so interested in their husbands and children as people, but whose lives revolved around their own menstruation and fertility.

In these and other psychologically disturbed women hysterectomy may be followed by depressive reactions requiring treatment (Ackner 1960; Barker 1968).

PROLAPSE

Sudden depressive or hysterical reactions have been seen after operations for prolapse in patients with previously disturbed personalities, and occasionally in those who have been perfectly well-adjusted.

Termination of pregnancy, sterilization and *infertility* are described later (see pp. 376, 382 and 261 respectively).

HABITUAL ABORTION

The causes of this are not yet properly understood but it is commonly held that emotional stress and sudden fright may sometimes play a part in bringing on a spontaneous abortion. An interesting animal experiment by Yaron et al. (1964) showed that female hamsters who, instead of having been handled gently in their own infancy, had been handled with forceps only, had a much higher rate of abortions later on than females who had received gentle handling when they were young, and in general they behaved more aggressively when grown up. Although one cannot, of course, draw firm conclusions on human behaviour from observations in animals, these findings lend some support to the theory that psychological factors, perhaps related to their own personality development and consequent physiological changes may play some part in habitual abortion in humans.

In any case, in treatment of women prone to spontaneous abortion the relationship between the patient and the obstetrician is especially important. The patient needs much reassurance and encouragement, and an opportunity to express her fears to the obstetrician so that she feels that he knows her particular problems. Attendance at ante-natal classes helps and only when the patient does not settle under such a regime is a psychiatrist required during pregnancy. Psychotherapy may be indicated at other times, especially as women are likely to get anxious and depressed after repeated miscarriages.

FURTHER READING

Ackner, B. (1960). 'Emotional aspects of hysterectomy, a follow-up study of fifty patients under the age of 40'. *Adv. Psychosom. Med.* 1, 248. Karger, Basel.

Barker, M. G. (1968). 'Psychiatric illness after hysterectomy'. *Brit. Med. J.*, 1, 91.

Kroger, W. S. and Freed, S. C. (1951). *Psychosomatic Gynaecology.* Saunders, London.

Wengraf, F. (1953). *Psychosomatic Approach to Gynaecology and Obstetrics.* Thomas, Springfield, Mass.

Wolff, H. H. (1966). 'Psychological reactions to gynaecological procedures'. *Medical World*, 104, 23.

Yaron, E., Chovers, I., Locker, A. and Groen, J. J. (1964). 'Influence of handling on the reproductive behaviour of the Syrian hamster in captivity'. In Groen, J. J. (ed.), *Psychosomatic Research.* Pergamon, Oxford.

The symptomatology of psychiatric reactions has already been discussed in the earlier parts of this book, under the classical titles of illness; and so has their treatment. It may, however, be helpful now for the GP or student to look at the matter from a different angle and to consider various stages in life, each with their own stresses, which most people have to meet; and to describe certain common reactions to these. The GP and student may thus be encouraged (as has been stressed before) to look at the total picture of the patient's personality and whole environment; and see that often it is the concatenation of many stresses, predisposing and precipitating, which causes illness, rather than any single factor. It may also be possible for the doctor to prevent some breakdowns by early recognition of the signs of stress, for example from lack of security in the family, from marital.tension, or from frustration at work.

37 Infancy and early childhood

The definition of behaviour disorders varies in different dictionaries and textbooks of psychiatry, reflecting the fact that this term is used very loosely to describe abnormalities of conduct occurring in children and thought to be due to environmental rather than organic causes.

PRIMARY BEHAVIOUR DISORDER

The pattern of behaviour described as abnormal is usually one which at an earlier stage of the child's life has occurred as a normal phase of his physical or emotional development. Thus the soiling and wetting that are an integral part of infancy, the temper tantrums which begin around eighteen months, and the need of the young child to be near his mother for much of the time he is awake, are all examples of normal behaviour. But if such behaviour *persists* until the child is well beyond the stage when he could normally be expected to have 'grown out of it' then it must be regarded as abnormal and should be investigated.

Such persistence of a behaviour pattern beyond the age at which it is appropriate can be referred to as a *primary behaviour disorder.*

SECONDARY BEHAVIOUR DISORDER

1 A child who has hitherto developed normally may, under strain, *regress* to a more infantile stage of development. Such regression will be seen in all children who are ill, but in most cases the children revert to their previous behaviour when they recover from the illness. However, some children subjected to severe trauma, e.g. a young child separated from his mother or mother-substitute for a long time, may regress to a more infantile stage and this regression will persist — indeed it may become more apparent when the child returns to his mother.

Regression of this kind appearing in a child who has previously developed normally can be referred to as a *secondary behaviour disorder.*

2 This term is also used to describe emotional disturbances, other than autism, superimposed upon the difficulties of mental or physical handicap in children.

AETIOLOGY

At present we do not know enough to understand why one child will succumb to a particular stress while another exposed to apparently similar stress will seem to develop unharmed. Also, while it is evident that from very early infancy individual babies show differing patterns of responsiveness and activity, we are not able to assess whether these differences are due to hereditary or environmental causes.

However, there is a large body of knowledge acquired from very different fields which demonstrate that, given a suitable environment, the healthy child will develop emotionally, physically, socially and intellectually in a manner which is predictable in broad outline, though the details will vary in each individual.

For the very young infant such an environment is usually provided by his parents, particularly his mother who lovingly supports his complete dependence. As the baby grows older he becomes able to see himself as an individual separate from his mother. His world widens to include his father and other members of his immediate circle. At each stage of his development his parents respond to his changing needs, encouraging his independence, helping him to tolerate frustration, while sheltering him from stresses which are beyond his strength.

This presupposes that the child's parents are secure enough in their relationship with him, and with each other, to support his total dependence in infancy and then to help him grow into independence without holding him in an infantile relationship to satisfy their own needs.

In every family, tensions occur at times as a result of the changing needs of the members or from pressures outside the family. The family equilibrium becomes upset — each member feels varying degrees of discomfort and tries to adapt his behaviour in an effort to restore the equilibrium and relieve the discomfort. The experience of dealing successfully with such situations is a part of every family's story and forms an important and necessary experience for all its members. Sometimes, however, the family are unable to adapt their behaviour successfully. The discomfort persists and increases until they may be forced to seek help from outside. Children who are members of families in this stage are often the first to show signs of disturbed behaviour, and persistent complaints of a child's difficult behaviour at home or at school may be an early signal of his family's difficulties. While every family differs in its ability to cope with stress, there are some situations which very commonly cause difficulties.

1 (a) The parents of a handicapped child may not recognize or, more commonly, cannot accept the fact that he is unable to learn as fast as his peers. The pressure on the child will add to his difficulties and he may well show signs of

disturbed behaviour as a result (see p. 58).

(b) If a young child's parents do not appreciate the effect that a prolonged separation from his mother will have on him, they may be bewildered by his disturbed behaviour when they are re-united and be unable to give him the support he needs.

2 Emotional difficulties may exist between the parents themselves, though this may not be apparent when they are first seen, and they appear to be complaining about the child.

3 Social pressures — poverty, poor housing, or the difficulties of adapting to an unfamiliar culture may combine with other factors to disrupt the relationships in families who might have coped under more favourable circumstances. Similarly the widowed or unmarried mother faces great difficulties when she has to bring up her children unaided.

DIAGNOSIS

When parents decide to seek outside advice about their children's difficulties, they often turn to the family doctor or the doctor at the Welfare Clinic, among others. Many parents can give a fairly clear account of what is worrying them, but for some the fear that their child will be found abnormal, or that they will be harshly judged to be 'failed parents', prevents them from voicing their worries openly. If parents — commonly the mother — repeatedly bring a child to the doctor with complaints of a wide variety of physical symptoms and are not reassured when investigations prove these fears to be unfounded, then the doctor should try to pick up from their remarks a clue to their real anxieties and help them to express these.

History

He will then need to take a detailed history covering details of the mother's pregnancy and delivery, of the child's social and physical development and of any illnesses or separations. He should enquire about other children in the family, their ages and state of health, and gather what he can about the parents' health, work, social and cultural background, housing conditions, and the part played by grandparents or others in the life of the family.

Traditionally, the mother brings the children to see the doctor. But when the latter is consulted about behaviour disorders in a child, he is wise to try and see the father also, preferably with the rest of the family, so that in addition to hearing the history from both parents, he can observe how they behave towards each other and towards their children.

Examination

In addition to a routine physical examination, the doctor should test the child's vision and hearing and assess whether he has achieved the appropriate physical and social milestones.

Organic causes for the child's disturbance must be excluded — for instance his enuresis may be due to frequency caused by a urinary infection, or his tantrums to the frustration resulting from partial deafness, etc.

If no physical cause can be found for the child's behaviour disorder and the doctor decides that the family need psychiatric help, he should explain the diagnostic procedure which they will encounter at a child guidance clinic. There the child will be seen for psychological testing, and will also be seen by a psychiatrist while the parents see a psychiatric social worker. In some centres, however, if the child is felt to be old enough to discuss his difficulties, the psychiatrist and psychiatric social worker may first see the parents and child together, later separating for individual interviews. At the end of the diagnostic interviews the parents with or without the child will meet the psychiatrist, psychiatric social worker and psychologist to discuss their findings and their recommendations for treatment.

TREATMENT

1 *Psychotherapy.* This is based on the principles of psychopathology and psychodynamics (pp. 19 and 307) — and the techniques used will vary with the age of the child. The young child expresses his feelings best by playing with toys, sand or

water provided, while the older child may play or may prefer to talk. In either case the child conveys how he perceives himself and the people around him, including the psychiatrist. The psychiatrist makes use of this information and of the relationship between the child and himself, to help the child re-experience his earlier difficulties and work through them to a more realistic conclusion.

Commonly the child will be seen once a week while one or both parents are seen by a psychiatric social worker. In some centres children who need more intensive treatment can be seen daily.

2 *Family therapy.* This involves treating parents and older children together. This technique was first developed for treating schizophrenic children and their families and some clinics are experimenting with its application to families with children suffering from behaviour disorders (Howells 1968).

3 *Behaviour therapy.* This depends on conditioning the child to behave in an appropriate fashion. The alarm bell apparatus which wakes the enuretic child when he begins to pass water is an example of this technique (see p. 331).

4 *Drugs.* Tofranil is used for the treatment of nocturnal enuresis (see p. 236).

Sedatives may be useful for young children who are wakeful at night, the rationale being that if the parents can get some sleep they will be less irritable, and better able to meet the child's needs during the day. Antihistamines such as phenergan are safe sedatives and can be given in doses of 5-25 mgm according to the age and size of the child. They should only be prescribed for 3-4 nights at a time as they are likely to become ineffective over longer periods.

Apart from these examples, drugs play little part in the treatment.

PREVENTION

This aims at avoiding or modifying situations which are liable to disrupt the relationships within a family and cause emotional disturbance in the children.

Perhaps the best known example is the change in the management of young children admitted to hospital which followed the publication of the findings of Bowlby (1965) and Robertson (1958) on the effects of hospitalization. These changes make it possible for mothers of young children to stay with their children in hospital, or, where this is not possible, to be with their children during the day (see p. 295).

Counselling of the parents of handicapped children aims at helping them to adapt their expectations to the child's limited abilities and to come to terms with their own feelings about the child. The counsellor will also ensure that the family receive whatever practical help is available.

The family or welfare clinic doctor who sees the family regularly is in a very favourable position to help parents who are having difficulties in the management of their children. If, at an early stage, the doctor is prepared to give the time to let these parents talk about their difficulties and to help them understand the pattern of their child's development he will find that many of them will be able to adapt to more appropriate behaviour.

At present one can only speculate about the long-term effect of such help in averting a more serious disruption of the family's relationships but this would seem to be a fruitful field for investigation.

ENURESIS

This is a common condition, previously often considered to be due to some physical defect, e.g. spina bifida occulta or urinary infection. It is now regarded as largely psychological; if secondary, that is when a child who has been dry becomes wet, it is generally due to factors which produce anxiety in him, such as separation from the mother — or from her affection; a situation which, ironically, the symptom itself may then make worse. Werry (1967) has given an excellent review. MacKeith (1968) considers it often due to an interference with learning at a sensitive period.

Other, primary, causes may be due to delayed maturation of the nervous system, and Hallgren (1959) showed a much greater frequency in both identical twins than in non-identical ones.

Treatment

This is an excellent example of the value of a combination of the points listed above.

Having ruled out physical causes for the complaint the doctor should see the child regularly to discuss his progress. The child can be asked to keep a chart on which the nights when he is dry are marked with a star; he can set his own alarm clock to wake him at night and he can be encouraged to hold his water for increasingly long periods in the day.

At the same time the child's parents can be helped to understand his difficulty and support him in his efforts. Such counselling should be tried in these cases before resorting to drugs or the alarm bell.

This instrument is an example of behaviour therapy (p. 331) and if the parents are co-operative and provide encouragement and reassurance, it is often successful.

Tofranil is currently popular for the treatment of nocturnal enuresis. There is a considerable success rate while the drug is taken but a high relapse rate when it is discontinued. It can be given in doses of 25 mgm nightly for children of eight years and increased to 50 mgm for older children. It should not be used when there is any history of convulsions.

FURTHER READING

Bowlby, J. (1965). *Child Care and the Growth of Love*. Penguin.

Erikson, E. H. (1950). *Childhood and Society*. Norton, New York.

Freud, A. (1965). *Normality and Pathology in Childhood*. Hogarth, London.

Hallgren, B. (1959). *Acta Paediatrica*. Suppl. No. 118, 66.

Howells, J. G. (1968). *Theory and Practice of Family Psychiatry*. Oliver and Boyd, Edinburgh.

Kahn, J. H. (1965). *Human Growth and the Development of Personality*. Pergamon, Oxford.

MacKeith, R. C. (1968). *Developmental Medicine and Child Neurology*, 10, 465.

Robertson, J. (1958). *Young Children in Hospital*. Tavistock Publications, London.

Soddy, K. (1960). *Clinical Child Psychiatry*. Baillière, Tindall and Cassel, London.

Stone, F. H. and Koupernik, C. (1974). *Child Psychiatry for students*. Edinburgh.

Werry, T. S. (1967). *Can. Med. Assoc. Journal*, 97, 319.
Winnicott, D. W. (1964). *The Child, The Family and the Outside World.* Penguin.
Winnicott, D. W. (1971). *Therapeutic Consultations in Child Psychiatry.*
Wolff, S. (1969). *Children Under Stress.* Penguin.
A brilliant description of play therapy is Axline, V. M. (1971). *Dibs: In Search of Self.* Penguin.

38 School problems

From the age of 5 to 15 or more a child spends a major portion of his life in school, and many of the problems of personal, social and cultural adaptation will necessarily present in a school setting. School can be considered as a microcosm of society in which a child tests or develops his ability to adapt to social necessities, to face frustrations and to achieve social satisfaction. At 5 years, a child is expected to relinquish many of the satisfactions of babyhood and in particular to begin to loosen the close links with, and dependence on, his parents. At school he must share his teacher's attention with 20 or 30 other children and learn to accept the rules of group living. If his early experiences in the family have provided him with adequate security he will regard new situations optimistically as sources of new satisfaction. If on the other hand his experiences have left him insecure, new situations will appear to him as a threat to what security he has, rather than as an opportunity to achieve more sophisticated and more mature satisfactions.

SCHOOL ENTRY

The situation introduced above is apparent in its purest form at school entry. Although tears are traditional on the first day, this separation anxiety soon settles in most children, as the advantages of the new situation begin to outweigh the frustrations. In a few, however, the tears continue, the child withdraws, making little contact with other children or the teacher, or he clings to the teacher claiming exclusive attention. There is of course a continuum between the child who is out of things for a while and the child who remains in a separation panic state.

In severe cases, the family must be investigated and help given, in particular to the mother who may herself be in a state of separation anxiety. At this age, and when mother-child symbiosis is intense, help can best be given to the child through his mother, by supporting her. Although the school entry hurdle is usually cleared, the same problem can recur when children move from junior to secondary school or under some other stress. (See School refusal, below.)

COMPANIONSHIP AND PLAY

School offers major opportunities for the child to find a balance between his need to express and gratify himself, and his need to fit in to a group with mutual support and some responsibility for each other. On this balance may depend his stability as an adult. It will be more difficult to find if he has been allowed to have his own way too much at home; or alternatively if every decision has been taken for him by his parents, whether they believe this to be for his benefit or not. The first step of getting accepted by a new group, whose support and approval he will need if he is to live with them, may be frightening, and the newcomer has to demonstrate that he wants to join and is neither threatening nor a trouble-maker; generally his anxiety makes him conciliatory and so he is accepted, but if he becomes aggressive he will be rejected and remain odd man out.

Generally some companionship with other children develops, with interdependence and yet some competitiveness. Some definition of function is worked out and an efficient co-operative group is formed, which presumably has its basis in the hunting group of primitive man. The special bond which then develops between the boys has thus a very ancient history. This relationship, with or without overt homosexuality, has been a source of strength in war (in various armies of the past) as well as in hunting. Some degree of rivalry still exists, and this can be met in games which allow self-expression within the over-riding needs of the team. The formation of in-groups may be seen even more obviously in adolescents (see p. 242). The companionship between girls has perhaps a rather different basis; their roles in primitive societies were very different and for them a relationship with a male became more important. Nevertheless friendship, more or less intense, satisfies a major need in nearly every human being.

In either sex, much misery and anger may be caused by the sense of not belonging to any group. The rejected boy or girl is isolated, and the temptation is to respond by despair or by anger — which will emphasise his 'difference' and provoke counter-aggression; he may well become a scapegoat. Even if this is minor and temporary it may condition him to the dislike and fear of other people in groups, and to becoming aggressive (or conversely over-conciliatory) to them. Without the basic satisfaction of belonging to a group, other satisfactions can scarcely be achieved.

BEHAVIOUR PROBLEMS AT SCHOOL

Aggressive, uncontrolled behaviour (or stealing) disrupting the school group may be reported by the school, though it may pass unnoticed or not exist in the home. In very rare cases a neurological disturbance is involved but most often the problem requires to be traced back to its origin in the family environment. The child has not been able to adapt socially and obtain acceptable social satisfaction. Discipline at home may be so rigid and ubiquitous that the child has no experience or understanding of social rules which develop spontaneously among his peers in the school group. On the other hand the deprived child may have developed an understandable philosophy of getting what he can, when he can.

Treatment consists of counselling, psychotherapy and/or welfare help. In some cases placement in boarding school is advisable and if the disturbance is severe, special schools for maladjusted children alone are equipped to tolerate persistent antisocial behaviour.

LEARNING DIFFICULTIES

Children may be referred at any age, but more especially about the ages of 7, 8, or 9 (according to school and family standards) when it is becoming clear that they are not mastering the basic subjects, especially reading and writing, which are essential for further progress.

Psychological assessment may indicate inferior intelligence, for instance an IQ between 60 and 80. It should be remembered that low intelligence affecting scholastic achievement may be masked by reasonably good social and practical competence and sometimes by denial and pressure of the child's parents. Remedial teaching can be organized in borderline cases, and special ESN schooling offers the child below an IQ of 70 the opportunity of progressing at the slower pace more suited to his possibilities.

In many cases however the child is clearly of average or even high intelligence. Physical handicaps may be responsible, such as hearing and visual defect, or more discrete mid-brain damage affecting, for instance, spatial orientation. A detailed history often reveals disturbances in essential learning areas during the pre-school period which may produce difficulties in communication and motivation for learning. Motivation is an important factor and may be at a low level. A child may react negatively to competitive situations and respond to failure by withdrawal. The social and educational standards of the family may offer little support for a child's scholastic efforts. Cultural and linguistic differences in immigrant families can also present problems.

Dyslexia is a specific disability in writing and reading, with letter reversals, associated with uncertain cerebral dominance expressed for instance by crossed laterality, and in some cases with a mild degree of paresis. Environmental factors are frequently involved and require investigation and consideration in treating the condition.

Treatment consists of correction, where possible, of physical handicaps, remedial teaching, welfare help for the family; and psychotherapy when learning is inhibited by a complex personality disturbance.

TRUANCY

The children involved are often of low intelligence and come from poor social backgrounds. They are absent only occasionally and tend to play in streets and parks, or go to cinemas rather than stay at home. This should be distinguished from refusal to go to school.

SCHOOL REFUSAL

Although the emphasis is put at first on the school situation, this is almost invariably a deeper problem involving the home. Bullying, or physical timidity or fear of a particular teacher, often associated with physical symptoms such as headaches or recurrent infections, are presented as the cause of the disturbance. Although these need to be taken into account the real problem is that the child does not so much avoid school, as cling to the parents, usually to mother; illness in the family may trigger off fears about the parents' health or safety. Treatment consists of counselling and psychotherapy with the child, and usually the mother, to remedy the disturbance in their relationship. It is important also to help the child get quickly back to school, or to an alternative establishment such as small tutorial groups.

DIFFICULTIES AT PUBERTY

The approach of puberty reawakens unsolved problems of the intensely emotional pre-school period, and often produces disturbances at school. Difficulties in study, rebellious disruptive behaviour, and indiscreet sexual activities may present at this period and may continue throughout adolescence. It is possible for personality disturbances such as hysterical and obsessional patterns to take on the characteristics of major neurotic disorders. At this stage help in dealing with anxiety is very valuable as it may prevent hardening of these neurotic defences against it. Early signs of schizophrenic breakdown must also be watched for.

In all cases, good relationships with schools, and education and welfare authorities, are essential and direct contact with the schools through the clinic's psychologist will smoothe many difficulties and avoid many misunderstandings.

FURTHER READING

Eibl-Eibesfeldt, I. (1971). *Love and Hate*. Methuen, London.

Hersov, L. A. (1960). 'Persistent non-attendance at school'. *J. Child Psychol. Psychiat.*, 1, 130.

Ingram, T. T. A. (1969). 'Disorders of speech in childhood'. *Brit. J. Hosp. Med.*, 2, 1608.

Rutter, M., Tizard, J. and Whitmore, K. (1970). *Education, Health and Behaviour*. Longmans, Green, London.

Rutter, M. and Yule, W. (1973). 'Specific reading retardation'. In Mann, L. and Sabatino, D. (eds.), *First Review of Special Education*, Butterwood Farms, Philadelphia.

Tiger, L. and Fox, R. (1972). *The Imperial Animal*. Secker and London.

39 *Adolescence*

NORMAL ADOLESCENT DEVELOPMENT

Adolescence can be defined as that period between childhood and adulthood which is marked by the physical and emotional changes associated with puberty and the gradual development of an independent personality. It begins somewhere between the ages of 12 and 14 and ends at about the age of 20.

Until quite recently the attitude prevailed that adolescence is a period of upheaval in the person's life, that it is of trouble to the person himself and to his environment, and that it is a relief to everybody when it has passed and the person has become 'mature'. But, as we learn more about adolescence as a period of physical, psychological and social development, we see that this period is crucial in the person's whole emotional development, and that what occurs during adolescence is valuable in its own right and affects future mental health and social relationships.

Every adolescent experiences psychological stress at some

period. It is possible, in spite of this, to isolate four common areas which are of special importance in affecting the adolescent's behaviour and where major changes must take place if the person is to develop towards 'psychological maturity'.

1 *His relationship to his parents.* By this is meant the ability during this period to change from dependence on the parents to greater emotional independence. The adolescent should learn to formulate and accept his thoughts and feelings as his own and to become less dependent on how his parents may react. This can be formulated as follows: Is the adolescent able to separate emotionally from the parents, even if this means that his parents may not approve of his way of going about it?

2 *The view which the adolescent has of himself as a physically mature person.* Included in this is the adolescent's acceptance of himself as a masculine or feminine person, capable of functioning sexually, as well as his ability to change his picture of himself from that of a child who was mainly in the care of his parents to becoming somebody who feels that he is the owner of his body with the right to choose and be responsible for his own actions.

3 *His relations with his companions.* He is likely at this time to change from an old group of friends to a new one; he will need their support even more if he is losing that of his parents. He will therefore need once again to try to 'belong' (see p. 238) as he did first at school, but the forms of behaviour here will be more complex: and at this stage many small 'in-groups' or gangs form (sometimes of one sex, sometimes of both): their own insecurity makes them more suspicious of outsiders, and elaborate rituals may occur firstly to test out, and secondly to celebrate the admission of a newcomer.

Most human groups therefore develop customs which do this. Greeting rituals throughout the world have this common basis, although they appear very different. The acceptance of the newcomer may be signified by some ceremony of initiation which provokes some pride in the initiate and some horror on the part of others if they hear about it. Similar customs occur later in life and interesting parallels have been drawn between Red Indians, primitive African tribes and more (or less) civilised universities of the Western World.

4 *His heterosexual status.* This develops at different ages in

different cultures, but is clearly an area of potential conflict and doubt. Casual testing-out relationships can only be regarded as natural; yet they are prone to leave one or other with a sense of rejection, resentment or despair, if they go badly. Moreover, in cultures which place considerable emphasis on the need for sexual satisfaction at this stage, girls and boys may be pressed to try to find it before they are emotionally ready or have any skill, and so suffer again from a sense of failure (see p. 106).

PSYCHIATRIC ILLNESS IN ADOLESCENCE

Minor symptoms

There are quite a number of young people who experience some stresses in one or more of these areas. Sometimes this stress is only temporary, but there are times when it is a sign of more serious psychological trouble and when the formula 'you will grow out of it' is completely meaningless. Often these difficulties are not entirely new but have in some form existed since childhood and have become more noticeable and troublesome as the result of the changes the adolescent has to deal with, causing him some degree of anxiety or depression or both. The adolescent may begin to feel more isolated, more worried about how he is developing physically and emotionally. It is as if the solutions which the child was able to call upon, especially from parents, are no longer of much use when he reaches adolescence, and trouble spots become more difficult to conceal.

It is very important to note if the adolescent is failing in any of the areas mentioned, partly because help given to adolescents at this stage can prevent more serious illness later on, and partly because the person is at a point in his life when major decisions which will affect his whole future life have to be taken, especially with regard to education, work, the family and sexual behaviour.

Sexual problems

1 *Masturbation guilt.* Masturbation only constitutes a problem if it is associated with excessive conflict, guilt or anxiety. We are

now a long way from the mistaken view that masturbation must not take place because it is wrong. We know that it is a normal activity which reaches its height during adolescence. In fact, masturbation contributes to normal psychological development in that it gives the person the opportunity to experience sexual feelings within the temporary safety of his fantasies and thoughts. But at the same time we know that some adolescents, usually those who are also disturbed in other areas, experience extreme guilt and shame, or even feel that they are harming their bodies and brain. Sometimes reassurance can be of help to such adolescents provided, of course, that one has made it as easy as possible for them to mention their problem; but in those in whom this is only one aspect of a wider disturbance, more formal psychotherapeutic help may be necessary.

2 *Homosexuality.* Again, a period during which adolescent boys and girls experience love and sexual feelings towards members of their own sex is almost universal and constitutes a normal phase of development. Sometimes, however, it causes them undue guilt, anxiety or depression, particularly if they fear that they may remain homosexual, or if they are subjected to an attitude of strong disapproval or even punishment, e.g. at school. In such cases reassurance may help to allay their fears but in some cases more formal psychotherapy may be needed, especially if there is an undue amount of guilt and depression. On the whole the less guilty the adolescent is, the sooner are heterosexual interests likely to appear (see also p. 249).

Identity crisis of adolescence

This is the commonest form of psychiatric illness in adolescents and it may present in many different ways. It has been described in detail by Erikson (1956, 1958). As the result of the changes the adolescent is undergoing, he may feel lost in almost all aspects of his existence and be unable to develop an identity of his own. Neither child nor adult; torn by the desire to rebel against the parents and invite their disapproval, and yet to retain their sympathy; unsure of his sexual role and often troubled by sexual guilt; without any ideas about his plans for work or career in the future, and often disillusioned by his present occupation, if any, perhaps at school or university;

afraid of close relationships and involvement and yet lonely in his isolation, he may break down more or less completely.

Such a breakdown may take on many forms. If he is fortunate enough to know whom to go to for help, and if he can overcome his reluctance to do so early on, he may present himself with one or more of these problems, e.g. his difficulty in deciding on a career, before he is seriously ill. Or he may present with depression, sometimes partly concealed, or so severe that he may have made a suicidal attempt; occasionally these are successful. And again, he may develop symptoms of acute anxiety, hysterical or obsessional symptoms; or he may develop a psychosomatic disorder, e.g. a duodenal ulcer, migraine or asthma, or less clearly defined physical symptoms which hide the underlying emotional disturbance. Occasionally he may appear completely withdrawn, or alternatively, in a state of acute excitement, confused, disorientated and unable to express himself coherently so that it may be difficult to distinguish between a severe, but temporary adolescent crisis and a schizophrenic illness. Observation over a period of time may be the only way of reaching a decision.

Lastly, the disorder may not have led to illness or suffering on the part of the adolescent himself but instead he may have developed a severe behaviour disturbance so that he causes distress or even danger to others, for example his parents; he may then be brought to his doctor or a psychiatrist, against his will, by parents, school authorities or the courts. Aggressive, violent and delinquent behaviour or drug taking are the commonest forms.

Anorexia nervosa in adolescent girls is dealt with separately (p. 196).

Rebellion against their parents or their elders must be regarded as part of normal adolescence, and a search for some independence; which hopefully for both sides may lead to an interdependent relationship between more mature people. But it is common enough for children to react in ways which outrage their parents — especially if the child chooses behaviour which the parents were never allowed to think of in their childhood: and antagonism, non-understanding, guilt and self-justification grow on each side. Parents who treat their children as toys are naturally hurt if the child criticises them — and feel it is very unfair 'after they've brought the child into this world solely for their own good, and sacrificed so much for him'. Children made to feel guilty respond by behaving more exaggeratedly, or worse by withdrawing. Parents who give too much independence to their children may seem not to care: those who give too much care stifle independence. Small wonder both parents and children feel they can't win. Yet each at this stage needs the other, perhaps as never before, and if earlier a good relationship has been formed, patience and the display of as much affection as can be accepted will get both through. Talking to friends may help both sides.

In other adolescents the search for independence may be less strong than the desire to remain attached to the parent or family; to which an over-possessive or over-dominating parent may have contributed. Here too behaviour disorders, generally masked, or indirect, passive aggression towards the parents may occur, but the disapproval which follows produces more fear, more sullenness and more confusion about identity. It is extremely difficult to break through this stage without professional help for both parents and the adolescent.

At this stage in particular, resentments and anxieties may become fixed and form the basis of future behaviour disorders, or psychoneurotic conditions.

TREATMENT

Psychotherapy

Here the GP may be able to persuade them to accept treatment, if he can gain the trust of both sides and help each to understand the other. But more skilled psychotherapy will often be needed.

Adolescents often resist the idea that they might need psychotherapy on account of their mistrust and unwillingness to reveal their feelings to anyone else, especially someone belonging to the generation of their parents. In fact, sometimes, they have to be allowed to find their own solutions. If they are not too seriously ill, a so-called psycho-social moratorium, i.e. a period in which they are left to themselves, may be the best way for them to solve their own problems and to develop an identity of their own. However, others do need regular psychotherapy and once they see that the therapist is on their side, and that instead of imposing his own views on them, he is there to listen and to understand their problems, they often form a useful psychotherapeutic relationship with him.

Work with the parents may be necessary, too, if only to help them, but it is often better for them to be seen by a psychiatric social worker or someone else who can make the parents understand their son's or daughter's problems better; otherwise the adolescent may begin to suspect that his therapist, if he sees his parents as well, may betray his confidence or even side with them against him.

Drugs

These may be necessary in addition to psychotherapy if the patient is seriously depressed, anxious or shows signs of frank psychotic or borderline schizophrenic symptoms; the choice of drug will largely depend on the nature of the symptoms.

Inpatient treatment

This may occasionally be the only way of handling a severe adolescent illness or behaviour disturbance, e.g. if the adolescent is suicidal, tries to mutilate himself, is so aggressive that he tries to damage others or is smashing windows, or if he is going through a psychotic episode. Such adolescents are best treated in special units for adolescents with staff who are used to working with them.

BIBLIOGRAPHY

Blos, P. (1962). *On Adolescence.* The Free Press, New York.

Erikson, E. H. (1956). 'The problem of ego identity'. *J. Amer. Psychoanal. Ass.*, 4, 56.

Erikson, E. H. (1958). *Young Man Luther.* Faber, London.

Freud, A. (1958). 'Adolescence', *Psychoanalytic Study of the Child.* vol. 13.

Laufer, M. (1966). *Danger Signs and Prediction in Adolescence.* Case Conference, vol. 13, no. 6.

Laufer, M. (1975). *Adolescent Disturbance and Breakdown*. Penguin.
Mead, M. (1949). *Male and Female*. Gollancz, London.
Miller, D. (1967). 'Family interaction and adolescent therapy'. In Lomas, P. (ed.), *The Predicament of the Family*. Hogarth, London.
Winnicott, D. W. (1965). *The Family and Individual Development*. Tavistock Publications, London.

40 Homosexuality

SOCIAL ATTITUDES

Homosexuality, both male and female, has existed in every form of society to a greater or lesser degree, some societies being approving, others disapproving. Female homosexuality or lesbianism has met with much less disapproval than male homosexuality, and both were widely accepted in Ancient Greece; thus the term lesbianism is derived from the Aegean island of Lesbos where the poetess Sappho expressed overt homosexual longings in beautiful poems, and male homosexuality was idealized in classical times.

In this country, on the other hand, male homosexuality was until recently a criminal offence, but the Act of Parliament which arose from the Wolfenden Report (1957) has removed these legal penalties and allows homosexual relationships between consenting adults. Much fear and blackmail has thus been removed, but male homosexual relationships with a person under the age of 16 are still a punishable offence. Female homosexuality has never been illegal. In spite of the change in the law there is, however, still a good deal of prejudice against homosexuality in our society; this may cause guilt in individual homosexuals and make it harder for them to feel accepted thus adding further problems to those which they may have already. In fact, problems in homosexual relationships are common, especially among males, just as psychosexual problems frequently occur in heterosexual relationships too. It is essential that doctors should treat patients presenting with problems connected with their homosexuality with sympathy and frankness and without condemnation or disapproval, as in the case of heterosexuals. It must also be realised that many people have a bisexual orientation and may at different times have relations with members of both sexes.

NATURE

As with heterosexuality, homosexual behaviour includes varying proportions of tender affection and physical passion. The emotional bond between the two partners may be as strong as between heterosexuals; this applies particularly to women whose lesbian relationships are often stable and long lasting; relationships between male homosexuals, though they can be equally stable and mutually emotionally satisfying, tend to be more casual and short-lived, especially if the homosexual orientation is associated with a personality disorder and emotional immaturity. In such cases the absence of any meaningful or lasting relationship is often a source of dissatisfaction, jealousy, loneliness and depression.

Homosexual attraction usually leads to overt sexual behaviour if both partners are willing, but conflict and guilt, partly engendered by social pressures, may prevent or limit physical expression. Orgasm between persons of the same sex is obtained by means of mutual masturbation, anal intercourse, fellatio (intercourse via the mouth) or cunnilingus (stimulation of the vulva with the mouth and tongue); these variations are, of course, also commonly used in heterosexual relationships. In both male and female homosexuality either partner may at times assume the more active or more passive role. In lesbian relations an artificial phallus may be used to effect penetration.

Incidence

The most complete studies have been the Kinsey reports on the sex-life of cross-sections of the white American population. In a sample of 4000 males it was estimated that 4% remained exclusively homosexual all their lives, and 37% had had some adult homosexual experiences leading to orgasm. Assuming that the figures in Great Britain are comparable this means that there are approximately 1,000,000 exclusively homosexual males in the population.

Available figures for women are less reliable but are lower than in men; Kenyon (1970) estimates that about one in 45 of the adult female population, just under 2%, is exclusively homosexual, about half as many as in the case of male homosexuals.

Origins of homosexuality

In spite of claims to the contrary there is no conclusive evidence that genetic or endocrine factors play a significant role in the origin of human homosexuality. Environmental influences in childhood and later life (see p. 105) seem to be the main determining factors. Homosexuality can occur in people who have a well integrated personality, often with creative and artistic gifts but, just as in people who are heterosexual, there may be an associated personality disorder or mental illness. It is best not to regard homosexuality as such as abnormal, and even less as an 'illness', but to regard it as a variation of the normal range of human behaviour, and to assess instead whether the personality as a whole is in some way or other immature or disturbed, or whether it is relatively stable and integrated.

All people are endowed from birth with bisexual instinctual drives, and all children and adolescents pass through various phases of being attached to and attracted by persons of either sex, the parents being the earliest and most important. The relationship of the child to its parents and their personalities will largely determine the child's development and its future predisposition to homosexuality. In the case of male homosexuals the following influences are especially important:

1 A dominating and seductive mother who encourages her boy to identify with her rather than with his father; and who by increasing his sexual attachment to her may cause him to feel guilty about his sexual feelings towards her and hence towards other women later in life.
2 Absence of, or weakness in the father which makes identification with him impossible or difficult to achieve; or a tyrannical father towards whom the boy can only adopt a

passive, submissive, feminine attitude. Other factors include guilt feelings concerning sexual attraction towards a sister, or excessive attachment to a brother which may lead to later attachments to other men. A persistent desire to fuse with someone who is as near as possible identical with oneself ('narcissistic object choice') may underlie the wish to choose a sexual partner of the same sex. Later in life fear of women and disappointments or failure in heterosexual relationships or an all-male background may reinforce a tendency towards homosexuality laid down at earlier stages of development.

SYMPTOMS DUE TO HOMOSEXUALITY

Anxiety about homosexuality may lead to an anxiety state or other psychoneurotic or psychosomatic symptoms, or it may lead to repression which can give rise to various difficulties and conflicts, e.g. extreme hostility to any manifestation of homosexuality in other people or excessive displays of masculinity, often associated with attempts at heterosexual promiscuity (the Don Juan type in the male, and nymphomania in the female). As in heterosexuality, disappointments in homosexual relationships are a common cause of depression, all the more so as being exclusively homosexual prevents marriage and having children which may create a fear of loneliness and isolation. Repressed homosexuality may also be a factor in causing a paranoid psychosis.

MANAGEMENT

Clearly, homosexuals will come to consult a doctor and ask for treatment only if they are in some way dissatisfied with their sexual orientation or if it has led to symptoms for which they need help; unless they have been referred by a court, e.g. in the case of homosexual relationships with children; as in heterosexuals this is almost always a sign of an underlying, severe personality disorder.

In many cases the aim of treatment will be to help the person concerned to come to terms with his homosexual or bisexual orientation and to help him overcome his guilt feelings and to establish more stable and meaningful relationships. In others who wish to achieve a heterosexual orientation more basic change in personality and behaviour is needed; in many instances it may not be clear at the outset of treatment how far this will be possible, and the aim of therapy will have to be more clearly defined as treatment proceeds. The two main forms of therapy in use are psychotherapy and behaviour therapy.

1 *Psychotherapy*. Depending on the aim and the presence or severity of an underlying personality disorder this will vary from supportive therapy or once weekly insight-directed psychotherapy, individually or in a group, to psychoanalysis which may last for several years (see p. 308). In order to achieve a change in sexual orientation treatment will have to be intensive and much work will have to be done on the patient's early childhood experiences and its consequences, and on his fantasy life and repressed conflicts. Even then a satisfactory outcome cannot be predicted.

2 *Behaviour therapy*. In some cases attempts have been made by means of aversion therapy (see p. 330) to decondition the patient to his attraction to male figures and then to condition him to develop an attraction to women. However, this is unlikely to be successful if there is a severe underlying personality disorder; and if the patient were to lose his attraction to men and fail to get attracted to women he might be worse off than before and get severely depressed. Alternatively, if fear of women is thought to be the main factor which underlies his homosexuality attempts can be made to desensitise him so that he overcomes his fears and becomes free to relate to women. Behaviour therapy is gradually becoming more integrated with psychodynamic concepts, and it is possible that a combination of both approaches may help some patients who are strongly motivated to change their sexual orientation.

REFERENCES

Bancroft, J. H. . (1970). 'Homosexuality in the male'. *Brit. J. Hosp. Med.*, 3, 168.

Freud, S. (1905). *Three Essays on Sexuality*. Standard edition, Hogarth, London, vol. 7.
Kenyon, F. E. (1970). 'Homosexuality in the female'. *Brit. J. Hosp. Med.*, 3, 183.
Kinsey, A. C., Pomeroy, W. B. and Martin, C. E. (1948). *Sexual Behaviour in the Human Male*. Saunders, Philadelphia.
Kinsey, A. C., Pomeroy, W. B., Martin, C. E. and Gebhard, P. H. (1953). *Sexual Behaviour in the Human Female*. Saunders, Philadelphia.

FURTHER READING

Baldwin, J. (1962). *Another Country*. Corgi, London.
Renault, M. (1959). *The Charioteer*. New English Library, London.
These novels beautifully describe the experience of homosexual relationships.

41 Marriage

Marriage in our culture is a social institution which lays the basis for family life and the rearing of children. From a psychological point of view it has both positive and negative aspects and its success or failure depends on a variety of factors. These include particularly the personalities of the two partners, their abilities or otherwise to allow each other sufficient freedom to retain their individuality, and at the same time to accept the limitations imposed by a close and monogamous relationship.

RESPONSIBILITIES AND DEPENDENCE.

Marriage implies the taking over of the roles and responsibilities which in childhood were felt to be the exclusive right and duty of one's parents and the whole 'adult' world. These include especially responsibilities for other people; firstly by entering into an interdependent relationship with one other person, the spouse, and giving up considerable independence in doing so;

and later possibly by protecting and caring for children — a role which later still would have to be modified as the children grow up. Earlier conflicts about dependence versus independence and security in relation to their own parents may be re-activated in one or both marriage partners.

One partner may feel very anxious in a situation where he is dependent on the other one for his needs as this activates memories of his experiences as a child when he was similarly dependent on his mother or father to satisfy earlier needs. This could, for instance, lead to fear of uncontrollable anger at any sign of possible frustration, or to overt outbursts of rage. Others may avoid this anxiety by choosing a partner who will seem to be dependent on them so that they feel the stronger of the two; and this domination may arouse resentment. The possible combinations are endless: the classic solutions of compromise or 'spheres of influence' do not always work.

SEXUAL ANXIETIES

At the same time the sexual relationship within marriage may lead to anxieties about one's sexual role and functions; for a woman her fears about being sexually attractive, responsive and feminine, for a man his masculine potency. These two aspects can easily get into conflict, as can be seen superficially by arguments between marriage partners as to how the responsibilities of running a home and family should be shared between them. A wife may feel rejected and devalued if her husband doesn't help with the housework, especially if she envies his male role; the husband may feel it as a demand for submission, and an infringement on his masculinity, if he accedes to her demands for help, especially if he is ashamed of, or not enough in touch with, his feminine side, or unsure of his male role. Because marriage implies dependency of each partner on the other for satisfaction of sexual and emotional needs, very real and deep anxiety within the relationship can be aroused by one partner in the other.

Further, one or other or both partners may have entered marriage with lack of knowledge, inhibition or fear of sexuality; on the other hand a partner may function well in a purely sexual role but may be unable to fuse sex with the affection necessary for a satisfactory marital relationship. Sexual satisfaction by itself is not sufficient but must be combined with tenderness, love and genuine understanding of the other partner's emotional and sexual needs. (As it has been put, 'many partners need to learn skill at the breakfast table, more than skill in bed'.) Hence it is a pity when at school only the physical side of sex is taught, divorced from the emotional side; it is worse if sexual 'success' becomes a status symbol.

FOCUS FOR CONFLICT

Temperamental differences and frustrations in sex may thus lead to emotional tension in many areas; it may be focussed on the children, the in-laws, the husband's job, the wife's career or hobbies, or an extra-marital relationship of either partner. And conflicts may lead to regression within the relationship; the feeling of becoming a child in relation to one's partner is present more in a marriage relationship than in most others. The degree of anxiety about oneself is related to the need a person has for reassurance and will be the measure of the demand which is made on the other partner to supply this reassurance. The anxiety may be mostly on a sexual level, i.e. 'Am I satisfactory in my sexual role?'. The conflict aroused may be due to the unrealistic ideals of sexual behaviour that have been set up in one person — e.g. sexual intercourse is only allowable at certain times or in certain places or in a certain manner, in order for that person to feel that it is 'normal' behaviour, and the suggestion or wish to break these rules is disturbing. Sexual failures easily occur (see p. 104), especially between people who have grown up with different 'rules' or patterns of satisfaction, often related to fantasy, or to previous sexual relationships with others before marriage.

These same conflicts may be expressed mainly through arguments, e.g. about money. The wife who criticizes her husband for not earning enough may be expressing anxiety about her husband's masculinity, or a wife's anxiety to earn some money of her own may be the expression of her anxiety at feeling dependent for all her needs on her husband. Most couples normally find ways of arranging their lives in such a way as to deal with these anxieties without help: but some fail to do so, and indulge in *constant* quarrelling about roles or money. Children and their upbringing or behaviour may be another source of argument and any serious problems there, violence towards a child by either parent, for instance, should be viewed as a symptom of trouble in the marriage. All this is particularly likely if the partners have chosen each other on a neurotic basis; e.g. a woman who after a childhood of emotional deprivation is still looking for a mother and therefore marries a gentle, maternal, somewhat effeminate man may later on, perhaps, after she has had her first child, wish that her husband were more potent and masculine. Under such circumstances she may begin to resent him and accuse him of weakness which may give rise to disagreements and rows as described. Much toleration of one partner by the other is needed, for every person has parts of him or herself that he feels ashamed of and feels are either signs of abnormality or of childishness. In marriage reassurance is sought that these parts of oneself are at least partly accepted by the other partner and that one is still loved and not rejected or despised because of them. In marriage we seek to recreate, unrealistically, an idealised childhood situation where the mother is supposed to love her child and to accept it totally despite its 'naughtiness', where all the old childhood fears of not being loved or of being rejected are thus reactivated in the relationship. If frustrated by the other one, each partner may make ever increasing demands leading to further frustration and mutual resentment and estrangement. They may often also project aspects of their own personalities on the other one and then accuse him or her of attitudes and behaviour which they dislike in themselves.

But this must not obscure the fact that some of these problems are real irritants in their own right. Children may provoke a split between their parents. Elsewhere we have seen the problems of a child's unresolved Oedipal rivalry. What of the father's jealousy and fear of his son's power over or attraction to his mother? What of the mother's fear of being surpassed by a beautiful young daughter?

The presence of a possessive or dominating mother-in-law can wreck a marriage from the start; the need to care for elderly parents produces anxiety and guilt — even, and perhaps more so, when the parents don't make obvious demands, but suffer in lonely silence. Housing conditions are often still appalling and may be further complicated by too many children to cope with.

Many jobs make demands which make the wife feel that the husband is married to the job (medicine is one of them: see p. 260). A career for the wife may satisfy part of her, but deprive her of some of the satisfaction of running a happy home and family; many women, particularly those who had a satisfying career before getting married, suffer from a conflict between wanting to be a wife and mother and wanting a career of their own. This may lead to envy of the husband's greater freedom, a tendency to criticise and attack him, and this in turn makes him angry and resentful of his wife, and more inclined to work longer, and go into his shell at home.

Apart from all these, there are differences of temperament, likes and dislikes on minor matters, which make living together a matter of patience and skill; solid affection from the start could overcome it, but many partners start not with solid affection, but with passion; and this may not last, nor does it always lead on to patience. Some partners of course have started without either, though less now than formerly.

Many couples are capable of working through such situations, with the help of strong physical attraction and the accompanying feelings of tenderness, and such conflicts are solved and anxieties reassured simply by each other's help. Even feelings of emotional or sexual dependence may be satisfactorily resolved by reaching partnership and a real interdependence; and the relationship may deepen with age and increasing respect and responsibility, even if occasional friction is inevitable. But in some marriages conflicts remain unsolved, friction gets worse, struggles for dominance ensue and interests diverge, and the danger of all this occurring is presumably one reason why civil and ecclesiastical authorities have produced very strict rules to protect the sanctity of marriage, however much they protest simultaneously that this sanctity is a natural state and should need no such protection. Keeping marriages together by such sanctions is seldom the best way to happiness and has in the past produced intense misery by no means redeemed by the opportunity for self-sacrifice given to the 'weaker' spouse. Professional help is needed.

TREATMENT

Patients with marital problems sometimes come to the GP for help; sometimes they are prepared to state their troubles openly, if onesidedly; more often they make an excuse to seek advice on some other less embarrassing subject, and then hesitantly broach the problem, if the GP gives them time and encouragement to do so. Patients in hospital, similarly, may confide in their doctor, nurse, or student. He or she must, therefore, be alive to this approach. Some patients, of course, are unaware of their true feelings towards their partner, and the indications they give will be more evident to the doctor than to themselves — though they may be obvious to the partner. Sometimes the patient will present with psychological or psychosomatic symptoms which are due to marital tension, even though the patient may be unaware of this, or a child is brought to the doctor with physical symptoms or behaviour disorder caused by the patient's own marital problems.

If the doctor is a close friend of either, he is less likely to receive their confidence than if he simply has a professional relationship; each partner appears to need to feel that the doctor is impersonal, but warmly sympathetic; utterly experienced in every sort of emotional or sexual problem but beyond reproach in his personal life; able to sense what is meant when it is not said, and to forget it when it wasn't meant — all with no sense of incongruity!

How much skill and experience will be required to deal with marital disharmony must of course depend on its depth, its duration, and, above all, the basic compatibility and love between the two, and their genuine desire to get closer. If these are strong much can be achieved. Unfortunately many couples have allowed petty irritations, rivalries and disappointments to fester, for they have repressed their feelings, perhaps at first for good reasons; but later one has adopted a pattern of behaviour and come to accept him or herself as a martyr, or a tyrant even, and take the slight satisfactions got from this as a substitute for the deeper satisfactions. Even so, it may be possible for a sympathetic listener to allow the two to regain their adjustment and get out of the vicious circles of antagonism which have arisen. Obviously the GP must be most careful to avoid taking sides. He may go so far as to use counselling techniques or to see husband and wife together. But he must avoid advice to precipitate action; he must remember that changes often occur in his patients' attitudes after they have left him, if he has done his job well, and that they may then get on better terms again. Occasionally they use him as an umpire to see that the other observes the rules: but this at least means their conflict has become more of a game, and less of a war.

While much misery can be helped by these simple measures by the GP, Marriage Guidance Counsellor, nurse, student or friend, it must be admitted that there are many problems which arise from deeper personality conflicts in one or both partners and need psychiatric help, and opportunities exist for marital therapy, singly or as a pair, at a few clinics. A behavioural approach has also been used to modify the partners' sexual interaction which offers considerable hope if this is the basic problem, and not a focus for other conflicts (see p. 109). If all these approaches fail both partners may need help to face the fact that the marriage has broken down and that separation or divorce may be the only solution.

WIVES OF PROFESSIONAL PEOPLE

Special problems exist for the wives, and less often the husbands, of professional people. Resentment at being left with a humdrum job, and at getting too little help with the chores and the children, jealousy that her husband has all the interest and glamour, disappointment at seeing too little of him, all these occur in many walks of life, politics, business, the services, industry, aviation, the law, the church and medicine. If it is the husband who has to take second place to a wife with a successful career it may be more difficult still for him to adopt a more masculine role at home and this may produce further problems in the family.

The GP's wife is an example of someone exposed to all these stresses, and others which are peculiar to her position. She is asked to play a series of different roles, mostly subordinate, throughout the course of the day, and night; and all under difficult conditions, which her husband may not fully understand, taken up as he is with everyone else's troubles. Besides this, she is faced with a number of quite conflicting expectations from his practice. How much does she know of the illnesses or personalities of the patients? Can she give her husband sympathy when he needs to let off his exasperation at his patients, or the government? Or would it be better if he told her nothing, so that she resents being left out?

The phrase 'are you married to me, or to your job?' must have been used in almost every profession which attracts conscientious people. Resentments are bound to occur, and some needs bound to be neglected. If these difficulties can be realised early, before patterns of disgruntlement become fixed, all will be well; but under pressure, they are easily ignored. In an attempt to bring them to discussion the College of General Practitioners has collected tape recordings (Tredgold 1974).

INFERTILITY

Many patients complain of infertility either to their GP or to an infertility clinic. Physical causes in both partners must be looked for, and treated if possible. Emotional tension in either or both partners can be a significant factor either by interfering with satisfactory sexual relationships or preventing them altogether, or possibly more directly by reducing the likelihood of conception. Infertility in turn often causes anxiety and depression. The psychological aspects need investigating and psychotherapy for the woman or the couple may be helpful. If the husband turns out to be infertile artificial insemination from a donor (AID) may be considered but it has its own psychological complications which need to be taken into full consideration and dealt with. Adoption is also a possible solution, but it too has its risks (see p. 380).

FURTHER READING

Crowe, M. J. (1973). 'Conjoint marital therapy: advice or interpretation?'. *J. Psychosom. Res.*, 17, 309.

Dicks, H. V. (1967). *Marital Tensions*. Routledge, London.

Friedman, L. J. (1962). *Virgin Wives: a study of unconsummated marriages*. Tavistock Publications, London.

'Medica' (1955). *Any Wife or Any Husband*. Heinemann, London.

Skynner, A. C. R. (1968). 'A group-analytic approach to conjoint family therapy'. *J. Child Psychol. Psychiat.*, 100, 81.

Tredgold, R. F. (1974). 'Jill of All Trades and Mistress . . .?'. Audiotape, cat. no. 74/491. Medical Recording Service Foundation, Chelmsford.

Van der Velde, T. H. (1953). *Ideal Marriage*. Heinemann, London.

42 Pregnancy, childbirth and parenthood

ANXIETIES IN PREGNANCY

Every woman experiences some degree of anxiety during pregnancy. This is natural in the state of medicine when we have only partially controlled the hazards which arise. Maternal deaths are extremely rare, but pregnant women are liable to various forms of morbidity, and at a teaching hospital where all the multiparae who are admitted are so because of their previous bad history, there is an inevitable perinatal death-rate.

During the first three months women do not know whether or not they will lose their pregnancy. The first trimester is also a time of intense physiological change and many symptoms which are not dangerous can seem frightening when encountered for the first time. Hence, women in early pregnancy are more emotional than at other times.

Teaching girls about sex and childbirth differs enormously from one individual family to another and is very confused. Unfortunately, a great deal that is taught about childbirth is frightening and many of the methods of introducing sex to, or of concealing it from, girls give rise to considerable degrees of sex-guilt and trauma. These have their effect not only on the patterning of sex in early marriage but also upon a woman's apprehensions of the functions of her pelvis at childbirth.

Acute mental disturbance can arise during the first trimester in women who combine a vulnerable personality with an adverse life situation and these can temporarily threaten her life or sanity. Even a medical termination of pregnancy can give rise to guilt or remorse, and a criminal abortion can have far-reaching effects on the personality. Later infertility or still-births can be blamed on an abortion, and the sense of guilt in the mother will need long and patient disentangling and re-assurance (see p. 379).

Vomiting occurs in one-third to one-half of all pregnancies. It is entirely outside the control of the patient. It is much more likely to arise in women who have a previous history of gastro-intestinal disturbances. Though there is evidence that women who are ambivalent about pregnancy are likely to vomit more severely than women who are not, interpretations and exhortations make this symptom worse. It is improved by understanding and by anti-emetics and tranquilisers; only Largactil and Phenergan have not been questioned as potential sources of foetal abnormality, however, and many widely used anti-emetic drugs are suspect.

ATTITUDE TO THE ANTE-NATAL PATIENT

Though students and doctors when they are themselves patients encounter the same anxieties as other patients, and become disturbed by their loss of status within the hospital hierarchy, their usual attitude to the hospital environment is coloured by the fact that it is the milieu in which they themselves are enjoying an exciting and satisfying career which has been the target of their ambitions for some time. Patients, on the other hand, inevitably associate hospital with the sights, sounds and smells of hospital derived from childhood, and their past experience of illness, both in themselves and members of their families, which have been unpleasant and frightening. The student can do a great deal to mitigate this by being prepared to listen and to receive the patient in a careful and friendly way.

In the ante-natal clinic many women are encountering vaginal examinations for the first time in their lives. Women are unused to being undressed and examined in what, sometimes justifiably, seems to them a public place. Primiparae are especially apprehensive and ashamed and even multiparae never really get used to it.

In addition, mothers notice the contradiction between our insistence on the normality of childbirth as a physiological activity on the one hand, and our request to them to submit to physical examinations and physiological tests in order to ensure their safety and that of their infants.

Having a baby is widely assumed to be the goal of a woman's ambition; its advent, however, can bring so many changes into her social and economic relationships that she experiences mixed feelings and may even reject her pregnancy. Rejection is, to a certain degree, normal in the present state of society and must not be regarded as something which has to be condemned. Gross ambivalence needs to be given free expression and the woman who has been allowed to 'blow her top' is found more likely to settle down in later pregnancy than one who has not been allowed to do so.

LABOUR

Just before and during labour, many patients feel extremely anxious as to its outcome and this anxiety may emerge in the form of guilt feelings. These are most likely to relate to sexual behaviour and pelvic functions, including early childhood experience. Bowel interference and previous gynaecological operations naturally make for apprehension in labour; this also applies to cases where there have been sexual assaults.

There are a number of ways in which the contractions of labour can be made less uncomfortable. Education in natural childbirth and the methods of relaxation taught in ante-natal classes are undoubtedly of far greater value if the labour ward staff, including the students, believe in them and are prepared to assist the patient by putting them into practice. It is also possible to reduce the discomfort of labour by hypnosis or by talking to the patient carefully during her labour. During labour and delivery, the woman's experiences become much more frightening if she is left alone and if she is made to feel that she is making a fuss about her pain. It needs to be clear that adequate efforts are being made to relieve her discomfort. Though some of the anxieties which women in labour express may seem irrelevant or trivial, they should all be dealt with equally seriously if the patient is to remain confident and co-operative. It is important to give the mother, and not her attendant, the credit for having produced her own baby. Hysterical patients in labour should never be hit or scolded, however much this is advised by older midwives.

MOTHER-CHILD RELATIONSHIP

A normal mother-child relationship does not develop auto-matically in hospital, can easily be interrupted, and is always upset by any delay in the mother seeing her baby after delivery. A mother who is warned of this will not feel guilty or abnormal that she does not at once love her baby. To mitigate the adverse effects of separation, mothers should be encouraged to see their babies as much as possible and to feed them as soon as the baby is fit. In spite of this a great deal of anxiety is engendered, and mothers whose babies are in a special care unit a long time may have difficulty in forming a normal relationship and feel that the baby is not really theirs. They are also sometimes shocked by the appearance of the baby, especially if premature, in his incubator and by the rubber tubes and other medical impedi-menta with which the child is surrounded.

We are also aware that excessive anxiety about breast feeding can make a mother over-anxious, self-conscious about her capacity to secrete milk for her baby and spoil what should be a normal, enjoyable function. Breast feeding is not an instinctual process and there are many physical difficulties which can intervene and be mistaken for a psychological problem; nor should a mother be made to feel guilty if, for one reason or another she is unable to breast feed.

Mothers who have been insufficiently re-assured during their pregnancies and insufficiently supported in labour, can project their anxieties into the belief that there is something wrong with their baby. The normal mother-child relationship may also be adversely affected by experiences in labour or pregnancy which have seemed particularly painful and distressing. Blame for this can be projected on to the husband or the baby and can affect the family relationships.

If the father is going to play his essential part in the early development of the child he should not be excluded from the process of labour and should have an understanding of pregnancy, puerperium and all his wife's and child's needs when they get home. This does not mean that every father has to be present at the birth of his child.

PSYCHOTIC AND PSYCHONEUROTIC
REACTIONS IN THE PUERPERIUM

In any situation which combines pain, drugs, dehydration and upset of electrolyte balance, patients become disturbed and confused. Labour and the puerperium are no exceptions to this rule and following delivery a patient may react by being depressed, anxious, withdrawn, apathetic or hallucinated. Infection can exaggerate these reactions, and the first line of defence is to treat the underlying pathological and physiological disturbance. Many acute reactions in the puerperium are transient, responding to treatment combined with sedation.

Severe ante-natal and post-natal mental illness is uncommon and seldom occurs in the absence of previous adverse psychiatric history. There is nearly always a difficult situation in the home and the final precipitating factor may be an abnormal pregnancy. A history of maternal deprivation and emotional insecurity in their own childhood is common in women who develop severe mental illness during the puerperium. They often feel that they are not emotionally ready to be mothers and want to regress and be treated as babies themselves. Psychotic reactions after delivery occur in about 2 per 1,000 deliveries; they usually commence soon after or within a few weeks of delivery. Symptoms are either depressive or schizophrenic or both may co-exist. Fear of harming the baby is a common feature. Treatment in a mother-and-baby unit may be required; the condition tends to clear up more rapidly than similar mental illnesses in women of the same age who are not puerperal.

Neurotic depressive reactions are more common and may persist unless treated early on; the woman's worries usually centre round her baby, her marriage and the family.

Patients who are already suffering from mental illness may or may not become more acutely disturbed in pregnancy and the puerperium. They do, however, need careful supervision throughout their hospital care, and liaison with the general practitioner and health visitor for long-term care and follow-up supervision. They have a higher peri-natal mortality than other women. In general a great deal can be done to *prevent* psychiatric illness during pregnancy and the puerperium by encouraging women to talk freely about their conflicts and fears, and by providing psychotherapy for those who are more seriously disturbed. From the physical angle, hormonal treatment for women who have suffered from premenstrual tension may prevent puerperal depression (Dalton 1971).

PARENTHOOD

The importance of ante-natal classes in dealing with natural anxieties in the mother and father has already been emphasised, but the arrival of a new child in the home still presents a challenge to parents and the other children. Even when there are no particular difficulties (as described on p. 229-32) and even when the child is entirely wanted, there are major changes in routine needed, and a series of chores which may entail more drudgery, more irritation and less glamour than women's magazines and fathers' fantasies have allowed for. Young parents are less helped by their relatives than previously and though plenty of books of a more scientific kind have replaced the old wives' tales about children's needs and dangers, they do not give as much emotional support as a grandmother might, though Dr. Spock has done his best. An excellent, still up to date account is given by Winnicott (1964). With more money needed the husband will be concerned to keep working, but the wife may want his help more at home. Tensions arise. Help by nurse or GP in listening and counselling may avoid resentments building up.

Besides the obvious difficulties, parenthood unfortunately falls into the group of social skills which do in fact take a lot of time and patience to learn but are regarded as a disgrace to be without. Consequently parents don't always welcome advice and may retaliate by pointing out that the nurse has no children of her own or that the doctor's children are well-known to be neglected. The old phrase 'You can't tell me anything about children, I've buried five' is fortunately less common, but the attitude persists.

All this is very much worse if the child was not entirely welcome or unwanted and if other stresses exist in the shape of overcrowding and poverty. At the worst infanticide and battered babies can occur (see p. 279).

REFERENCES

Brooke, E. (1963). *A Cohort Study of Patients first admitted to Mental Hospitals in 1945 and 1955.* HMSO.
Dalton, K. (1971). 'Prospective study into puerperal depression'. *Brit. J. Psychiat.*, 118, 689.
Douglas, G. (1968). 'Some emotional disorders of the puerperium'. *J. Psychosomatic Res.*, 12, 101.
Jansson, B. (1964). 'Psychic inefficiencies associated with child-bearing'. *Acta psychiat. Scand.*, 39, Suppl. 172.
Pond, D. A. (1973). *Counselling in Religion and Psychiatry.* OUP, London.
Tylden, E. (1952). 'Psychiatry and the maternity unit'. *Lancet*, i, 231.
Tylden, E. (1968). 'Hyperemesis and physiological vomiting'. *J. Psychosomatic Res.*, 12, 85.
Winnicott, D. W. (1964). *The Child, the Family and The Outside World.* Penguin.
Winnicott, D. W. (1971). *Playing and Reality.* Penguin.

43 Work

THE DOCTOR'S ATTITUDE

There is a nice paradox in the attitude of many general practitioners — and medical students — to work (other than their own). On the one hand, they know it is essential for their patient, and they accept the responsibility of saying whether he is fit for it or not; on the other hand, they seldom bother to find out what it consists of, and so make elementary mistakes in their recommendations (such as light regular meals, or no lifting) when these are quite impossible to fulfil. Worse, they often ignore what work means to their patient, or to his family; it is all too common for otherwise excellent medical histories to dismiss the patient's occupation in one word, e.g. secretary — which logically can range from a filing clerk who can't type to a Secretary of State — or technician with its technique unspecified. Yet work occupies a third of our waking hours for much of our lives, and the satisfaction we get from it — or don't get — may make all the difference to our health, as well as to our happiness and our efficiency.

Any doctor, then, whether in general practice or in hospital, must have some understanding of the meaning of the patient's work to him. This is the more difficult in that doctors are luckier than most: mostly they have chosen their own career, and enjoy it; the satisfactions are many, some material, some emotional. They do not always remember that others may have had less choice and been pressed by economy or geography or by their families into something with less intrinsic satisfaction and a serious risk of unemployment.

SATISFACTIONS IN WORK

Understanding is made no easier by the use of the same words in different senses which makes definition inexact. Work to one may mean high creative satisfaction, to another painfully boring drudgery. Nearly all jobs contain some of both; but the proportion varies widely from job to job, and even in the same job from day to day.

There are certain basic satisfactions needed by every worker (using that term to mean anyone working, and not, as often, a manual worker alone). Money, being necessary to all, is a convenient reward for a job, and an apparent measure of its value to the community. It is easy to visualize, easy to argue about, easy to strike for – or to think one is striking for. Unfortunately, these advantages prevent us from seeing the corresponding disadvantages; that it is easy to ignore a job's other strong but less tangible satisfactions, that money means very many different things to different people, and that too great a pre-occupation with it leads to miserliness, or worse, to envy of any neighbours who may have been more highly paid; hence comes a narrow outlook which hampers an industrial solution even when this has been specifically designed to break the vicious circles of collective bargaining, leap-frogging and inflation. But people in any case need more than money; there are emotional satisfactions as important.

Few people work in isolation; their relations with their fellows, subordinates and superiors are vital to them, and if these are poor, recognizable symptoms of deficiency may follow. The essential needs are threefold.

1 The need to belong. This need is generally satisfied imperceptibly, but a few people fail to be accepted by their group — at home or at work, temporarily or permanently. To be 'odd man out' is unpleasant. Customs generally demand that a newcomer fits in with the group: if he does so, he is accepted: but if not he will feel unaccepted, isolated, anxious and depressed. Sometimes he may become aggressive, and if so, he will provoke overt hostility in turn from the group, until he is effectually walled off, and perhaps discharged. His only value to the group then has been as a scapegoat, temporarily uniting them in their hostility to him; an intelligent and skilled worker may be wasted, simply through lack of social know-how.

2 The need to express one's personality by doing a useful job and doing it well. Unfortunately many routine jobs do not seem to provide much sense of achievement. Other jobs have more than is apparent at first sight, and the satisfaction they provide can be enhanced by a knowledge of their value and of the group's appreciation of it. For this, open appreciation may be necessary, the more so at a lower level where the worker's intelligence, knowledge of his work's value, and inherent job satisfaction are all less; but appreciation is uncommon in most industries — and in other walks of life. Lack of praise and lack of achievement lead to apathy, resentment, and a desire to get away with the minimum.

3 The need to exercise some responsibility. If the first two needs are met, it is human to respond by being more responsible, at whatever level. Yet many workers are given too little responsibility; like some medical students (temporarily). The result is irresponsible self-centredness, and lack of identification with the firm.

If these needs are met, the people working together form a strong, healthy, cohesive and productive team, and respond constructively to appeals for better or longer work, or to threats from outside. Their morale is high, and in general, sickness, absenteeism, and labour-turnover are low.

But often none, or not all, of these satisfactions are available; some people are not capable, because of their up-bringing, of fitting into any group, and some groups are already so much under tension that they can tolerate no newcomer. On a far wider scale, many people have less sense of achievement in their work than they need; there are not enough creative jobs to go round, and many people have to be content with something below their level and some have no work at all. Some people think this situation may improve with automation, others fear it will get worse. Besides this, the spread of education — admirable in itself — leads many people now to expect they have a right to be given a job, once they are educated, and if no such job exists their disappointment and anger against society are the greater. And in a social structure where opportunities for satisfactory jobs are by no means equal, it is no surprise that much envy occurs of those who are more fortunate. People dissatisfied in their jobs or because of a lack of responsibility become disgruntled and unhappy and in need of some outlets for their frustrations. This may lead to self-centredness and self-interest, or interest only in a small group at the expense of society, and therefore to social disharmony or anarchy.

Expressions of aggression in sport or creative hobbies or even social crusades may be beneficial, but it is something of a toss-up which way they go (see p. 277).

The physical environment of the job is clearly important too. But it was paradoxically the classic Hawthorn experiment, which set out to study its effect, which ended by emphasizing the value of emotional factors. Though its findings have been criticised since, a weight of evidence suggests that physical factors can be tolerated if morale is high, but are at once blamed if it is not.

These reactions only concern the doctor indirectly; some of the consequences may need medical help. Other reactions are more his direct concern insofar as frustration, anxiety and the internalisation of aggression may lead to various types of neurotic illness.

INDUSTRIAL NEUROSIS

Considerable research has taken place in most industrialized, and developing countries, on the problems of job satisfaction, motivation, absenteeism, accidents, inefficiency, group antagonisms — to name only a few headings. The problem has been approached from the angle of a manager interested in productivity, of a trade unionist interested in satisfaction and security at work, or of a doctor interested in maintaining health: though these three aims are interlocked, the three sides collaborate all too seldom. Studies of behaviour as such are undertaken by psychologists and sociologists — as well as by politicians. There is a wealth of literature. A very useful introduction is given by J. A. C. Brown (1954).

The GP or hospital doctor may feel that the problem is beyond his scope: but he should realize its existence and should be prepared to collaborate in matters concerning the health of his patients with his colleague in the factory or office — the industrial medical officer, who is generally skilled in early recognition and treatment of the neurotic.

The cost each year to industrial efficiency from absenteeism, whether due to sickness or other causes, is much greater than the cost of strikes. In absenteeism, neurosis plays a large part: the classic work of Russell Fraser (1947) estimated that neurosis was responsible for 25-33% of cases of sickness absence, or more striking still, for 20-25% of all absence cases. This figure shows no signs of having diminished since.

But the cost does not end there, for there are many people working at less than full efficiency, for neurotic reasons, who do not actually go off sick. And there is the cost in time, temper, and health to those whose job it is to cope with such people's behaviour disorders, and who may themselves break down in the process.

Conley and others (1973) have made an assessment of the total cost to the USA of mental illness in industry there: 20,000 million dollars a year. In Britain in 1971 medically certified absence lost 324 million working days (*Brit. Med. J.*, 1974).

The form of neurosis

The symptoms of industrial neurosis are much the same as those of neurosis elsewhere, and specific occupational diseases (e.g. miner's nystagmus) are uncommon. But certain conditions in industry, e.g. danger, competitiveness or boredom, may easily provoke exaggeration of symptoms: thus some anxiety and failure of concentration may occur from the stress of overwork and over-responsibility: to this may be added fear of further inefficiency and loss of earnings, so that a vicious circle develops. Physical symptoms may enhance this, especially if it is known that stress may precipitate a coronary attack or a peptic ulcer.

The special problems of the executive meeting ever-increasing stress, with ever-diminishing outlets, deserve much study in this respect (see p. 274).

Compensation neurosis is a hysterical phenomenon: if an injury is caused at work, or in other circumstances, e.g. a road accident, which make litigation and compensation likely, the patient has a vested interest in remaining disabled until his claim is discharged: if this is unconscious, he is quite sincere in his (conscious) determination to get back to work as soon as possible, but his symptoms prevent him. Psychotherapy is most unlikely to succeed as long as his case is unsettled: once this has been done, it *may* not be necessary, but, since few claims are met in full, some ventilation of resentment may be valuable once the final payment has been made. Naturally other factors, loss of confidence and of pride, and fear of other risks, may complicate the issue.

It must be remembered that after a severe emotional shock — such as a train accident — a period of heightened suggestibility occurs, in which the behaviour of those around the patient is very important: the same has been seen in battle. The GP's attitude is therefore vital: and he must beware of letting his natural sympathy with his patient overcome him, and of encouraging him to press more than any just claim he has against an apparently impersonal and inexhaustibly wealthy industry — or government.

ACCIDENTS AT WORK

Accidents on the roads receive great publicity, though their prevention remains difficult. Industrial accidents, less news-worthy, are also mounting. Attempts to prevent them obviously depend on knowing their causes, and these are often obscure. The human factor is blamed in many, and it seems likely that although only a few people are consistently 'accident prone' (and these include some subnormals), most people have phases of temporary accident proneness. These consist of a feeling of tension, a desire for aggressive outlets, and a weakened control:

a complex which may also produce psychosomatic conditions under other circumstances (see p. 174), and traffic accidents.

Industrial accidents may also provide a way out of an intolerable situation. Hirschfeld and Behan (1963) in a retrospective study of American workers have demonstrated this. Individuals may well be promoted beyond their capacity to their 'level of incompetence' (the 'Peter principle'). They can neither cope nor admit their incapacity. Conflict may be avoided by staging (unconsciously) an accident, avoiding protective devices and then delaying recovery from the physical results of the damage — which is clearly a hysterical mechanism. Compensation may add to the difficulties of treatment. Good selection for jobs and for promotion at all levels is obviously a possible means for prevention.

TRAVEL STRESS

Travel is associated in many people's minds with holidays and pleasure, and the physical risks may thus be cheerfully accepted. It has, however, considerable psychological risks when it is part of working efficiency. Long journeys are today taken with such apparent ease, and the stimulus of new surroundings is so attractive, that the actual fatigue is masked: until its effects on concentration and judgment may have become irretrievable (Wright 1960).

A special danger, which is likely to increase, is that known loosely as 'transatlantic syndrome'. The executive who crosses the Atlantic and steps at once into totally different timings — as well as other stresses — may suffer gross fatigue, with impaired judgment and concentration on his second or third day. Other physiological effects follow the derangement of his 'internal clock'. Changes in Circadian rhythms have been shown due to the activity of the adrenal cortex (Mills 1966) while more recently Fröberg and others (1972) have shown that the loss of efficiency may be due partly to sleep deprivation and partly to change in the rhythm of the adrenal medulla as measured by catecholamine excretion.

Stringent medical warnings are often ignored, the more so by the more senior executives, accustomed to trust their own judgment in all matters and to override opposition. Dietary changes also have their risks.

Travel psychosis has been described, but it is rare, and far less important than the above milder syndrome.

FURTHER READING

British Medical Journal (1974). Editorial, 'Sickness absence'. ii, 249.

Brown, J. A. C. (1954). *The Social Psychology of Industry.* Penguin.

Conley, R. W., Conwell, M. and Arrill, M. B. (1973). Noland, R. (ed.), *Industrial Mental Health and Counselling.* Behavioural Publications, New York.

Fraser, R. et al. (1947). *The Incidence of Neurosis in Factory Workers.* HMSO.

Fröberg, J., Karlsson, C.G., Levi, L., Lidberg, L. *Internat. J. Psychobiology*, 2, 23.

Hirschfeld, A. H. and Behan, R. C. (1963). 'The accident process'. *J.A.M.A.* 193-9, 300-6 and (1966) 85-9.

Jaques, E. (1951). *The Changing Culture of a Factory.* Tavistock Publications, London.

Jaques, E. (1961). *Equitable Payment.* Heinemann, London.

Levinson, H. et al. (1962). *Men, Management and Mental Health.* Harvard University Press.

McLean, A. A. (1973). 'Occupational mental health'. In Noland, R. (ed.), *Industrial Mental Health and Counselling.* Behavioural Publications, New York.

Mayo, Elton, (1933). *The Human Problems of an Industrial Civilisation.* Harvard University Press.

Mills, J. N. (1966). 'Human circadian rhythm'. *Physiol. Rev.*, 46, 128.

Tredgold, R. F. (1963). *Human Relations in Modern Industry.* Duckworth, London.

Wright, H. B. (1960). *Business Travel: The Health of Business Executives.* Chest and Heart Association.

44 Leisure, creative activity and violence

In these words lies the whole problem of how each person is to use his creative gifts, express his personality and reach some satisfactory relationship with his group; or fail to do so — and need medical help for himself or others.

From childhood, each of us meets threats to security or obstruction to his wishes, and reacts by anxiety or anger, or both. The strength of emotion depends not only on the strength of the stimulus but also on his personality and past history. How he then reacts to his emotion depends not only on these factors but also on his understanding and control, and the support of others. He may be overwhelmed by extreme emotions; but generally, as a child he learns to modify their expression, and with his parent's help to canalize them into constructive or harmless activity; although the amount of aggression which may be displayed and the channel chosen depend a great deal on the customs of his contemporaries and of course on the standards of his parents and teachers. In some cases he is taught to repress his aggression and even to be ashamed or afraid of it; or even to deny its existence, and he shows the facade of calm, a stiff upper lip under all circumstances, as was so much an ideal a generation ago. Certainly it had its virtues then and still does, provided an outlet can be found of an acceptable kind so that his equilibrium is preserved.

There are, of course, many outlets possible; satisfactions in work have been discussed in the last section; but many cannot find these and seek some leisure pursuit instead.

Leisure is important for all; for many as a change and relaxation, but for others whose lives are sheer drudgery perhaps as a main interest. It may allow drudgery to be carried out without complaint. Increasing automation may diminish the time spent on work, as many hope, or remove the interest of many jobs, as many fear; either way satisfaction in leisure will become more necessary. It has been said paradoxically that the greatest task of industry in the next ten years will be to consider the healthy use of leisure. The value of this after retirement has been discussed elsewhere (see p. 302) but it is important throughout the lives of many people. For if leisure becomes as passive and mass-produced as work, it leads to apathy, and if companionship is lacking, loneliness and depression become acute. Hence activities such as television-watching may add insidiously to isolation, and passivity: whereas 'do-it-yourself' pursuits allow a sense of achievement.

CREATIVE AND HARMLESS ACTIVITY

Those who lack satisfaction at work may find it instead in creative activity, in drama, art, music or hobbies, which may of course provide some of the most sublime human experiences: and which must be a major factor in maintaining mental health, at lower levels, for those who act in it, look at it, or listen to it. Naturally such pursuits can also be used in helping sick people express themselves and resolve conflicts: and art and music therapy both have proved their worth (though they have developed more slowly than might have been expected) as part of comprehensive occupational therapy, which (it is not always realised) has progressed far beyond the stage of filling time for bored chronic patients.

Others' aggression may be satisfied in sport; most children learn in their family or at school to divert some of their aggressive energies away from the people that provoke them (which include parents and teachers as well as companions) into some game or sport, approved by society, and sanctioned by strict rules; competitiveness is encouraged, and channelled, losing or injury come to be accepted with resignation or good humour; the team spirit is learnt; fresh air and exercise are no doubt beneficial. What is even better, though curiously seldom admitted, is the chance of a harmless outlet for aggression. And those who do badly in one field may succeed in another.

Injuries in sport seldom have hysterical exaggerations, except for momentary gamesmanship, for heroes don't exaggerate, and financial compensation does not apply, as it does in industry. There are however interesting psychological states to be seen *before* important events, at sport, on the stage, etc. and these symptoms of getting the 'needle' (as it was known before drug addiction came in) can be used constructively by an experienced coach or captain.

On the whole then sport is a useful safety-valve, and even international rivalries can be canalized by the Olympic Games, or World Cup — with occasional lapses.

Some sports such as mountaineering involve accepting a challenge by nature, and the considerable risks involved. Clearly enormous satisfaction is gained in the achievement of climbing a mountain just because it is there and of overcoming the risks by forethought, skill and courage. Here the psychological sequels of accidental injuries are few, and probably psychological illness in those who take part is well below average.

Other outlets still are needed for many adults, who have little else to shine in, or to be aggressive in. Hitting unoffending balls about may be a conscious or unconscious substitute for attacking one's boss — or others. Even vicarious expression of feelings, by watching rather than participating, may help; and fit in with some identification with a special 'hero' in sport, or in the fantasies of a thriller on TV or in a book or film. Though occasionally these stimulate outbreaks of violence, and appear to condone extremes of it, on balance they do more good than harm, if the distinction between reality and fantasy is clear.

DRIVING AND TRAFFIC ACCIDENTS

For some, driving a car fast is an outlet, combining the thrill of speed, power, competitiveness, and high skill, with the acceptance of risk; all well fostered by the advertizers. Inevitably judgment is sometimes lacking, the unforeseen occurs, mechanical or physical faults arise, and accidents 'happen'. All of us are capable of being 'accident-prone' if tense or angry; yet pride in our skill prevents us from admitting this, or heeding anyone's advice at the time — and of course there are back-seat drivers, whose interference really is dangerous. A certain class of habitually furious driver — the Jehu syndrome — may be recognized but, for obvious reasons, is difficult to study scientifically.

Traffic accidents have received great publicity although their prevention remains very difficult. Research into the emotional factors preceding an accident is clearly extremely hard, for the patient may be dead, amnesic, or have a vested interest in evading the truth; nevertheless the evidence is mounting (Wilson, 1974) that many accidents are associated with unexpressed aggression, impaired judgment, a weakened control and a desire for an outlet. It is of course noteworthy that alcohol, which in some circumstances is an attempt to reduce the tension felt, may on the roads contribute seriously to the risk of driver, passenger or pedestrian.

The above may be seen as attempts to find creative or

(nearly) harmless outlets: but a person may be unable to find one and so remain frustrated; and to this may be added anxiety from external insecurity, and fears of his own mounting feelings. He still tries to repress these. But later anxiety or aggression may break through either in an entirely uncontrolled outburst (as terrifying to him as to others) or onto a legitimate target if one exists, or if he can find something which he can convince himself is one. Here the influence of others is important; if at that moment he is in a state of heightened suggestibility, he may accept strong suggestions from others towards impulsive violence or flight, or rumours of disaster or triumph, and act on them without exercising his own reason or responsibility.

It is therefore easy to see how an increase of anti-social and especially anti-authoritarian feeling mounts in any group of frustrated, insecure people who are dissatisfied with their own way of life, yet see no change possible by any other means than violence. This may be the major reason for the growth of violent crime, of which 'mugging' in big cities is now notorious, though scarcely new; or of other types of violence: for example violence within the family, which is as old as Cain; and wives have been beaten by alcoholic husbands for years. Many wives have retaliated: either parent may vent their feelings on the children instead.

BATTERED BABIES

Battering babies deserves a special note: although it too has probably occurred for years, much more notice has been paid to it lately and its real incidence may be rising (Smith et al. 1974). The essential feature is collusion between parents in concealing the truth of the injury which the baby has received from one or other, apparently under considerable tension. The discovery of unexplained physical injuries in a baby should lead to urgent investigation of the family situation. Marital disharmony, illegitimacy, and personality disorders in one or other or both parents are common factors. Obviously treatment must consist of trying to get both parents to get some relief by expressing their real feelings and in so doing trying to develop more control and focus their energies on dealing with the situation in which they are trapped, rather than set up a vicious circle which endangers the baby and themselves. To protect the baby legal action may be essential and the child may have to be taken into care.

GROUP VIOLENCE

Group violence also seems to be increasing. Although watching sport may provide for some a satisfactory outlet for aggression, it has become notorious that other spectators are not in fact purged of their emotions during a football match, but are led to pour them out later at some quite inoffensive target, and very destructively and irresponsibly; often of course helped by the just-empty bottle in their hands. The words hooliganism and vandalism are used to describe destructive actions to property or to people of a senseless irresponsible kind, which have been serious enough to warrant a special enquiry directed by the Minister for Sport (*Lancet*, 1968), which however dealt more with controls than with causes; though it is. significant that teenagers with too little outlets or interest elsewhere were held partly to blame. Discussion since has tended to ignore the latter, and focus on more complicated fortifications for restricting violence.

Violence which seems at first sight more rational occurs in 'popular' demonstrations, which in theory support a noble cause but inevitably come to be directed against the police (whose job it is to allow free speech, to prevent provocation, and to tell which is which). A study by Stewart (1969) of student riots showed that these were organised by privileged groups, but were focussed on the grievance of the under-privileged, and often protested more than the grievance really warranted; they stressed the need for 'do-as-you-please freedom', to the point of anarchy, were anti-authority, professedly pacific, but easily became violent. Again, they were easier to describe than to solve. It seems likely that the combination of altruistic motives with aggressive outlets, sanctioned and perhaps even glorified by one's inner circle, is the root; many people need a crusade, or holy war; and if heroism is the crown for success, and martyrdom for failure, it is not surprising that violence is spreading; especially as the targets, which it must have, are likely to hit back (and sometimes too hard) so that patterns of antagonism are formed, which last for years. Race prejudice at immigrants is described below (see p. 285). Religious beliefs may provide even more apparent justification, and even higher sanction.

In the same way, international war has in the past provided a legitimate outlet of aggression for many people, and politicians and generals have appealed to their best feelings of patriotism and altruism as well as to the worse ones of fear and cruelty; atrocity stories play their part. With all this many people do undoubtedly feel more useful and so happier in wartime, in spite of all its horrors and personal griefs. Suicide is said to diminish.

THE DOCTOR'S PART

There is thus a problem for the doctor in violence. Besides having to deal with its victims he may have to see the aggressor and decide whether he is likely to repeat his violence in the future, or can be helped not to do so. As it can be seen that not only wars but other kinds of violence 'begin in the minds of men', so with some understanding of the frustrations and conflicts which lead to violence, the doctor may be able to help the patient either to control it or to release it harmlessly. In many cases skilled psychiatric help in a mental hospital will be needed: and it is interesting that violence in the latter has been considerably reduced by less restrictions, by more under-standing staff, by outlets for physical energy and for creative occupational therapy, and perhaps by better food.

BATTLE

Quite a different problem exists for the individual compelled to take part in violent actions which conflict with his upbringing and personality: as in the Armed Services. Moreover, battle contains threats of death, mutilation, or captivity, and physical exhaustion for all.

It is therefore not surprising that there are many psychiatric casualties as well as physical ones. In the First World War, these took the form of 'shell-shock', which was later realized to be hysterical. In the Second World War, hysteria was far less common, for which there were various reasons; but there were many acute anxiety states (battle or combat fatigue, or exhaustion states). The doctor's part here was to ensure that these were treated quickly, as near the fighting as possible; and remarkable success was achieved. The chronic sequels of invalidism, depression, and gross hysterical symptoms of the First World War were largely avoided; rapid recovery was usual.

Such treatment was only part of the work of the Army Psychiatric Services (fully described by Rees 1945). Prophylaxis was also successful. In training for battle (battle inoculation), methods were successfully used which allowed the soldier to understand and accept and control his own anxiety and aggression, at the same time as he learnt the more obvious skills and quick reactions in handling weapons, and machinery. Thus the fear of being afraid, i.e. of being a coward, was replaced by an acceptance and control of normal anxiety. Courage is of course the conscious mastery of fear, not its absence.

The application of psychology and psychiatry in the fighting services also included job selection, tests for promotion, studies of the basis of morale, and the reasons for military crime, such as absence without leave.

Civil Defence Services have also been taught that, similarly, after major civil catastrophes, there may be a period of shock, amounting at times to apathy and paralysis, and a total inability to help oneself; later, there is a phase of suggestibility, with some power to co-operate, and later the release of anger, grief or fear. First-aid workers can do excellent work if they realise these phases will occur, and provide appropriate treatment.

RESEARCH AND EDUCATION

Studies of the behaviour of different groups under the stress of war has also contributed to sociological research; and it is interesting to recall Trotter's philosophic speculations (1916) on the likeness of certain human groups to animal herds, and to compare them with more recent and more detailed observations on the instinctive and learnt behaviour of certain animals and birds made by Lorenz, from which he draws highly important conclusions on human reactions to certain stimuli. His three books (below) are to be recommended for this, as well as for their general interest.

The influence of the size of the territory defended by animals, and their methods of doing so have been studied by Lorenz (1966), and Lack (1943). Such lessons may be more important for the human race, as it increases. The defences of man against his own aggression have been excellently described by Storr (1968): and the resulting vicious circles in individual and social behaviour are of profound importance.

These have been discussed elsewhere under various headings, especially for asthma, ulcerative colitis and depressive illnesses and suicide (v.s.): and their medical importance is obvious. But social illnesses, in the shape of chronic patterns of antagonism, e.g. in industry, or between races, are also examples of dangerous vicious circles due to a failure to handle aggression: and indeed a correlation has been found between poor mental health, low job satisfaction, and high racial prejudice.

The understanding and control of aggression is thus of vital importance to society, and perhaps even to the survival of the human race: yet very little formal education exists at present: and the psychological resistances to discussions on it are manifold and very strong; which is rational in that they stem from our own childhood feelings and their repression.

The doctor can then play several parts in handling violence. He can press for more research on its causes; he can help train first-aid workers to deal with its effects; and he can do something to prevent its expression by some individuals who consult him, and whose threatened outburst he can get them to divert into other, harmless, channels.

FURTHER READING

Kornhauser, A. W. (1965). *Mental Health of the Industrial Worker*. Wiley, New York.

Lack, D. L. (1943). *The Life of the Robin*. OUP, London.

Lancet, 1968, Editorial 1, 406.

Lorenz, K. (1952). *King Solomon's Ring*. Methuen, London.

Lorenz, K. (1954). *Man Meets Dog*. Methuen, London.

Lorenz, K. (1966). *On Aggression*. Methuen, London.

Rees, J. R. (1945). *The Shaping of Psychiatry by War*. Chapman and Hall, London.

Smith, S. M. et al. (1974). 'Social aspects of the battered baby syndrome'. *Brit. J. Psychiat.*, 125, 568.

Stewart, G. T. (1969). 'Student riots'. *Lancet*, i, 617.

Storr, A. (1968). *Human Aggression*. Allen Lane, London.

Trotter, W. (1916). *The Instincts of the Herd in Peace and War*. T. Fisher Unwin, London.

Wilson, C. R. M. (1974). 'Psychology of an accident'. *Care in the Home* 1, 14.

Wolff, H. H. (1969). 'The role of aggression in the psychopathology of illness'. *J. Psychosom. Res.*, 13, 315.

45 *Expatriation*

There are four large groups of people who are to be found living abroad, workers, students, soldiers and refugees. Doctors should be aware of the special psychological stresses involved, and their reactions to them. They may of course be in any one of these groups themselves.

FOREIGN WORKERS

Special problems arise over the use of foreign workers of two types; those who are attracted by higher wages and an apparently higher standard of living to another more industrialised country (generally known as immigrants or migrants); and those who are attracted, conversely, by artificially high salaries, to move to a special unit in a less developed area (often called expatriates). Both groups have more in common than the obvious difficulty of adapting to a foreign country. Since the newcomers of either kind have generally left their families behind they tend either to become isolated or to live in small communities of their own, and either way may develop antagonism to the local people, so that absorption is slow, and even slower if the migrants are clearly there simply to send money home, or are obviously 'different' in behaviour and colour.

The migrants have moved to work which may be essential, such as public services, hospitals or mines, but which has been despised by most of the locals and does not always carry a high social status. The expatriates feel socially superior, but cause other criticisms; they generally earn a higher salary because of their special expertise or perhaps because a parent company prefers employing them to locals; but such a start provokes antagonism and envy, which is made worse by arrogance, impatience and insecurity on their part, with sensitivity and resentment against 'imperialists' on the other. It is then easy enough for a community which needs an outlet for its hostility to focus on the other side as a scape-goat, and to behave in such a sensitive way that race prejudice soon develops if it was not there to start with.

The picture is easily recognisable in Britain; a recent working party (Verhaegen 1972) described similar problems in other European countries. Such complaints have been reported throughout the world in primitive cultures such as Papua New Guinea (Pulsford and Cawte 1972), and studies in highly sophisticated managers transferred to backward areas (Kearns 1973).

Sainsbury (1973) has demonstrated that there is a higher incidence of suicides in immigrants to Australia and to the USA as compared with the countries they come from: and a similar picture exists for people who move from the country to London boroughs. If it is realised that the psychological problems are basically loneliness, insecurity and frustration in work and personal relationships, something can be done by counselling and support, whereas logical arguments about paranoid antagonisms and race prejudice are a waste of time.

But some syndromes need special description.

European expatriates in the tropics

Personality factors. The manifestations of the psychiatric disorders seen in the tropics depend greatly on the personalities of the people serving there and their ability to adapt to the stresses of the tropics, which are themselves considerable. Most of the patients referred for psychiatric opinion will be found to be markedly more obsessional than normal, show more anxiety, and be more likely to be depressed and to have more difficulties with authority figures. In a study carried out at the Hospital for Tropical Diseases, London, in 1971 an overall psychiatric morbidity of 45% was found (Wilson 1974). It is clear that personality disorders are rife among people going abroad, for one of the ways of attempting to escape from oneself is to move frequently, hence the flight of many people who see the tropics as a means of escape from themselves, to overseas jobs lasting two to five years. It may also offer a chance to escape authority for those whose aggressive problems make it impossible for them to work in a structured European environment. The others are those who are sent overseas by their Companies or go abroad because they are unlikely to gain promotion at home. They are unable to express their feelings about being trapped abroad and unable to come home because this is financially damaging. Unfortunately, all these people are far more prone to breakdown when things go against them. A different group consists of those in missionary work who try to avoid their own problems by helping others; they are especially prone to isolation, overwork and tend to be idealistic, rigid and un-yielding. On the other hand those workers who have come to terms with themselves before going abroad are a very outgoing and stable group.

Environmental factors. Tropical countries have different cultural norms from Europe; and as mentioned above, Europeans tend to stick together and not to mix with the indigenous population. Married women are the group most at risk. They do not often want to go abroad, but do so to avoid being separated from their husbands. They are not encouraged to work and it is the usual thing to have servants. There is lack of privacy and also lack of communication. Wives often report that they feel they cannot talk to their husbands because they are so busy. If children are taken abroad, the fear of disease is often a worry. Sending children home for schooling brings damaging separation.

Work conditions are often very frustrating. The tempo of work is different, there are language difficulties, and a constant struggle to get local workers to conform to European standards. Frequently, excessive demands are made on the man on the spot by his superiors back in Europe who fail to understand the situation so that he dare not risk mistakes. He is often isolated.

Heat and humidity are often profound, producing lassitude, insomnia, anorexia and loss of libido, and so often marital tension: hence degrees of depression are common as is memory loss. Other climatic factors include the monotony of unchanging weather and the lack of twilight. The local insects and reptiles are often terrifying to newcomers and there is the constant fear of tropical disease.

Symptomatology. Although depression is not often the presenting symptom, tiredness and vague symptoms of abdominal pain and diarrhoea, or sexual and gynaecological problems, may reveal its existence. It seems to be commoner among young single women. Intense anxiety may be the first sign of a depressive illness; headaches are often found among women. It is usually free floating but may become fixed to a particular part of the body, giving a hypochondriacal picture, with the fear of having contracted a particular tropical illness.

Hysterical manifestations, contrary to popular belief, often occur in people who appear mature and capable; they are the typical 'stiff upper lip' types who show little emotional reaction to stress until they break down. Symptoms are often based on an original tropical infection. This is cleared by treatment but the symptoms generally return after a short gap.

Diarrhoea and abdominal pain are the commonest physical symptoms seen. Often changes in diet have led to some gastro-intestinal upset on meeting new bacteria; in the past this was dignified by many alternative titles — Bombay Belly, Cairo Colitis, Delhi Diarrhoea, gyppy tummy; the infection is normally soon over, but many people, notably soldiers, have pinned their anxiety, e.g. from home-sickness, on to the yearning emptiness caused by their abdominal complaints and made the latter chronic, convinced that they will never recover where they are, but would at once do so on return home.

Headaches, dizziness and paraesthesiae are common. Alcoholism or drug addiction may complicate the picture. Patients are usually invalided home for investigation for medical rather than psychological reasons and there is thus considerable secondary gain in removal from the source of stress and the avoidance of loss of face. Hysterical manifestations seem to be equally common among European men and women. But all these symptoms may be associated with, or mask, a depressive state.

Treatment. Physical complaints must first be ruled out, after which a combined psychotherapeutic and pharmaceutical approach is necessary. The depressive element is usually amenable to tricyclic anti-depressants. However, it is supportive therapy with perhaps a little superficial interpretation which will allow the person to show his real feelings, thus helping the symptoms. Hysterical symptoms are more difficult to treat as they serve a distinct purpose and the patient tends to cling on to them, but the nature of the symptoms must be explained to the patient and an attempt made to bring underlying problems to the surface.

Asian and Africans in Western culture

Unfortunately, less attention has been paid to the psychiatric problems of Asians, West Indians and Africans migrating to Britain than to the political overtones, but the number of immigrants has gathered momentum since the 1950s. Although all groups tend to show an incidence of psychotic and neurotic illness similar to that of the world population, there are some special problems. Asians are usually urbanized and most illnesses are contained within a very strict family circle which is all-embracing, and which may prevent some of the family, especially the wife, from local contact. Depression is common and usually hides behind physical symptomatology. Complaints such as faintness, dizziness, sweating attacks and abdominal pain are seen and are thus commoner in women than in men. Some Asian customs clash sharply with those of the West and much illness is caused by this, especially in the young, who fall firmly between two cultural patterns. Arranged marriages are still the rule in India and it is common for a girl of eighteen to be sent to Europe to marry a man she has never seen. No Indian woman would ever mention marital problems, as this would stain the honour of her husband. Hysterical acting out may occur.

Treatment. Except perhaps with the West Indian group, language presents enormous difficulties, especially with Indians and Pakistanis, and to a lesser extent with Africans. Although the doctor and patient may be able to communicate at a superficial level, it will often not be possible to use the emotion-laden words which are essential for psychotherapy, so treatment must mainly rely on drugs. In this case these must be given by the doctor with absolute conviction that they will work and precise instructions to the letter for taking them. The patient must be reassured that his symptoms will completely disappear; thus the authority of the doctor is established and his priest-like role emphasized This usually has a marked therapeutic effect.

FOREIGN STUDENTS

A special group of immigrants consists of students: their particular problems should be mentioned. The student arrives to study and is often disillusioned. His first problem may be that his learning ability seems slower than that of the European students so he finds it difficult to keep up, having been considered clever in his own country. Sometimes this is simply because he has not yet acclimatized or is not familiar with the colloquial language: he may also encounter problems in finding accommodation, and race prejudice and loneliness. Most Africans are used to group living and the isolation of European cities is difficult for them. To return home without the desired qualification would be intolerable as it would mean loss of face for him and the family; the student is usually one of a greatly favoured minority, either chosen by the Government or financed by the local community to study in Europe, so the prossibility of failing is unthinkable. He may then present to the doctor with a physical complaint, thus avoiding the need to take the feared examination and the risk of failing it. Although this pattern of symptom presentation is hysterical, there is often a strong depressive element in it, which can be treated; and if support and understanding are forthcoming, the student will usually succeed in getting his exams provided his intelligence is in fact adequate.

If, however, this is impossible it is likely that he will not only retain his symptoms, but blame the doctors for not being able to cure him; and also blame the culture which appears to be rejecting his value.

SOLDIERS

Soldiers sent abroad may be exposed to stress very similar to those of workers, with the additional anxiety over the safety of their families at home, and the threat of battle for themselves (see p. 281); the whole subject of military psychiatry has been well described by Rees (1945).

In the services great attention was paid to the emotional needs of the soldiers returning after long service abroad, and even more to the released prisoner-of-war. It included re-education about current affairs and rehabilitation into a job, and a redevelopment of a sense of responsibility which often had been lost by the need to kill, and to survive. Physical illness and addictions added to the difficulties.

REFUGEES

Traditionally both Britain and North America have been proud to accept and absorb many refugees from many countries and have benefited from their skills and their stimulus. Today tragically the world has thousands of refugees who can be accepted nowhere, and are driven to die — or kill — in desperation. But many still do arrive and present special problems for the doctor in their new home.

They face the climatic, dietetic and social changes already described (see p. 284): they are isolated, often unemployed, homesick and anxious for their relatives; they tend to join compatriots which may keep them alienated from their hosts: they may form a scapegoat for any hostility around.

Small wonder a few develop markedly paranoid attitudes, besides the reactions of the expatriate worker already described.

Treatment is therefore extremely difficult: sometimes all the doctor can do is to prevent the patients' condition worsening, which it is likely to do if he feels the doctor (of another race) is yet another hostile person: and yet this is very likely to be the case, when his own unhappiness, anger and isolation have impinged on the doctor and made the latter in turn feel helpless and irritated.

Great patience may be needed to get across to the refugee some reassurance and some sense of being understood.

FURTHER READING

Kearns, J. L. (1973). *Stress in Industry.* Priory Press, London.

Macek, O. and Meyer, B. (1972). 'Yugoslav workers in an Austrian textile factory'. In Verhaegen, P. (ed.), *Mental Health in Foreign Workers.* Acco, Louvain.

Pulsford, R. L. and Cawte, J. (1972). *Health in a Developing Country.* Jacaranda Press, Milton, Qld.

Rees, J. R. (1945). *The Shaping of Psychiatry by War.* London, Chapman Hall.

Sainsbury, P. (1973). *Proc. Roy. Soc. Med.,* 66, 579.

Wilson, C. R. M. (1974). 'Psychiatry in the tropics'. In Woodruff, A. W. (ed.), *Medicine in the Tropics.* London.

46 Illness, injury and operation

From the start the student has been urged to consider two aspects of the patient's history — his emotional state at the onset of his illness and his emotional reaction to its symptoms. Each may obviously affect the other: the first has been discussed under the heading of psychosomatic disease (see p. 173), the second needs consideration here.

The full impact of severe illness, injury, operation or other treatment procedures on a previously healthy person is often not realized by his GP or by the hospital staff or by the students. This is partly because doctors tend to minimize the psychological effect and to focus their interest on the obvious physical aspect, and partly because patients are shy of being thought cowardly or fussy if they admit to their natural reactions. But failure to express them can enhance their disability and must not be ignored. They often need early supportive treatment.

A surgical operation provokes reactions which need special comment: they vary considerably. Patients may enter hospital hoping to be relieved of their urgent distress when they are admitted for a surgical emergency or they may enter for a routine operation after weeks or months on a waiting list. Although the word 'operation' does not have the frightening

overtones it had fifty years ago it is still a very anxious time for
the patient when he comes into hospital, the place of mystery
with customs all its own. He may well be handicapped by
having no idea at all of the magnitude of the surgical procedure,
the gravity of the operation or of the surgical and nursing care
behind it. He does not always know what is expected of him.
Many patients find being in bed in a public ward and submitting
to medical and nursing ministration very embarrassing. Pre-
operative investigation and preparation may make considerable
demands on the patient, both psychological and physical. A
great deal of this can be prevented if the likely psychological
effects of such frightening treatment procedures are considered
in designing these special units and if the doctors and nurses are
aware of them.

INTENSIVE CARE UNITS

There are special problems which may be caused by intensive
care units. Kornfeld (1969) reported acute confusional states
after cardiotomy; these were generally separated from the
operation by a lucid interval, which suggested that the
atmosphere of the intensive care unit, with its frightening
equipment and difficulty of sleeping, was itself responsible. A
change of its procedure, coupled with a pre-operative psychiatric interview, halved the incidence of such confusion (Lazarus
and Hagens 1968). Reassurance can also help the anxiety bound
to be felt by the staff.

Similar complications in patients undergoing renal dialysis
were reported by Kaplan De-Nour et al. (1968), and an
excellent study of the effects of dialysis has been made by
Cramond (1970); he describes how new psychological stresses
have arisen from the dependence of the patient on a machine,
or on someone to work it, and mentions the tendency to deal
with his feelings by denial and projection; it is therefore
necessary to select patients for such treatment who can be got
to discuss their feelings, and of course equally necessary to
provide opportunity for them to do so. But the psychiatrist
involved may well become the target of the hostility of the
patient as well as that of his medical colleagues under some
stress. Over all this is the shadow of the patient's anxiety about

the possibility of receiving a kidney by transplantation from a living donor or from someone recently dead, whose relatives have not yet come through their period of mourning.

PLASTIC SURGERY

There are, of course, people whose physical handicaps, especially facial, may provoke shyness, shame, depression, isolation and so more pre-occupation with their disfigurement. If there is a significant physical deformity, e.g. of the shape or size of the nose, rhinoplasty may offer considerable relief, provided the patient's expectations from surgery are realistic. There are unfortunately other patients who focus their emotional problems on some major, minor, or even fancied physical abnormality, and convince themselves that plastic surgery and nothing else will cure this. They may put intense pressure on their GP or on a surgeon to operate. Since a major emotional conflict is not to be solved in this way, they gain nothing from the operation and either at once blame the surgeon for his failure, or try to persuade him to operate yet again. This applies, for example, to men who in spite of minimal nasal deformity insist on a rhinoplasty and become depressed or paranoid after the operation. By then it is nigh impossible for psychotherapy to give them insight. Such cases are very difficult, but a few can be helped by appropriate psychiatric treatment if given early, and then by asking a surgeon to consider what he can do solely on the merits of their physical abnormality. Throughout close consultation between GP, plastic surgeon and psychiatrist is essential.

SPECIAL RISKS

There are special risks in certain conditions which may exist before operation:

1 *Old age.* With the increasing expectation of life, more old people are undergoing major surgery. With lessened powers of adaptation they find hospital admission difficult and may show nocturnal confusion. Here, if possible, it is wise to take things

slowly and to give the patient a few days to become adapted to hospital life before embarking on exacting investigatory procedures or operation itself. Good post-operative co-operation and good surgical results are then much more likely.

2 *Alcoholism.* If the patient is known to be a heavy drinker, the risk of his developing delirium tremens can be diminished by tranquillizers and parentrovite injections, preferably pre-operatively, but if not possible then, post-operatively. No harm can result from such treatment and the danger of post-operative delirium can be reduced.

3 *Depression.* Another surgical pitfall is to undertake surgery in a patient whose physical symptoms are in fact due to a depressive illness or to operate while he is seriously depressed (see p. 75). Unless there is a surgical emergency, treatment of depression takes priority over surgery.

4 *Past trauma.* Patients who have already had traumatic experiences in hospital in childhood may react badly.

EMOTIONAL REACTIONS

The emotional reactions which can occur may be listed as follows:

1 *Anxiety.* Anxiety is natural about the outcome of illness or operation, about pain, about relations who may be left uncared for, about a job to be lost. If the patient can talk about his feelings and get sympathy he is generally relieved of some tension. Anxiety is often based on ignorance, and can be helped by information – about the future, the type of treatment, including the extent of any operation proposed, and the amount of pain to be met and how it can be controlled. A patient in hospital is often puzzled by the number of staff and by the various hospital rules: it is helpful to know who is who, who is responsible for what, and why the various regulations exist. Most of this can be told him by the nursing staff; but they often need doctors' support. Before operation a particular fear is of 'mutilation' – a word seldom used by staff but occasionally in the mind of the patient. This can be helped by exact information, and, even more, by the attitudes of doctor, nurse and student. To accept, for example, a colostomy is a task

which needs courage and resolution in the patient and sympathetic help from staff and relations. A hysterectomy has special problems (see p. 226), and so has cardiac surgery. Fears of death are discussed elsewhere (see p. 303).

2 *Aggression.* Anxiety is not always displayed as such: it may make the patient aggressive, and if his behaviour presents as an attack on the doctor or establishment, especially if he picks on legitimate grievances — he will not be popular nor will he meet sympathy or relief. Criticisms provoke exaggerated defence and possibly retaliation by overworked staff and the patient risks being given that most damaging (and enduring) label 'a difficult patient'. But if this aggression can be harmlessly ventilated, and met by patience and understanding, it can usually be tolerated.

3 *Resentment and anxiety at separation.* This has happened too often in the past to children who have been isolated and deprived of visits or contact with parents, for all sorts of reasons — to avoid infection spreading, to keep the ward peaceful and clean, to reduce the load on parents; some of these reasons may have been understandable but they ignored the damage to the child's security (see p. 234). Many patients today owe their present anxiety to such 'hygienic measures' (others owe it to evacuation to unwelcoming homes in the war — which may have saved some deaths from bombing but left chronic invalids).

4 *Depression* is particularly likely when severe disability hits someone in middle life who has never been ill before. It is then possible for the symptoms to become the focus of gloomy interest, and for the patient to become more and more demanding, hypochondriacal, and self-centred. Some secondary gain may be obtained in the shape of more attention, but the overall picture is one of loss of friends, interests and reputation. This is partly a hysterical condition (see below) but there is a basic depression which is easily missed: yet if it is recognized and treated this tragic deterioration can be saved.

5 *Regression* to a childish dependent level may occur in any sick person and may even be useful if it makes him more amenable to treatment. It is therefore encouraged by the nursing staff over a period of crisis in illness or after operation. But if the nurses persist — and it isn't easy for them to know when to alter their attitude — then the patient may remain helpless, self-centred and demanding: and he may become

'hospitalized', which is anything but helpful to the staff, and provokes their criticism (spoken or not); the patient in turn resents this, and may respond by being aggressive or hysterical.

6 *Hysterical* exaggeration of disability due to illness or injury has been mentioned elsewhere (see p. 101). This is particularly likely if compensation is in question (see p. 273) or if the onset of the disability has been sudden and shocking and so led to a period of marked suggestibility. The reasons for this reaction must be carefully sought, and handled. Condemnation will simply increase symptoms.

7 *Confusion*, sometimes amounting to a psychotic confusional state is not uncommon after operation, especially after cardiac surgery, or injury, or in acute or chronic illness for a variety of physical reasons, which are described elsewhere (see p. 149).

Several of these emotional reactions may be combined in a patient suddenly faced with major changes in his pattern of life, from grave illness such as a coronary or a stroke. His capacity to work, to earn, to enjoy himself, even to think or to communicate as he did may be very limited and he may find himself humiliated by being temporarily or permanently dependent on someone else's care. Even if his helpers nobly accept the burden of care for him, he may still feel guilty; if they are less noble much friction may occur for their pattern of life has also had to change. A further risk then is that one or other in this position may take refuge in drink or drugs.

THE RELATIVES

Besides the patient's feelings, the relatives' reactions also need consideration. At home, they will have much longer influence on the patient than his doctor's views: even in hospital their comments while visiting may undermine confidence in the staff. Some attempt must then be made to assess the relatives' influence, their attitude to the patient, and his to them, and where it seems desirable and possible, to give them some information and support.

As discussed elsewhere, there are many conditions where this is especially important, e.g. depression (see p. 81) and certain psychosomatic conditions (see p. 178) for various patterns of antagonism, isolation or despair may follow and interfere between the patient and those who could help him. In particular, relatives need help in learning to tolerate, accept and relieve occasional aggressive outbursts from the patient: it is by no means easy to see that these are seldom directed at anyone but are really expressions of the patient's anger or guilt at himself, at his own failure or inadequacy. He feels helpless, so that his behaviour is often directed towards making others feel equally so. This is bad enough for his doctors, far worse for his wife or family. They badly need help.

Who is best suited to give this help? Unfortunately the answer is often 'someone else' and many relatives are thus left without help; this makes them resentful and anxious and if things go wrong perhaps litigious. In any case their attitude may in the long run cause more work for the doctor and delay the patient's recovery. While a conversation with Ward Sister or Houseman (always with the patient's approval) may be easier than one with the consultant, it must be the latter's responsibility to see that it is made possible. Clearly the GP can help enormously here, either when the patient is in hospital or on discharge. But often he complains he gets information too little and too late from the hospital staff. Too often the latter complain that the GP does not seem to care. The major sufferers of this lack of communication remain the patient and the medical profession's reputation.

REFERENCES

Baxter, S. (1974). 'Psychological problems of intensive care'. *Brit. J. Hosp. Med.*, June, 875.

Cramond, W. A. (1970). 'Psychological problems of renal dialysis'. In Hill, O. W. (ed.), *Psychosomatic Medicine* 2. Butterworth, London.

Hay, G. G. (1970). 'Psychiatric aspects of cosmetic nasal operations'. *Brit. J. Psychiat.*, 116, 865.

Kaplan De-Nour, A. et al. (1968). 'Emotional reactions of patients on chronic haemodialysis', *Psychosom. Med.*, 30, 521.

Kornfeld, D. S. (1969). 'Psychiatric view of the intensive care unit', *Brit. Med. J.*, 1, 108.

Lazarus, H. R. and Hagens, J. H. (1968). *Am. J. Psychiat.*, 124, 1190.

Olley, P. C. (1974). 'Aspects of plastic surgery'. *Brit. Med. J.*, ii, 248, 322.

47 Getting old

We are all aware of the difference in outlook between the middle aged and elderly on the one hand and the younger generation on the other. In the course of a life-time everyone passes, often imperceptibly, from the attitudes of one stage to those of the other. With the passage of years one's mental mechanisms and ways of dealing with problems become more and more firmly set, so that however difficult the problem on hand may be, the elderly usually keep on with the same approach, no matter how unsuccessful it has been.

MIDDLE AGE

Intellectual and emotional changes

It has been said that all creative original research has been started by the time the investigator is 35. This may well be true and it serves to underline how early in life one's mental processes and reactions become fixed.

But few people regard themselves as even middle aged at 40: and in general they disregard their handicaps cheerfully, blaming their contemporaries and even more the younger generation for any incompatibility. In many walks of life too, their experience, social confidence and judgment will outweigh any slowness in learning; though technical advances make this less easy. There may therefore come a time when the first ardour for life, career, family and hobbies loses some of its lustre. Successes have been gained and are not to be repeated. Sights need lowering a little and the fact that there is a great deal of drudgery in most jobs, and some disharmony in most families has to be accepted.

Problems may come to the surface as their children become adolescent. It is unfortunate that this happens — in societies where marriage is far later than sexual maturity — at the same time as the mother becomes menopausal. Irritations and antagonisms, overt or repressed, easily develop and may result in a complete breakdown of the family, even splitting husband and wife as well. It has been pointed out that the problems of the middle-aged have attracted far less study than either paediatrics or old age. But two publications have remedied this: Ellis (1961) has written a popular account of Mediatrics, whose lightheartedness makes many painful truths palatable: and a most detailed and comprehensive study has been produced by Soddy and Kidson (1967).

THE INVOLUTIONAL PERIOD

At the involutional period in either sex — the menopause in women, and the fifties in men — there may be a sense of disappointment and failure; not all hopes have been achieved, and it has to be realized that many never will be. Physical changes impose some restrictions, and so some diminution of emotional outlets. This may pass as the person accepts 'going into a lower gear', or it may lead to a severe involutional depression (see p. 76) especially if there has been previous psychological disturbance.

Two special dangers exist here:

1 An early, sometimes the first, symptom of a depression is lack of sexual desire. This may lead to shame and not therefore be openly discussed even between husband and wife. Secretiveness hurts: and one partner, insecure and resentful, may suspect that the other is having an 'affair'. Vicious circles of bitterness and despair, ending in the divorce court, or in suicide, have begun in this way.
2 A physical illness starting at this time may undermine confidence so much that depression and anxiety become focused on the symptoms to the exclusion of other interests, and the patient becomes a totally different person (see p. 295).

OLD AGE

For the purpose of retirement the age of 65 is regarded as the time when people may be classed as elderly. But many people are still vigorous and active at that age, while others show the marks of ageing before then.

In 1970 about one in seven of the population was 65 or over. Because of the increased expectation of life more people are living into the period when the diseases of degeneration, e.g. cerebral arteriosclerosis, attack them. This inevitably means an increasingly heavy demand on psychiatric and geriatric services — especially as many of these patients make great calls on nursing time and skill. (The psychiatric diseases of old age are described on p. 165).

The world of the young child is a developing, ever-expanding one in which he continually enlarges his contacts and experiences; the world of the elderly person is an ever diminishing one which may easily contract down to the individual himself. So, in the elderly person the claims of outside activities, of friends and finally of family, become less important and disappear. In the emotional sphere this is often shown by a lack of normal emotional response to events which would formerly have moved the patient, e.g. the death of a near relative. There comes in fact a poverty of emotional response.

Concurrently with this comes the failure of recent memory. This results in repetition of conversation to the boredom of the patient's companions and a tendency to dwell on and talk about the past rather than the present. If this failure of recent memory persists it is an important factor in leading to confusion and disorientation.

Isolation due to physical factors

The normal person is kept in contact with the world and his fellows especially by the twin special senses of sight and hearing. Unfortunately both are liable to undergo degeneration with age. Normally hearing is at its most acute between the age of 5 and 10; thereafter the maximum audible frequency gradually declines. Similarly the near point for the emmetropic eye is at infinity at the age of 45.

Both these changes occur normally and to them may be added the many degenerative conditions affecting the ear and eye. It is probable that deafness is the more serious threat to the integrity of a patient's personality. He often passes through a stage of mishearing or misinterpretation to a stage of severe deafness, and so is cut off from the correcting force of other people's views, as by no other illness. It has been shown that the incidence of deafness and/or blindness are many times greater in senile psychiatric patients than in comparable groups outside mental hospital care. Besides this, lack of teeth may lead to malnutrition, and lack of warmth to hypothermia; both lead to loss of energy and of confidence. Special disabilities, such as arthritis, may add to their loneliness.

Isolation due to social factors

The isolation of old age may be increased by other factors:

1 The longer one lives the fewer relations and contemporaries there are to bear one company. The death of the husband, wife or supporting child may be a particularly devastating blow.
2 Retirement, with the loss of the friendly interest and stimulation of fellow workers.
3 Loss of status from being 'Mr. X who works in the City' to 'the old man' hanging around the house in his wife's way.
4 Financial stress — resulting in old people living in top back rooms, virtually prisoners, because of the difficulty of negotiating stairs.
5 Urban isolation in large cities.

Prophylaxis

The gradual deterioration of one or more physical systems, and in particular of the central nervous system, is to be expected at some time in every human being. There is, however, an enormous range of variation; and much energy, health and happiness remain for many elderly people. There is certainly no reason for the GP to be defeatist at the first sign of breakdown — for many are temporary, and some compensatory functions by other parts, even of the brain, are remarkable. In general, good nursing and medical care will help enormously (see p. 169), but dementia cannot be cured. Prophylaxis offers more help.

What can be done to prevent degenerative illness? Quite a bit. Unfortunately the arrangement of the working life of many people is the worst possible preparation for a healthy retirement and old age. One day a person is fully employed with all the self-respect that brings; the next day he is pensioned with a greatly reduced income, no work and a fall in self-respect and morale. Retirement is still largely unplanned and too many people look upon it simply as a kind of long holiday with freedom from the necessity of regular timetables and work. In fact work plays an essential part in the life of all of us in making us feel important members of the community; take this away and we are thrown on our own resources. Indeed it may be said that retirement, and the way we use it, shows what kind of person we really are.

The essential of retirement is that it should be planned so that we can continue to use our skills. For some people, e.g. the manual labourer who earns his living by sheer physical labour, this may be impossible. If the person can find part-time work (professional or skilled), it eases him gently into retirement and maintains his morale. Some large firms do employ older workers in special workshops where they are found to be good at skilled and semi-skilled work, particularly if not suffering competition from younger men. Old people's voluntary workshops are particularly useful. This enables old people to meet together to exercize their skills from the very simple to the quite complex.

Retirement also demands the development of hobbies carried over from earlier life. The retired person who feels he will occupy himself by not getting up to catch the early business train, pottering in the garden and doing the shopping, is courting disaster; old people's clubs, like old people's workshops, have a valuable place in the life of the elderly in making them still feel members of the community.

'Meals on wheels' for the elderly also ensure that they get one dietetically adequate meal a day and so diminishes the risk of developing a confusional state due to vitamin deficiency.

Finally, bearing in mind the importance of sight and hearing, in keeping in touch with their fellows, it is important to remember the value of spectacles, opthalmic surgery, hearing aids and plastic otological surgery.

FURTHER READING

Amulree, Lord (1951). *Adding Life to Years.* Nat. Council of Social Service.

Chisholm, C. (1954). *Retire and Enjoy Life.* Phoenix House, London.

Ellis, H. F. (1961). *Mediatrics.* G. Bles, London.

Office of Health Economics (1968). *Old Age.*

Ogilvie, Sir Heneage (1962). *Fifty.* Max Parrish, London.

Soddy, K. and Kidson, M. (1967). *Man in Middle Life.* Tavistock Publications, London.

48 Death and dying

Many criticisms have been made that doctors are never taught, as undergraduates or postgraduates, how to deal with the attitude of patients, relatives, and themselves, to death and dying. A conspiracy of silence surrounds the whole subject. Even experienced GPs find it impossible to give the help they feel they should in their embarrassment and fear.

Patients, relatives, nurses and doctors therefore suffer more than they need. Yet it has been said by Jung that a doctor's main job is to prepare patients for death. (A similar conspiracy of silence is admitted in other professions, e.g. the clergy.)

Obviously this is not solely a psychiatric problem: nearly all other consultants have a clear responsibility to teach their students, and even more their housemen and registrars. But students often voice their uneasiness on this score to psychiatrists ('death is not on our programme, but it is on the patient's') and as the attitudes to be met depend often on unconscious factors and personality traits, some comments may be made from a psychiatric angle.

The responsibility of discussing impending death with the patient and his relatives must vary according to the authority given by the consultant to his registrar, houseman and student; and according to the questions asked of each by the patient.

These questions present a very difficult problem. Ideally,

surely, a doctor should give an honest answer to a sincere question. But in practice, many patients ask questions to which they do not want a true answer; others do not ask direct questions, but wish to know. It is essential therefore for the doctor to give his patient the opportunity to voice his anxieties and to understand what his real need is before he can decide what to tell him. The diagnosis of the patient's need is as important as any other diagnosis in medicine (Balint 1968).

It is probable that there are more doctors who fail to give answers when wanted than there are who give unnecessary answers. To fail here may be to deprive the patient of his confidence in his doctor and the chance of establishing stronger personal relations with his family and setting his affairs in order. This risk must be assessed by the doctor responsibly.

Besides him, in practice, two other people are very often closely involved: the ward sister, whose task in helping patients meet death is not always helped by frantic belated efforts at resuscitation ('the dignity of death', as one said, 'has disappeared'): and the chaplain, who is ready to discuss the problem, but would much prefer to get to know patients as a routine, and not be called in, so to speak, as a vulture-like harbinger of death.

DIFFERENT REACTIONS

Human reactions to the knowledge, or suspicion, of impending death are enormously varied and have been described in innumerable writings, religious and lay, prose and poetry. Few doctors can be familiar with more than a fraction of this literature; yet many doctors are asked for help. An account of the common reactions may therefore be of some value.

1 *Fear of the unknown*, including pain in dying. This is more often felt than openly expressed, from shame at being thought a coward; the doctor can certainly help by reassuring the patient, by his behaviour as much as by his words, that he will watch his needs and meet all of them that he can.

2 *Fear of extinction*. To some, the extinction of their personality is intolerable — especially to the young, energetic, egocentric; and some analysts have held that this has led, as a

compensation, to a belief in an after-life, and indeed in God. Others are upheld by a sure and certain hope of a fuller, happier, personal survival, though accounts of this vary from the childish to the ineffable. The idea that the dying person will not reach 'heaven' unless he dies in one particular faith, notorious in the middle ages, is still held by some today. But it may be thought that such last minute conversion is no part of a doctor's profession, nor indeed that it fits with any concept of a beneficent Almighty.

3 *Fear of damnation* still occurs, though out of keeping with modern theological (or lay) thinking; for many people have been brought up with these ideas, and they recur as death approaches, none the weaker for having been repressed through life. They present a problem of diagnosis as well as of treatment for the doctor. Some are rational and respond to rational discussion: others are frankly part of a depressive state, which may be accompanied by intense guilt, and even by hallucinations and delusions. If so, anti-depressant measures, physical as well as psychological, should certainly be used. But it must be remembered that a period of loneliness and isolation from God has also been experienced by the most saintly (and sane) people, as a phase of their mystical experience: described as the 'Dark Night of the Soul' by St. John of the Cross.

The minister may clearly help religious crises as much as, or more than, the doctor: but he is unfortunately untrained, at the present, to recognize psychiatric conditions.

The treatment of guilt is a subject on which priests and psychiatrists largely agree, though their advice is couched in different terms. Confession, penance and expiation, atonement, and forgiveness: all have their psychological counterparts.

4 *Anxiety for others.* Any patient with love for his family and friends feels anxiety for their future and is helped if he believes that he can go on helping them by his legacy (financial or emotional): if they will in fact be exposed to much hardship, the doctor and welfare services can provide reassurance of help.

5 *Relief.* Even without severe pain, old age isn't much fun and the effect of medical science in prolonging life without the capacity to enjoy it is two-edged. It is hard to blame the patient for wanting to escape: paradoxically those who most count on a joyful after-life are the more deterred from suicide by their religious views.

It may be asked whether or not a doctor should help a patient to the means of suicide, which raises enormous ethical and social problems (see Euthanasia, p. 386).

6 *Courageous resignation.* This is perhaps the commonest attitude: strengthened by religious faith, consideration for others' grief, or pride in showing no feelings: so that the patient appears to need no help. But occasionally this attitude may be a façade concealing one or more of the above: and the doctor should be sure that he is not misled.

It is tragic if the doctor's life of service to the patient should fail at this moment of crisis and he should therefore fail to give needed help.

7 *Acceptance of death* and the end of existence may also be reached as one of the tests of living by many rationalists as part of their belief or as an inevitable and final outcome of life (see Paul Tillich).

8 *Joyful welcome.* Those who have reached this stage will need no help but instead give it to their doctor, and, through him, to other patients.

The reader will have noted that it is, in the writer's view, not the doctor's job to impose his own religious views, unasked, on a dying patient: he may also have noted (here) that it is very hard to prevent those views from seeping through.

FURTHER READING

Balint, M. (1968). Personal communication.

Bright, P. (1962). *The Day's End.* Macgibbon and Kee, St. Albans.

Hinton, J. (1967). *Dying.* Penguin.

Kastenbaum, R. and Aisenberg, R. (1974). *The Psychology of Death.* Duckworth, London.

Kübler-Ross, E.(1970). *On Death and Dying.* Macmillan, London.

Platt, Lord (1963). 'Reflections on ageing and death'. *Lancet*, i, 1.

Tillich, Paul (1962). *The Courage to Be.* Fontana, London.

Toynbee, A. et al. (1968). *Man's Concern With Death.* Hodder and Stoughton, London.

49 Psychotherapy

INTRODUCTION

Treatment methods used to help psychiatrically ill and emotionally disturbed patients can be divided into (1) physical methods, using drugs (see p. 316), or ECT (see p. 326) or surgical procedures (see p. 341), and (2) psychological methods which rely on various psychological, verbal and non-verbal, methods of influencing the patient.

Psychotherapy is by far the commonest form of psychological treatment and will be considered next. Other psychological methods like behaviour therapy (see p. 327) and hypnosis (see p. 325) will be dealt with separately. (It should be noted that nowadays the term psychotherapy is sometimes being used generically to include all psychological treatments but the disadvantage of this is that it leaves no term to describe psychotherapy proper, as defined below).

The term psychotherapy is being used here to describe a psychological treatment method employed in a professional context which relies on psychological understanding of the patient's problems, symptoms and behaviour and in which personal communication between therapist and patient and the relationship between them is of central importance. It is important to distinguish between (1) *supportive psychotherapy* and (2) *formal psychotherapy*. The former relies essentially on the personal influence of the doctor or other professional worker on his patient and on his humane, non-judgmental understanding of his difficulties. Its aim is to support the patient rather than to bring about major changes in his attitudes and behaviour. It plays a part in the treatment of most patients independent of their particular illness and alongside any other physical or psychological treatment they may be receiving at the same time (see p. 321 and p. 347). Formal psychotherapy, on the other hand, is based on deeper understanding of the patient's personality and the reasons underlying his symptoms and disturbed behaviour; its aim is to bring about changes in his personality and to promote personal growth through insight into underlying conscious, unconscious and interpersonal problems and through emotional experience in the therapeutic relationship. Although Freud's work on the nature of mental processes has laid the basis for most of the formal psychotherapeutic procedures used nowadays, it must be emphasized that psychoanalysis as developed by Freud and his followers is only one, highly specialized and time consuming, method of psychotherapy, with very limited clinical applications. Some of the contributions made by Freud and other workers in this field and some of the psychotherapeutic procedures commonly used will be described below. They can be sub-divided according to three criteria:

1 *Depth of understanding aimed at:* ranging from exploration at a deep level in full-scale analysis through more limited exploration in analytically oriented psychotherapy to 'superficial or minor' psychotherapy, mainly supportive in nature and conducted at a conscious level (see p. 312).
2 *Frequency of treatment sessions:* ranging from 5 sessions a week in psychoanalysis, to only one a week or fortnight or even less often in supportive therapy.
3 *Setting of treatment:* ranging all the way from individual psychotherapy, or joint interviews (for example, for married couples or families) to small groups, large groups and whole therapeutic communities of a ward or even a hospital.

It should be noted that these various methods are used not necessarily by doctors but by other professionals, such as psychiatric social workers, lay psychotherapists or nurses, provided they have been trained in psycho-therapeutic practices.

PSYCHOANALYSIS (Sigmund Freud, 1856-1939)

Usually five sessions of 50 minutes each per week; treatment lasts from one to five years or longer, average two or three years. The patient usually lies on a couch with the analyst sitting behind him and uses free associations; special emphasis is put on exploring unconscious mental processes, on instinctual problems connected with sexuality and aggression, on dream analysis and ego-defences. Of particular importance is the development of the *transference* by which is meant that the patient relives in relation to the analyst past experiences and strong feelings, for example of dependency, of love and hate which he previously experienced in relation to other important persons in his life such as his mother, father or siblings. Transference phenomena play a part in all psycho-therapeutic relationships as well as in ordinary life but in psychoanalysis their development is actively encouraged and interpretation of the transference phenomena is one of the most important therapeutic tools in psychoanalysis. The analyst has to know and control his own 'counter-transference', i.e. strong feelings towards his patient which are at least in part the result of his own past experiences now re-lived in relation to his patient. He interprets the meaning of the patient's associations and communications to him keeping, at least according to classical psychoanalysis, his own personality and value systems and beliefs out as far as possible.

The use of psychoanalysis as a treatment method is limited not only by social and economic factors but also by the patient's suitability for analysis; this depends particularly on his motivation to undergo such treatment, a reasonable degree of intelligence, his capacity for reality testing and the absence of gross psychiatric, somatic and behavioural disturbances. Hence, psychoanalysis is useful particularly in the treatment of psychoneuroses and character disorders in reasonably young, well motivated, intelligent patients and borderline cases and in some psychosomatic conditions. It is a unique method for research into mental phenomena and for the training of psychotherapists. A great deal of our knowledge of other methods of psychotherapy is ultimately derived from psychoanalysis.

Post-Freudian modifications

Freud's daughter, Anna Freud, has since drawn particular attention to the importance of the mechanisms of defence employed by the ego in mental functioning and she has also been responsible for the development of child psychotherapy using analytical concepts.

Melanie Klein has laid special emphasis on the formative influences of the infant's earliest experiences, especially in its relationship to its mother, including the importance of primitive, aggressive and persecutory fantasies, schizoid mechanisms of projection and introjection and the development of a sense of concern, of guilt and of feelings of depression. These concepts have laid the basis for her method of analysis of children, using play therapy, and have also led to important modifications in the psychoanalytical treatment of adults.

The neo-Freudians (Karen Horney, Erich Fromm) have laid particular emphasis on the patient's total personality and on the influence of his interpersonal relationships and his social environment.

OTHER SCHOOLS AND METHODS

Carl Gustav Jung (1875-1961): *analytical psychology*

Jung was a colleague of Freud's until 1913, then established his own separate school of analytical psychology. Patients are usually seen three or four times a week; the couch is rarely used but free association and analysis of the transference and of dreams are used as in Freudian psychoanalysis. Jung paid less attention to sexuality and emphasized instead the importance of spiritual, including religious, problems and of symbolism. He introduced the concept of a 'collective' as opposed to a personal unconscious and of so-called 'archetypal images' supposed to be common to all cultures and races thus accounting for similarities of mythological, religious and individual human concepts and symbols found in different societies and at different stages of development. He saw treatment through psychotherapy essentially as a process of integration and 'individuation'.

The gap between Freudian and Jungian methods of analysis is narrower than it used to be although the two schools use different concepts, and Jungian ideas are often difficult to comprehend by those used to thinking in biological and scientific terms and are less easy to apply in practice.

Alfred Adler (1870-1939)

Adler was another pupil and colleague of Freud's who left the psychoanalytic movement in 1911. He paid less attention to the unconscious and to sexuality and stressed instead the desire for power and the establishment of a sense of personal achievement and superiority in one's social setting.

Existentialist concepts (Binswanger, Boss, Laing)

These have developed mainly under the influence of the European school of Existentialist philosophy (Heidegger, Sartre). Emphasis is placed particularly on the patient's actual conscious experiences in relation to the world in which he lives, and on the real, as opposed to the transference relationship between himself and his therapist in the 'here-and-now' situation. Particular attention is paid to the need in human development to establish a firmly rooted sense of existence, to be true to oneself and to develop an identity of one's own. Problems of uprootedness and alienation are of particular interest to existentialist psychiatrists, and so is the need to accept anxiety, guilt and conflict as essential aspects of human existence. Therapists influenced by existentialist concepts, whether they are aware of this or not, allow themselves to bring into the treatment situation more of their own personality and of their own value systems, and to get more directly involved with their patients than more orthodox psychoanalysts and psychotherapists.

Analytically orientated (dynamic) psychotherapy

Here, the same concepts, especially those of unconscious and transference phenomena, and similar methods are used as in psychoanalysis and related schools but treatment is often more limited in its aims. Treatment sessions are usually less frequent, from one to three sessions a week, the couch is used less often and treatment may only last a few months to a year or two. This is probably the commonest method of formal individual psychotherapy in use under the NHS at present. It can be used for patients with personality disorders, psycho-neuroses, psychosomatic disorders and even psychoses provided the patient shows sufficient motivation and his reality testing and behaviour are not too seriously disturbed.

Supportive psychotherapy

Here, the emphasis is mainly on conscious problems and the psychotherapist's main task is to help the patient to talk about his problems and to express his feelings by being prepared to listen and to accept him without bringing judgment to bear, and at times to reassure and support him. A great deal of the work of psychiatrists, GPs and social workers consists of this type of therapy, not necessarily in formal sessions but as part of their everyday contact with patients with psychological problems or psychiatric or psychosomatic symptoms (see p. 347).

Joint interviews and family therapy

While in classical psychoanalysis the analyst only sees the patient and avoids having contact with relatives, nowadays techniques of treatment are being developed in which husband and wife, and sometimes whole families are seen together. This development is in keeping with our increasing awareness of the importance of interpersonal, in addition to intra-psychic phenomena.

SMALL GROUP PSYCHOTHERAPY

Six to eight patients, both men and women, are treated together in a group by the therapist, the group leader, for 1½ hours once or twice a week. In closed groups the composition of the group remains constant for the duration of treatment — usually about two years. In open groups patients who leave or are discharged are replaced by others and the group can thus continue indefinitely. Patients are asked to talk freely about themselves and their problems and about their feelings towards each other and the group leader. The latter mainly adopts a listening role, except when he draws attention to problems of individual patients, to their interaction and to what goes on in the group as a whole (Foulkes and Anthony 1957, Walton 1971).

There has been a good deal of discussion whether group psychotherapy should be used for the analysis of the individual patients in the group or whether the therapist should restrict himself to interpretations of the behaviour of the group as a whole. Best results are obtained if the therapist adopts a flexible attitude; if by his own relative inactivity he encourages interaction between the group members; if he is prepared to make individual as well as group interpretations and to pay attention to each individual patient's past and present problems as well as to the here-and-now situation in the group. Occasionally it is useful to see a patient in individual sessions as well as in the group. Some groups are run by two co-therapists.

Group psychotherapy has not only got the advantage of being an economical method of treatment — hence it is widely used in National Health Service outpatient departments — but it also provides a very effective therapeutic experience for the group members. They learn to speak about topics which they have hitherto kept strictly to themselves, and the multiple interactions between each other and with the group leader and the changing attitude of the group as a whole all form the basis for often highly charged emotional experiences, as well as for interpretation by the therapist. Groups can be used for patients with a large variety of disorders, including personality disorders, psychoneuroses, psychosomatic diseases and occasionally border-line cases and psychoses, the latter usually being treated in separate groups. Apart from this exception patients with different disorders can be treated together in one group provided the age and intelligence range are similar. Patients who have never had a satisfying relationship with one other person and paranoid patients are better treated individually, but may subsequently benefit from group therapy.

Psychotherapeutic communities and large groups

The principles of psychotherapy can also be applied to larger groups of patients, for example, all the in patients in a ward or in one hospital (Jones, 1968). The patients and staff have regular meetings in which all the members of the group are encouraged to express themselves openly, the aim being to encourage better communication and mutual understanding. This method has been found particularly useful in the management of seriously ill neurotic and psychotic, particularly schizophrenic inpatients and in the treatment of psychopaths. It is also used in Day Hospitals.

Encounter groups

The encounter group or 'growth' movement from the United States is gaining recognition in this country and elsewhere. Patients meet, sometimes only on one occasion or at regular, say, weekly intervals, either for several hours or for a whole weekend ('marathon groups'). The emphasis is on generating intense emotional experiences in the individuals and the group. Bodily contact through touching, active bodily movement ('bioenergetics'), role playing, Gestalt therapy (Perls et al. 1973), and psychodrama (acting various parts which are of emotional significance to one or more group members) are among the various means which are used to help the participants to get in touch with aspects of their personality previously suppressed. Such intense here-and-now experiences may liberate members from life-long over-control and out-of-date habitual and maladaptive behaviour. It is probably most effective when it is combined with insight-directed psychotherapy either in the group itself or by undergoing one or other of the more conventional forms of psychotherapy on separate occasions.

CONCLUSION

The field of clinical psychotherapy, therefore, now constitutes a large discipline of its own. Supportive psychotherapy now plays a part in the management of almost every patient who consults a doctor. Even if the doctor is not aware of it, his personal approach and his attitude to his patients are bound to have an important psychological effect in addition to whatever physical treatment he is carrying out. The more aware he is of this, the greater the chances that his personal relationship to his patients will have a useful therapeutic effect. In fact, one important influence which psychotherapeutic thinking has had on medicine as a whole is that it has made doctors more aware of the role of their own personality and of their personal relationship to their patients. Balint's groups for GPs have played an important part in promoting this development.

Apart from this development, however, the different major or 'formal' methods of more intensive psychotherapy described above play an important part in the treatment of selected patients with personality disorders and psychiatric or psychosomatic illnesses. In clinical psychotherapy a flexible approach is essential, the method of treatment and the concepts used will vary with the patient's needs and the facilities available, and the different concepts and forms of psychotherapy can be combined with each other as well as with other methods of treatment, for example drugs, ECT, leucotomy, behaviour therapy, in-patient care and rehabilitation.

FURTHER READING

Balint, M. (1964). *The Doctor, His Patient and the Illness.* Tavistock Publications, London.

Bennet, E. A. (1966). *What Jung Really Said.* Macdonald, London.

Brown, J. A. C. (1963). *Freud and the Post-Freudians.* Penguin.

Caine, T. M. and Smail, D. J. (1969). *The Treatment of Mental Illness.* University of London Press, London.

De Maré, P. B. and Kreeger, L. C. (1974). *Introduction to Group Treatments in Psychiatry.* Butterworth, London.

Dewald, P. A. (1964). *Psychotherapy, a Dynamic Approach.* Blackwell, Oxford.

Foulkes, S. H. (1964). *Therapeutic Group Analysis.* Allen and Unwin, London.

Foulkes, S. H. and Anthony, E. J. (1957). *Group Psychotherapy: The Psycho-Analytic Approach.* Penguin.

Freud, S. (1949). *An Outline of Psycho-Analysis.* Hogarth, London.

Hill, D. (1970). 'On the contributions of psychoanalysis to psychiatry: mechanism and meaning'. *Brit. J. Psychiat.,* 117, 609.

Jones, M. (1968). *Social Psychiatry in Practice.* Penguin.

Jung, C. G. (1963). *Memories, Dreams, Reflections.* Routledge, London.

Kreeger, L. (ed.) (1975). *The Large Group.* Constable, London.

Laing, R. D. (1960). *The Divided Self.* Tavistock Publications, London.

Lieberman, M. A., Yalom, I. D. and Miles, M. B. (1973). *Encounter Groups: First Facts*. Basic Books , New York.

Mintz, A. L. (1973). *Encounter Groups and Other Panaceas*. Reprinted from Commentary in *Vesper Exchange*, 2147.

Perls, F., Hefferline, R. F. and Goodman, P. (1973). *Gestalt Therapy*. Pelican.

Reich, W. (1973). *Character Analysis*. Vision, London.

Segal, H. (1964). *Introduction to the Work of Melanie Klein*. Heinemann, London.

Stafford-Clark, D. (1965). *What Freud Really Said*. Macdonald, London.

Stewart, H. (1972). 'Six months, fixed-term, once-weekly psychotherapy'. *Brit. J. Psychiat.*, 121, 425.

Tarachow, S. (1964). *An Introduction to Psychotherapy*. Hogarth, London.

Walton, H. (ed.), (1971). *Small Group Psychotherapy*. Penguin.

Wolff, H. H. (1972). 'Psychotherapy: its place in psychosomatic management'. *Psychother. Psychosom.*, 22, 233.

Wolff, H. H. (1973) 'The place of psychotherapy in the district psychiatric services'. In *Policy for Action*, OUP, London.

Wyss, D. (1966). *Depth Psychology: a Critical History*. Norton, New York,

Yalom, I. D. (1970). *The Theory and Practice of Group Psychotherapy*. Basic Books, New York.

50 Psychotropic and other drugs

PSYCHOTROPIC DRUGS

In the preceding pages various drugs have been listed under the treatment of each clinical syndrome and their indications, dosage and side-effects have been discussed. The following pages tabulate the main psychotropic drugs in clinical use at present:

Mechanism and site of action of psychotropic drugs

Knowledge of the exact site and mechanisms of action of these drugs is still incomplete.

1 *The phenothiazine group of tranquillizers*. These appear to act mainly on such sub-cortical structures as the reticular and

limbic systems and the hypothalamus, in contrast to the barbiturates whose effect is mainly on the cerebral cortex. The sub-cortical structures mentioned are mainly responsible for the state of awareness, for emotional reactions and for the control of the autonomic nervous system and this may account for the fact that the phenothiazine group of drugs are of most use in the control of the major emotional, cognitive and behavioural disorders of psychotic conditions without interfering with consciousness. One of the actions of these drugs is to block the effect of catecholamines and serotonin which are found in high concentration in sub-cortical structures of the brain.

2 *The anti-depressant drugs.* Both the tricyclic compounds and the mono-amine oxidase inhibitors raise the level of available mono-amines at the synapses in the central nervous system. The discovery that reserpine when used as a hypotensive agent could produce a severe state of depression and that it causes depletion of mono-amine levels in the brain led to the hypothesis that a lowering of mono-amines might be the biochemical mechanism responsible for depressive illnesses. The fact that iproniazid which inhibits the enzyme mono-amine oxidase can lift depression and lead to a state of mental over-activity and excitement lent further support to this hypothesis. Since then various other mono-amine oxidase inhibitors have been found to be effective anti-depressants. The tricyclic compounds also increase the availability of free mono-amines at the synapses, not by preventing the breakdown of mono-amines but by preventing their re-absorption after their release from the nerve endings.

3 *Stimulants.* Amphetamine is the one best known and it acts by lowering the arousal threshold through its effect on the reticular activating system.

4 *Hallucinogenic drugs.* The occasional clinical use of lysergic acid diethylamide to overcome resistances during psychotherapy has been mentioned. Mescaline is another hallucinogen which has been used mainly in research on psychoses on account of the fact that like LSD it can produce temporary psychotic manifestations. Both these drugs act on the reticular system and increase arousal thus leading to greatly increased awareness.

5 *Abreactive drugs.* These are various but their mode of action is generally to produce unconsciousness, followed by a trance-like state (see p. 324).

TABLE III: *Psychotropic and other drugs*

Group	Official Name	Trade Name	Daily Dose		Indications
(1) TRANQUILLIZERS					
(a) Phenothiazine Derivatives	Chlorpromazine	Largactil	Low:	75 mg	Low dose: Anxiety and tension
			High:	600 mg	High dose: Disturbing symptoms and behaviour in schizophrenia
	Promazine	Sparine		150 mg	Anxiety and agitation
	Trifluoperazine	Stelazine	Low:	3 mg	Low dose: Anxiety and tension
			High:	30 mg	High dose: Schizophrenia, especially for apathy and paranoid symptoms
	Perphenazine	Fentazin	Low:	6 mg	} as above
			High:	60 mg	
	Thioridazine	Melleril	Low:	30 mg	} as above
			High:	600 mg	
	Fluphenazine decanoate	Modecate	25 mg fortnightly		Chronic schizophrenia with hallucinations
(b) Benzodiazepines	Chlordiazepoxide	Librium		20-30 mg	Anxiety and tension in psychoneuroses
	Diazepam	Valium		10-20 mg	Anxiety and tension in psychoneuroses
	Oxazepam	Serenid D		45-90 mg	Anxiety
	Medazepam	Nobrium		15-30 mg	Anxiety
(c) Butyrophenone derivatives	Haloperidol	Serenace		3-9 mg	Mania and hypomania
(d) Others	Meprobamate	Equanil, Miltown		1200 mg	Chronic anxiety
	Oxypertine	Integrin		30 mg	Anxiety and depression
(2) ANTI-DEPRESSANTS					
(a) Tricyclic compounds	Imipramine	Tofranil		75-200 mg	Depression
	Amitriptyline	Tryptizol		75-250 mg	Depression
	Nortriptyline	Aventyl		30-150 mg	Depression
	Protriptyline	Concordin		15-60 mg	Depression
	Dothiepin	Prothiaden		75 mg	Depression
	Trimipramine	Surmontil		50-100 mg	Depression

(b) Mono-amine oxidase inhibitors	Phenelzine	Nardil	15-75 mg	Depression
	Isocarboxazid	Marplan	10-30 mg	Depression
	Nialamide	Niamid	75-150 mg	Depression
	Tranylcypromine	Parnate	10-30 mg	Depression
(c) Stimulants	Amphetamine	Benzedrine	5-15 mg	Depression } Rarely used on account of
	Dextro-amphetamine	Dexedrine	5-15 mg	Depression } risk of addiction
(3) HALLUCINOGENS	Lysergic acid diethylamide	—	—	To reduce resistance in psychotherapy; dose 50-150 µg. Rarely used on account of side effects
	Mescaline	—	—	
(4) ABREACTIVE DRUGS	Thiopentone sodium	Pentothal	5-15 mg 2½% i.v.	Nitrous oxide, carbon dioxide, ether and other drugs have been used for the same purpose
	Methylamphetamine hydrochloride	Methedrine	15-30 mg i.v.	
	Amylobarbitone sodium	Sodium amytal	1 ml of 10% sol. per min. i.v.	Inadvisable from risk of addiction
(5) HYPNOTICS (a) Barbiturates	Barbitone sodium	Medinal	300-450 mg	Smaller doses of barbituates, e.g. sod. amytal can be given by day as a sedative
	Amylobarbitone sodium	Sodium amytal	200-400 mg	
	Quinal barbitone	Seconal	100-200 mg	} These two are combined as Tuinal,
	Butobarbitone	Soneryl	100-200 mg	} 100-200 mg
	Pentobarbitone sodium	Nembutal	100-200 mg	
(b) Non-barbiturates	Glutethimide	Doriden	500 mg	
	Dichloral-phenazone	Welldorm	650-1300 mg	
	Nitrazepam	Mogadon	5-10 mg	
	Methaqualone	Combined in one tablet as Mandrax	250 mg	
	Diphenhydramine		25 mg	

NOTE: Parstelin is a compound of parnate and stelazine, Drinamyl of dexedrine and amytal; Limbritol is librium and tryptizol.

OTHER DRUGS

Besides the psychotropic drugs, there are others used in psychiatry.

1 *Sedatives and hypnotics* to allay anxiety including its somatic manifestations; and to promote deep and untroubled sleep. The best known are barbiturates: but many non-barbiturates exist (see Table III) and are safer, in that addiction is less likely.

2 *Vitamins*, especially Vitamin B complex, are used in confusional states, especially if associated with alcoholism. A course of intramuscular injections of parentrovite is the most effective method.

3 *Insulin* was used in the past to produce insulin shock or coma (see p. 327); as 'modified insulin' in small doses it promotes appetite and well-being, especially in anorexia (see p. 199).

4 *Lithium carbonate* has been used for mania and depression (see p. 84).

5 When organic changes are present, e.g. anaemia, electrolytic disturbances, the various drugs appropriate to the organic condition must be used.

6 The anti-convulsants have been referred to in the section on Epilepsy (p. 164).

REFERENCES

Marks, J. and Pare, C. M. B. (1965. *The Scientific Basis of Drug Therapy in Psychiatry*. Pergamon, Oxford.

Sargant, W. and Slater, E. (1972). *Physical Methods of Treatment in Psychiatry*. Livingstone, Edinburgh.

Shepherd, M., Lader, M. and Rodnight, R. (1968). *Clinical Psychopharmacology*. English Universities Press, London.

51 Drugs, psychotherapy and hypnosis

THE COMBINED APPROACH

Recent advances in psycho-pharmacology have had a profound effect on the treatment, course and prognosis of many of the more serious and incapacitating psychiatric disorders, especially the psychoses and depressive illnesses and, to a lesser degree, of conditions with anxiety as the predominant symptom. On the other hand, drugs alone cannot alter the personality disorders underlying many of these conditions, nor can they affect the psychological factors which so often play an important, and sometimes the major role in the origin of psychiatric illness, especially problems of interpersonal relationships and of adjustment to difficult life situations. These aspects of psychiatric illness will have to be dealt with by one or other form of psychotherapy, and by various social manoeuvres aimed at changing the environment and at rehabilitation.

In clinical psychiatric practice all these procedures, physical, psychotherapeutic and social can and should be used, singly or in combination. The choice depends on the patient, his illness, his particular circumstances and also on the facilities for treatment available. It is unfortunate therefore that there are still some psychiatrists, those with a predominantly organic orientation, who believe almost exclusively in the use of drugs and belittle the importance of psychotherapy, whilst others, especially some psychoanalysts with an exclusively psychological orientation, believe only in the value of psychotherapy and are antagonistic to the use of drugs in the treatment of any psychiatric patient.

The reasons for this unnecessary and out-dated division are several. Treatment with drugs is the usual procedure in other branches of medicine and doctors are therefore more used to prescribing drugs than to realizing that psychological methods of treatment may be equally, or in some cases more important for a particular patient. Moreover, many patients expect to be treated with drugs and may be very resistant to the idea of being treated with psychotherapy only.

On the other hand, it is true that by prescribing a drug too readily both the doctor and the patient may overlook the relevance of important psychological aspects and the patient may thus be denied psychotherapeutic help which he may badly need in order to resolve underlying emotional and/or inter-personal problems which have led to the development of his illness. Sometimes it is the doctor who lacks the time or interest to deal with these psychological problems, even when the patient feels that what he really needs is understanding and not physical treatment. On other occasions the doctor may realize that the patient needs psychotherapy but the patient may insist on being treated with drugs because he is unwilling to accept his doctor's advice. In clinical practice it is just as wrong to withhold psychotherapy when this is indicated as it is wrong not to prescribe drugs when the patient's condition demands it, and in many cases both will be needed either in succession or simultaneously.

Some psychoanalysts and psychotherapists have been re-luctant to accept that while their methods of treatment are very valuable for patients with psychoneuroses and personality disorders who are relatively free from gross disturbances of behaviour and are more or less in touch with reality, many psychiatric patients who come under the care of the general psychiatrist are quite inaccessible to psychotherapy because of their disordered behaviour; they may be threatening suicide, assaulting others or taking drugs or alcohol, or suffering from gross delusions and hallucinations. Such patients need treatment with physical methods of treatment, often in hospital to begin with, and it is here that modern drug treatment has brought about the greatest change. It should be noted, however, that under such conditions a drug to calm down a patient is sometimes given less because the patient needs it and more in order to protect others, to preserve peace in the ward, or to allay anxiety in the staff (including the doctors). One also tends to overlook the unpleasant effect of certain drugs such as large doses of phenothiazines or anti-depressants; these are partly due to their side effects, but they may also make the patient feel that his feelings, thoughts and actions are no longer his own but are influenced by the drugs.

Once the acute symptoms have been brought under control the patient may be ready for some form of psychotherapy; in fact the advances in psychopharmacology, far from having reduced the demands for psychotherapy, have increased it by making patients accessible to a psychotherapeutic approach who would without drugs not have been able to co-operate in a psychotherapeutic relationship. Treatment with drugs and psychotherapy can then be usefully combined and, later still, treatment with drugs can sometimes be discontinued while psychotherapy continues to help the patient to resolve his problems sufficiently to prevent relapses in the future.

Even in less seriously disturbed patients drugs may be used initially to control acute symptoms; but, especially in psycho-neurotic patients, the condition should be re-assessed as soon as the crisis is over and the possibility of psychotherapy considered. It is often useful to take such patients into one's confidence by telling them that they are given a drug for relief of symptoms but that as soon as possible an attempt should be made to understand and deal with the psychological problems which have caused the illness.

Once a patient is in psychotherapy he may get temporarily more anxious or depressed when he becomes aware of the underlying reasons for his symptoms. Occasionally he may need treatment with drugs at this stage but usually it is preferable for him to work through such periods of anxiety or depression in treatment as this constitutes an important part of insight-directed psychotherapy and psychoanalysis. If in doubt, close co-operation between the GP and psychotherapist is essential.

If the patient is inaccessible to psychotherapy, or if he is chronically ill, or if no psychotherapeutic facilities are available, a combination of drug treatment and supportive psychotherapy may be the best practical method of helping him, particularly in crises or with exacerbation of his symptoms.

THE DOCTOR'S ATTITUDE

It must be remembered that the effect of a drug will not only depend on its pharmacological properties but on the attitude of the doctor, his belief or lack of belief in its efficacy; the patient's attitude to his doctor will also influence his (the patient's) response. The placebo effect of drugs and the effect of suggestion and counter-suggestion are well known. This often makes it difficult to assess the effectiveness of a particular drug accurately in the individual patient. We are even more uncertain about the exact effects of the different forms of psychotherapy although in an individual patient one may have no doubt about its effectiveness. In clinical practice in psychiatry, as in many other branches of medicine, we often have to do the best we can with what we have available and we cannot refuse to use drugs or psychotherapy or both because as yet the scientific proof of their exact value is lacking or incomplete.

DRUGS FOR ABREACTION

Drugs may also be used in combination with psychotherapy for abreaction techniques, that is, to break through the patient's resistances and allow him to recover repressed memories and emotions, and express them with the therapist present. Such procedures have their dangers, but they have also considerable advantages, e.g. in saving time, and so can be used for patients for whom psychotherapy is not available.

Many drugs have been used for this purpose — alcohol, carbon dioxide, ether, methedrine, lysergic acid, and barbiturates. Hypnosis has also been used for the same purpose (see below): abreactions have also been found to occur more easily after cortical undercuts (see p. 344).

Of the drugs, intravenous pentothal (in a 2½% solution) is most useful: it is safe, easy to give, and generally reliable; even if no abreaction occurs, the patient gains a temporary sense of relaxation and well-being: and in some conditions, e.g. ulcerative colitis (see p. 204), this benefits psychosomatic symptoms.

Methedrine has unfortunately led some patients to become addicts, and must be used with caution. Opinions vary considerably on lysergic acid: its use has certainly led some patients to *overcome* deep resistances and to abreact violently with subsequent improvement of insight and symptoms: others have become unmanageable, terrified with vivid hallucinations which may persist or recur, and become psychotic or suicidal.

HYPNOSIS

Hypnosis has a long history in psychiatry; and it seems to have been used in classical Greece with or without the aid of drugs. States of extreme suggestibility, release or repressed emotion, and impulsive, often violent action, with abrogation of personal responsibility have all been recorded. They were sometimes attributed to divine influence; sometimes studied scientifically, and sometimes used for therapeutic purposes.

Sargant (1957) draws a parallel between the states of collapse, suggestibility and sometimes ecstasy produced by such (apparently) diverse procedures as Bacchic frenzy, Voodoo, brain-washing, revivalist teaching and psychotherapy: music, the herd instinct, physical exhaustion, drugs and all the mechanics of staged demagogy can all play their part in different circumstances. Scientific discoveries of techniques and drugs have undoubtedly been used to damage as well as to heal.

More specific interest in therapeutic hypnotism stems from the work of Mesmer, which was mainly concerned with neurotic patients. Freud used hypnosis, under the influence of Charcot, to treat hysterical symptoms before he developed the technique of psychoanalysis. Since then its use has fluctuated with fashion: and today there are some psychotherapists who use it as part of their treatment and have considerable skill in it and in selecting suitable patients.

THERAPEUTIC USE

In practice there are two main uses of the hypnotic state: a patient may be able (1) to express hitherto repressed material and (2) to accept strong suggestions which may help him to overcome special fears or habits, or some physical symptoms. Both may clearly be useful in psychotherapy. A few people respond very well to hypnosis to overcome fears, e.g. stage fright, or asthmatic attacks (Magonet 1955; Maher-Loughnan 1962). It can also be used to prevent pain during labour or dental treatment. Patients can also be taught to use auto-hypnosis, e.g. asthmatics.

To obtain abreaction, when necessary, hypnosis is often

valuable. But although stage shows indicate that a few people are very easy to hypnotize, it is not easy to detect in advance who these are, and an attempt to hypnotize a patient which fails undermines his confidence. Some, for this reason, and others because they fear hypnotism may produce dependence, prefer to use drugs, such as pentothal (see p. 324). Symptom substitution has also been recorded, for example asthma may be replaced by dermatitis (Black, 1965).

FURTHER READING

Black, S. (1965). 'The use of hypnosis'. In Hopkins, D. and Wolff, H. H. (eds.), *Principles of Treatment of Psychosomatic Disorders.* Pergamon, Oxford.
Chertok, L. (1966). *Hypnosis.* Pergamon, Oxford.
Magonet, A. P. (1955). *Hypnosis in Asthma.* Heinemann, London.
Maher-Loughman, G. P. (1962). 'Controlled trial of hypnosis in symptomatic treatment of asthma'. *Brit. Med. J.*, 2, 371.
Sargant, W. (1957). *Battle for the Mind.* Pan, London.
Stewart, H. (1963). 'A comment on the psychodynamics of the hypnotic state'. *Int. J. Psychoanal.*, 44, 372.
Stewart, H. (1966). 'On consciousness, negative hallucination and the hypnotic state'. *Int. J. of Psychoanal.*, 47, 57.

52 Shock therapy

Two methods of treatment, convulsions and coma, both loosely described as 'shock therapy', owe much to the inspiration of von Meduna, in Budapest. Believing schizophrenia and epilepsy to be antagonistic diseases, he gave epilepsy, artificially, to his patients by injecting camphor preparations. Some success in this led him to do the same for depressives, who did better. But his method was risky, inaccurate, and unpractical and was soon superseded by electroconvulsant therapy.

Electroconvulsion therapy (Electroplexy or ECT), was introduced by Cerletti and Bini (1937), who designed a machine where electrodes are placed one on either side of the head in the posterior frontal regions: the passage of the current produces a major convulsion. This, however, was distressing and dangerous, from fractures, often of transverse processes of the spine, occasionally of the femur. Now, therefore, an anaesthetist gives pentothal and a short-acting muscle relaxant beforehand. Oxygen is required while the consequent respiratory paralysis lasts. The patient recovers consciousness in a few minutes, but may be confused and forgetful, especially of names. An average course consists of treatment given twice weekly 6 to 12 times. This can be carried out as an outpatient if relatives are co-operative. Light work the same day is possible.

ECT is of proved value, especially in depressions, and its risks are now negligible with the above procedure. It is, however, sometimes difficult to arrange, and interferes with work. Drugs are therefore generally tried first; but its use should not be delayed if these are ineffective. Its mode of action is still obscure. In some cases of recurrent depression it appears to be rather less effective in each attack, and patients tend to get progressively more afraid of treatment with ECT. Unilateral ECT appears less likely to produce side effects.

Insulin shock (insulin coma) was developed by Sakel in Vienna, and consists of giving the patient increasing insulin daily till hypoglycaemic coma occurs; this was stopped by glucose after an hour or so. It was used for many schizophrenics, but was dangerous, and required many and very well trained staff. It has now been superseded by drug therapy with or without ECT.

53 Learning theory and the behavioural therapies

Behavioural therapies comprise a variety of psychological techniques which aim to treat patients' problems directly by psychological means. Some of these techniques differ widely from one another both in their method of application and in their clinical indications. Each of these techniques aims to modify a limited aspect of the patient's disorder, and has to be used within the broad context of overall clinical management. Some of these techniques are based upon principles derived from experiments on learning. The most important techniques in use at the moment are as follows:

1 DESENSITIZATION

(Synonyms: deconditioning, counterconditioning, reciprocal inhibition.)

Technique

Desensitization is a method to reduce phobias by slowly accustoming the patient to the phobic situation while he is relaxed. Before desensitization is begun the patient draws up a list of all his phobic situations from the least to the most frightening stimuli. Desensitization is usually applied first in imagination (a method introduced by Wolpe) and then in practice. During desensitization in imagination the patient is relaxed systematically in a comfortable chair and is asked to visualize repeatedly a mildly phobic situation until he can tolerate that image without fear. Then he is asked to imagine more frightening fantasies until finally he can tolerate all his phobic situations in fantasy. He is then asked to rehearse in real life what has already been dealt with in imagination.

Desensitization is effective in selected cases, and the technique itself can be learned quickly. However, it can be a boring and lengthy procedure. On average 18 or more sessions are required to produce worthwhile improvement. To reduce the labour involved patients with similar phobias are sometimes treated by group desensitization, and recently workers have used tape recorders to simplify the procedure.

In the desensitization of children where it is difficult to counteract phobic anxiety by relaxation, one can instead use other pleasant stimuli such as sweets or social rewards. In phobic children desensitization can also be done by modelling — the children (singly or in groups) watch fearless models slowly engage in increasingly intimate contact with the phobic situation.

Indications

Desensitization is most useful in circumscribed phobias which are not complicated by multiple other symptoms. It can also be helpful in other conditions where focal anxiety is a problem, e.g. in asthmatics whose attacks are triggered off by particular recurrent stresses, in functional diarrhoea or urinary frequency with definite environmental triggers, and in sexual fears which may produce frigidity or impotence.

Mechanism of action

Several ingredients are combined in the desensitization procedure, each of which play their part. These include:

1 The relaxation procedure.
2 The habituating effect of repeatedly seeing the same phobic stimuli.
3 The counterconditioning effect of simultaneous relaxation and presentation of the phobic stimuli.
4 Suggestion, expectation of improvement and other cognitive variables.

2 AVERSION

(Synonym: negative conditioning.)

Technique

While desensitization helps a patient enter a situation he previously feared, aversion tries to do the opposite, viz, to stop a patient from engaging in particular behaviour by associating that behaviour with noxious stimuli.

In the past chemical aversion was often used, the noxious

stimulus usually being nausea and vomiting induced by apomorphine injections. Recently electric aversion has supplanted chemical aversion because it is safer, less unpleasant, easier to administer and more precise in its application.

Electric shocks are given to the arm or leg from a battery driven shock box while patients carry out their deviant behaviour in imagination and in practice, e.g. a transvestite will receive shocks while he has a fantasy about cross-dressing, and later while he actually puts on women's clothes. From 10 to 30 sessions may be necessary to reduce or eliminate his problem behaviour.

Indications

These are not yet clear. Theoretically any patient who wishes to lose a given behaviour could be given aversion. Patients must be fully co-operative and highly motivated. So far aversion has been most useful in patients who wish to lose their sexual attraction for certain objects or situations, e.g. transvestites, fetishists, sadomasochists, homosexuals. Experimentally, aversion has also been given in alcoholism, drug addiction and smoking, but results so far are inconclusive.

Mechanism of action

Aversive conditioning acts by pairing the problem behaviour with a noxious stimulus. Suggestion, satiation and other non-specific factors are inevitably present, but play a smaller role.

Aversion relief

A method of treatment by which the cessation of shocks is made to coincide with behaviour which it is desired to encourage, e.g. a phobic patient may receive a series of shocks which are terminated by his entering the phobic situation. The method is still purely experimental.

3 OPERANT CONDITIONING

(Synonym: instrumental conditioning.)

Technique

A method of shaping a patient's behaviour by reinforcing his behaviour with appropriate rewards or punishments, e.g. delinquents have developed social and learning skills by systematically being given graduated set tasks which lead slowly towards the desired behaviour, rewards being given for completion of each part of a sequence of behaviour — the reward may be points, money, social approval, aversion relief or other reinforcement. The theory behind this technique is discussed later in this section.

Indications

These are still unclear. Useful results have been obtained in developing skills in defective and autistic children, in delinquents, and in institutionalized patients such as chronic schizophrenics. It has also been used in obsessionals.

4 OTHER METHODS

Bell and pad treatment for nocturnal enuresis

The enuretic patient sleeps on a bed which contains special apparatus which rings a loud bell to wake him up when he voids urine in the bed. This method has been used extensively; it is bound to be associated with encouragement and interest, which may themselves be of therapeutic value (see p. 236).

Assertion training

A method in which patients are taught to assert themselves at appropriate moments when previously their shyness had prevented them from acting realistically; this can be done singly or in groups.

Negative practice

(Synonym: massed practice.) A method of eliminating behaviour by getting the patient to carry out that behaviour very repeatedly in a short space of time. Has been used in tics and facial spasms with tenuous results.

Behaviour modification

In this method, the patient's interactions with other people are analysed in detail to determine the source of some of his difficulties. He is then helped to modify those behaviours which are inappropriate and instead to develop more fruitful modes of social interaction. This method is indistinguishable from more conventional active psychotherapy. Behavioural therapists use this approach in patients with personality problems.

Implosion

Here a phobic or obsessional patient may be exposed with maximum intensity to the situation he fears. This causes severe acute anxiety which may be followed by diminution of his original symptoms.

Relationship between patient and therapist

As in any therapy the patient's relationship with his therapist may influence the results of treatment. A good working relationship is necessary for success and best results are obtained with active encouragement of progress although it has been reported that desensitization has been applied successfully with a tape recorder in the absence of a therapist. Patients may become dependent on the behaviour therapist and negative transferences may develop and may lead to interruption of treatment. In behaviour therapy, unlike psychotherapy, such transference phenomena are not interpreted; a certain amount of discussion of the patient's personal problems and emotional conflicts is, however, carried out by some behaviour therapists in addition to the other techniques: in general, there is an increasing tendency to integrate behavioural techniques with dynamically oriented psychotherapy. The importance of this is being increasingly recognized, as the removal of a symptom by one or other behavioural techniques, helpful though this undoubtedly is, not infrequently brings into the open underlying problems which may lead to the development of new symptoms or to difficulties in the patient's interpersonal relationships; for example the husband of a woman who, after having lost her agoraphobic symptoms, has become independent, may become jealous of her, and marital therapy may be needed to deal with the resulting marital problems.

THE ROLE OF LEARNING THEORY

Behavioural therapists often claim that their techniques derive from learning theory. Learning theory is that system of ideas and principles which attempts to describe and predict the observed phenomena of learning in all organisms.

Learning is usually held to mean a relatively permanent change in potential behaviour which occurs as a result of practice. We can only observe this change in potential behaviour by studying actual performances of an animal or man, and performance may reflect the level of learning relatively accurately or inaccurately, as every examination candidate knows. Learning is the hypothetical process which underlies the observed change in performance.

Learning may be reinforced by certain conditions which are very varied and which have no obvious common element beyond their ability to favour learning.

We have defined learning as a permanent change in behaviour which occurs as a result of practice. The term 'practice' need not refer to any observable event. Learning can take place when stimulation of the central nervous system is substituted for the usual external stimuli, and in the absence of any overt motor response. This suggests that the critical event in practice is some unknown process in the central nervous system.

Learning and conditioning

These two terms are often used interchangeably. Conditioning refers to the process of training which results in the formation of new links between stimuli and responses. The term learning in fact includes conditioning, but is much broader since it covers a wide range of processes from the simple classical conditioned reflex to complex human problem solving. There are two main forms of conditioning, classical and operant conditioning.

1 *Classical conditioning example* (synonym: contiguity conditioning, Pavlovian conditioning). A meat pellet placed in the mouth of a dog will produce salivation. If, several times, a bell is sounded shortly before the meat pellet is placed in the dog's mouth, the bell eventually also produces salivation even when it is sounded alone. Salivation to the sound of the bell is the new link which has been established — this is the classically conditioned response.

2 *Operant conditioning example* (synonym: instrumental conditioning, Skinnerian conditioning). A hungry rat is placed in a sound-proof compartment which contains, say, a lever which can be pressed down. The animal will wander around the cage and by chance eventually will press the lever, whereupon a small food pellet is delivered into the cage. Gradually the rat learns to press the lever repeatedly to obtain food until his hunger is sated. The rat is instrumental in making the new response to obtain food by operating on his environment, hence the terms for this process.

Classical and instrumental conditioning have certain differences but recent evidence suggests a fundamental unity in the two processes. Because the conditioning situation is simple and well-controlled, it is a fruitful source of postulates from which deductions can be made concerning complex learning. However, conditioning principles are still much too simple to account for most human behaviour, and there is as yet no agreed theory which adequately describes all facets of learning from the simplest conditioned reflex to complex human problem solving and creativity.

RELEVANCE OF LEARNING THEORY
TO PSYCHIATRY

Learning theory is relevant in psychiatry to the extent that psychiatric disorders are learned or psychiatric treatments employ learning principles. The extent to which this is true is not easy to decide on.

It is hard to identify which psychiatric disturbances can usefully be regarded as disorders of learning. Some neurotic disorders can be understood partly as disorders of learning. For example, focal phobias not uncommonly are acquired in situations analogous to those of classical conditioning. Some personality disorders can also be seen partly as maladaptive behaviour due to faulty social learning. On the other hand, it is hard to see how it is useful to regard an obsessional fear of harming one's child as a disorder of learning. Learning plays some role in certain psychiatric conditions, usually in conjunction with other variables as well.

Which psychiatric treatments employ learning principles? There are many different principles of learning, and some behavioural techniques do seem to employ some of these principles. For example, operant conditioning methods by which new skills are taught to delinquents or autistic children seem to be based upon operant principles originally worked out in laboratory experiments. In contrast, other techniques like desensitization only acquired their learning theory veneer after they had already been suggested and used without learning principles in mind. Nevertheless, once the technique was developed ideas from learning theory did suggest ways in which desensitization could be improved upon.

REFERENCES

Gelder, M. G., Marks, I. M. and Wolff, H. H. (1967). 'Desensitisation and psychotherapy in the treatment of phobic states'. *Brit. J. Psychiat.*, 113, 53.
Marks, I. M. and Gelder, M. G. (1966). 'Common ground between

behaviour therapy and psychodynamic methods', *Brit. J. Med. Psychol.*, 39, 11-24.
Meyer, V. and Chesser, E. S. (1970). *Behaviour Therapy in Clinical Psychiatry*. Penguin.

54 Collaboration with psychologists and others

TREATMENT BY PSYCHOLOGISTS

In psychiatric departments, psychologists participate in the various forms of treatment, in particular those based on psychological theories which have been developed within their own academic discipline. The treatments there in which they are directly involved are those built according to a learning rather than a medical model, including those based on learning theory, e.g. behaviour modification, and those derived from the study of inter-personal relations and group processes, which provide the theoretical background for group psychotherapy (see pp. 312 and 327).

In child psychiatry departments most psychologists undertake remedial education with children whose attitudes to learning need modification, or those with unusual cognitive difficulties.

Vocational advice may be given by the clinical psychologist to school-leavers who have difficulty in deciding upon a suitable career, or to adults who have to change their occupation because of physical or mental ill-health or deterioration. On the basis of a full assessment ranging over abilities, achievements, personality, preferences and aspirations, suggestions as to suitable types of occupation, and comments on the situations in which the patient may function fully, or those he would do well to avoid, can be discussed with him and reported to occupational therapists, rehabilitation units or employers.

Rehabilitation of patients after mental or physical illness again involves psychological skills in analysing the demands of work or activity, working out the adaptations needed in relation to the patient's residual assets and setting up for them a new learning situation which can be discussed also with workshop supervisors, occupational therapists, day centre staff and others involved. At present this is an underdeveloped field of work but one of considerable importance to the mental health of those passing through a recovery period and of the handicapped.

Certain adults and children may respond well to a supportive type of therapy, the objectives of which are to give the patient some self-knowledge with a view to strengthening his ego and his capacity for decision making. Counselling along these lines is sometimes undertaken by psychologists.

Some clinical psychologists, especially those with experience in social psychology and in management are developing work in relation to ward management and communication problems. They see various ways in which they can help other staff in the identification of problems, in their analysis of these problems and the solution of some of them referring to patient management and communication between staff. This is an area of increasing importance under new management systems and where frequent staff changes occur. Among the objectives is that of ensuring that all services provided for patients whether they relate to welfare, training, use of leisure or anything falling into these categories are used in such a way that their therapeutic effect is maximized. Advantageous as this may be for patients, it also promotes staff co-operation and mutual support, thus improving morale.

Assessing results of treatment

The extent and kind of change that has followed treatment is much more difficult to assess in psychological medicine than most other branches of medicine. But changes in the patient's responses to projective tests or tests of intellectual functioning can be of use in assessing, e.g., whether the patient is really 'better' or whether his conflicts remain although the original symptom has disappeared, perhaps having been replaced by another; or what has been the most important factor responsible for improvement.

RESEARCH

Psychologists are trained in research design and methodology. They often cooperate with non-psychologist colleagues, or advise them on planning research, as well as initiating their own projects. Some research by clinical psychologists is concerned with devising and refining psychological techniques of investigation, e.g. to explore thought processes, to predict suitability for treatment of various forms, to assess the extent and nature of changes following treatment.

Where research units have been formed, programmes of a more ambitious nature are undertaken to study, e.g. the characteristics of particular patient groups, the effects of controlled social change, or the epidemiology of mental illness. Generally these are collaborative studies with colleagues of other disciplines.

Special problems arise in the use of classical experimental methods in psychological research in the clinical field because of the difficulty of controlling the large number of variables involved, and of obtaining control groups (e.g. an 'untreated' group to match a 'treated' group). A good deal of research is being done on ways of evaluating treatment procedures and relating patients' expectations of treatment to their response to it. The results hopefully will lead to better discrimination in the choice of treatment in relation to personality as well as condition.

TEACHING

Psychologists participate in many of the teaching functions of a psychiatric department. In addition to the training of junior psychologists, this may include seminars and discussions with doctors preparing for post-graduate qualifications, medical students, social work students and nurses.

Their particular part in this teaching has enormously increased in recent years as the body of knowledge in psychology has grown very rapidly. Cover usually includes the psychological aspects of growth and development, studies of processes involved in the acquisition and use of skills and of influences on the integration of individual and social behaviour.

Within the considerable range of function for clinical psychologists it is impossible for one psychologist to undertake all the types of work described above. Where staffing arrangements permit there is usually some specialization. It is seldom that the research and the clinical needs of psychiatric departments are both adequately met, and the single-handed psychologist usually concentrates either on the clinical or on the research side, according to his own training, abilities and interests, and to the special demands of the department.

Although they give priority to the departments of psychiatry clinical psychologists are increasingly consulted by other departments in general hospitals, in particular those of neurology, geriatrics and paediatrics. The inclusion of more psychology in medical education and the increasing availability of clinical psychologists is likely to hasten this development. The wide relevance of psychological studies to general medical problems is resulting in research reports on a variety of subjects, e.g. on pre-operative medication and memory (Hetherington 1962), the stress of surgery (Briskin 1965), psychological reactions to illness and hospitalization in a group of medical inpatients (Spelman and Ley 1966), emotional disturbances in burned children (Woodward 1959). These are bound to proliferate. Changes in patient care, the growth of community services and reorganization of the National Health Service will all affect the psychologists' roles and lead to broader application of their skills. Further impetus to development may well result from a report to the DHSS from a committee set up to enquire into the role of psychologists in the NHS (the Trethowan Committee) presented early in 1975.

ANCILLARY THERAPY

Some types of therapy may be called ancillary in that they are seldom used alone, but in conjunction with psychotherapy and/or drugs. They are certainly not to be despised, and give most valuable help to some patients, and their exponents have a long skilled training in their profession.

Occupational therapy

This aims at enabling patients to express thoughts and feelings, and to gain insight into their conflicts by providing a task to fulfil, and a group to join, and so, personal relationships to handle. Some occupational therapists take part in running psychodrama and encounter groups (see p. 314). It is therefore far more than enabling a disabled and bored patient to pass the time, though even this may be of value in preventing or alleviating depression and withdrawal. A good occupational therapy department is essential for any psychiatric unit.

Art therapy and writing

This has similar aims, and many patients can express feelings in paint, chalk, plaster or clay, even if they have had no technical training in drawing or sculpture. Once this has been done, verbal expression may be easier. It may thus be a valuable means of getting the patient to communicate at a time when he feels able to do so (but when the doctor need not be present): and for some it seems easier than expressing their feelings in words, perhaps because the interpretations of pictures could (if necessary) be denied, though they seldom are.

For some of these reasons, some patients will prefer to write to their doctor, in verse or prose, and communication can well develop in this way once a first contact has been made — or often without it, to judge from the success of the help columns in daily and monthly papers.

Music therapy

Composing, playing or even listening to music may have similar value. Curiously little work has been done on the use of music, though nearly everyone recognizes its effect on moods, either in listening or in playing an instrument, and its success in treating the recurrent depression of King Saul by David was recorded.

Physiotherapy

Set programmes generally exist in a psychiatric unit, for it can be of great assistance in relaxing the chronic tension of anxiety which may have produced not only muscular tension but also a faulty posture, which in turn needs re-education. This applies, for example, to faulty head-neck posture, which may produce headache and a painful neck. Physical relaxation also leads indirectly to mental relaxation and patients can be taught how to practise relaxation by themselves.

REFERENCES

Briskin, P. (1965). 'The stress of surgery'. *New Society*, 24 June 1965.

Caine, T. M. and Smail, D. J. (1969). *The Treatment of Mental Illness*. University of London Press, London.

Eysenck, H. J. (1961). *Handbook of Abnormal Psychology*. Pitman, London.

Hetherington, R. R. (1962). 'Pre-operative medication and memory'. *Psychol. Reps.*, 11, 352.

Hetherington, R. R., Miller, D. H. and Neville, J. G. (1964). *Introduction to Psychology for Medical Students*. Heinemann, London.

Spelman, M. S. and Ley, P. (1966). 'Psychological reactions to illness and hospitalization in a group of medical in-patients'. *Social Work*, 23, 1.

Woodward, J. (1959). 'Emotional disturbances in burned children'. *Brit. Med. J.*, 1, 1009.

55 Psychosurgery

Brain surgery has been used for a variety of conditions, the best-known being comprised under the general heading of leucotomy, but other approaches have been successful and will be first considered.

TEMPORAL LOBE OPERATIONS

Patients with personality disorders associated with temporal lobe epilepsy have improved as the result of removal of temporal gyri, or temporal lobectomy, especially if there is a focal macroscopic lesion, but also where there is hippocampal sclerosis. Drug treatment for such cases is often unsuccessful. If so, operation should be considered. It is a highly specialized operation (Wilson 1973). Amygdalotomy may also be successful (Kelly 1973a).

CINGULECTOMY

Various procedures involving the cingulate gyrus have been developed including ablation bilaterally of its anterior half (by Cairns in 1931). Although the results are less likely to be sustained there is some evidence that this procedure has a more definite effect on patients with obsessive features.

Recently it has had some success in selected cases of schizophrenia: tension and impulsive action having been considerably relieved (Knight 1967).

LEUCOTOMY

Leucotomy means literally 'cutting white matter'. The term (or 'lobotomy' in the US) is used to describe operations on the frontal lobes of man which, by interfering with the interplay of activity between the cortex of the frontal lobes and certain parts of the thalamus and hypothalamus, cause changes in 'emotional tone'. The operation may thus be used to advantage for patients suffering from a wide variety of psychiatric disorders in which severe depression and anxiety are prominent symptoms. It will be appreciated that the extent and location of the surgical lesion will clearly have a bearing on the degree of change produced. Earlier operations were radical in nature and had many disadvantages and poor clinical results. In the past 20 years the operation has been modified in a variety of ways, refined and reduced in extent so that serious adverse effects are now seldom encountered. Many doctors, remembering the earlier procedures and their adverse effects and ignoring recent improvements, still tend to generalize about 'leucotomy' with the result that suitable patients may be denied the benefits of the modern procedures.

History

The first operation was conceived by the Portuguese neuro-psychiatrist Egaz Moniz who persuaded his neurosurgical colleague Almeida Lima to operate on the frontal lobes of some 20 patients suffering from severe schizophrenia. Their first report appeared in 1936. (Moniz was a remarkable man. He had introduced cerebral angiography into neurology in 1927 and had represented his country as Finance Minister at the Treaty of Versailles in 1919.) Moniz based his ideas on the experimental work on the frontal lobes of chimpanzees of the physiologists Fulton (1951), Jacobsen and Kennard (1944) and the earlier work of Victor Horsley, who had shown, in ablation experiments, that a profound reduction in the animal's emotional responses was produced by bilateral frontal lobectomy. The so called 'standard leucotomy' was developed by Freeman and Watts in 1942 in the USA and by W. McKissock in Britain. This was an extensive incision of the pre-frontal white matter (bilaterally) just anterior to the tip of the anterior horn of the lateral ventricle, carried out through laterally placed burr holes at the coronal sutures. Though encouraging results were obtained in many patients, this procedure was too often associated with unsatisfactory sequelae: apathy, irresponsibility, lack of judgment, incontinence and sometimes seizures. From this, as indicated above, opposition on moral and ethical grounds developed in medical, religious and lay circles.

Recent modifications

Since the late 1940s many modifications of the original operation have been carried out. All these have attempted to be more selective, with gradually increasing information concerning the neuro-anatomy and neuro-physiology of the frontothalamic and hypothalamic pathways in man. It was soon observed that the desired clinical effects were obtained with the least adverse sequelae when the lesion was made in the medial half of the prefrontal white matter and particularly in the inferior medial quadrant. This appeared to interrupt fibres radiating to and from the thalamus and hypothalamus to the grey matter of the orbital surface of the frontal lobes. Certain other radiations to the cingulate gyrus (above the corpus callosum) were also found to be important.

Several procedures incorporating these observations are now current but all probably depend for their success and lack of adverse sequelae, not only on their location, but upon the *quantity* of white matter divided.

The operations most frequently carried out at the present time are:

1 The 'Bimedian' section of Poppen. Section of the upper and lower medial quadrants of white matter. Virtually the medial half of the original operation of Freeman and Watts.
2 The 'Rostral' operation of McKissock. This is similar to Poppen's operation but carried out rather more obliquely forward but still involving the medial part of the frontal white matter.
3 The 'inferior quadrant' operation of Jackson. This approaches the fibres of the medial inferior quadrant and the lateral quadrant from a burr hole placed laterally as in the Freeman and Watts operation. A more extensive procedure surgically was devised by Grantham in USA to divide the inferior medial quadrants only.
4 'Orbital undercutting'. This operation was devised in 1949 by Scoville in USA and practised extensively in Britain by Knight since that time. It involves the division of the fibre projections to and from the orbital, or inferior surface of the frontal lobe. The operation is carried out under general anaesthesia via two large trephine discs sited parasagittally immediately above the frontal air sinuses.
5 A few years later Knight developed a stereo-taxic procedure to insert a palisade of Yttrium 90 seeds just anterior to and below the head of the caudate nucleus to create a lesion at the zone of outflow and inflow of fibres passing to and fro between the thalamus, hypothalamus and the orbital surface of the

frontal lobes and the cingulate gyrus. The results are at least comparable to those obtained from open operation in states of emotional tension (Knight 1969), with even less risk.

6 Limbic leucotomy, also carried out stereotactically, is directed at several areas in the lower medial quadrant and the cingulate gyrus.

Results and indications

The results of these modifications are very encouraging. In all of the latter three operations, immediate results are often remarkable. Many patients who have been ill and miserable for years, and untreatable by psychotherapy and by other physical means, have responded dramatically and have again been able to enjoy life and perform their previous jobs, without any sign of emotional, intellectual or moral deterioration. Some describe themselves as 'freed' and their friends and relations concur.

Several long-term surveys have been carried out. These show very similar results. After orbital undercut (Sykes and Tredgold 1964) an improvement rate of some 80% was recorded, both symptomatically and in working capacity; even though the patients concerned had failed to respond more than temporarily to any other means of treatment. Depressive of all types formed the majority of the group, and did better than the average: endogenous depressions did not recur; reactive depressions, chronic anxiety states and obsessions improved; but some were still in need of later psychotherapy and support. Hysterics, psychopaths and schizophrenics derived little or no benefit, except in the loss of some emotional tension. After Yttrium implants (Ström-Olsen and Carlisle 1971) improvement occured in some 73% in a roughly similar group of patients. Limbic operations have been more successful on obsessionals than the other two (Kelly 1973b).

In these conditions, therefore, surgery should certainly be considered if other treatment has been unsuccessful; but it is essential before operation to discover how much psychotherapy and social support will be required afterwards, and to arrange that this will be available. Further, the risks must be assessed; they are rather greater in orbital undercuts, but complete recovery is also more likely from these than from Yttrium.

Ill effects

Though these have been exaggerated (see above) they may occur after undercut:

1 The mortality rate is about 1.5%.
2 Personality deterioration, as described above, rarely occurs.
3 Increase of appetite and weight is common.
4 Epileptiform convulsions may occur in the five years after operation, generally in a group of several together; they can be controlled by anti-convulsants.

Patients suffering from (3) and (4) almost unanimously regard the operation as worthwhile in spite of this, in view of their general improvement.

Such ill effects have not been recorded after Yttrium.

Relapses

These have occurred in small proportion; they are seldom permanent. They occur under stress and generally respond to psychotherapy or drugs, even when the original illness did not do so. Occasionally, relapses have been successfully treated by a second leucotomy.

The future

It is possible that leucotomy will be superseded by the further advances in drugs which are being made. It seems also likely that with increasing surgical precision we shall be able to recommend leucotomy for carefully selected patients at a much earlier stage in their illness than we do at present, and with less fear of ill effects.

REFERENCES

Freeman, W. and Watts, J. W. (1942). *Psychosurgery, Intelligence, Emotion and Social Behaviour following Prefrontal Lobotomy.* Springfield, Mass.

Fulton, J. E. (1951). *Frontal Lobotomy and Affective Behaviour*. Morton, New York.

Kelly, D. (1973a). 'Psychosurgery and the limbic system'. *Postgrad. Med. J.*, 49, 825.

Kelly, D. (1973b). 'Stereotactic limbic lcucotomy'. *Postgrad. Med. J.*, 49, 865.

Kennard, M.A. (1944). In Bucy, P.C. (ed.), *The Precentral Motor Cortex*, University of Illinois Press, Urbana, Ill.

Knight, G. C. (1964). 'The orbital cortex as an objective in the surgical treatment of mental illness'. *Brit. J. Surg.*, 51, 114.

Knight, G. C. (1969). 'Bifrontal stereotactic tractotomy'. *Brit. J. Psychiat.*, 115, 257.

Knight, G. C. (1969). 'Stereotactic surgery for the relief of suicidal and severe depression and intractable psychoneurosis'. *Postgrad. Med.*, 3, 45, 1.

Levinson, F. and Meyer, V. (1965). 'Personality changes in relation to psychiatric status following orbital cortex undercutting'. *Brit. J. Psychiat.*, 111, 207.

Moniz, E. and Lima, A. (1936). *Lisbon Med.*, 13, 152.

Scoville, W. B. (1949). *J. Neurosurg.*, 6, 65.

Ström-Olsen, R. and Carlisle, S. (1970). 'Bifrontal stereotactic tractotomy'. *Brit. J. Psych.*, 118, 241.

Sykes, M. K. and Tredgold, R. F. (1964). 'Restricted orbital undercutting'. *Brit. J. Psychiat.*, 110, 60.

Wilson, P. J. E. (1973). 'The surgical treatment of epilepsy'. *Brit. J. Hosp. Med.*, February, 161.

56 Psychotherapy in general practice

Psychiatric cases form a large proportion of any general practice (Hopkin 1955), and only a determined GP can shut his eyes to it. Estimates range from a tenth to a third of patients (see p. 49), with a high peak for middle aged women. This is mostly minor illness: it will certainly occupy much of the GP's time: whether this is frustrating or constructive will depend on his ability to select cases he can help and to develop his own skill in handling them.

There is no doubt that many general practitioners, as well as many consultants in various specialities in hospital, carry out superficial psychotherapy with great success, but sometimes without much awareness of what they are doing. Their experience and personality have developed in them a sensitivity to the patient's needs and a skill in meeting them which has been part of the art of medicine much longer than there has been formal psychotherapy.

Nonetheless, some doctors have unfortunately been less successful, and their attitude to the subject has produced misery and resentment in the patient and more work for themselves (or, more often, for their colleagues or neighbours).

Yet the GP, in many ways, is in a very strong position to help the patient and in some, he has the advantage over the psychiatrist. He knows (or should know) the patient's background. He has opportunities for informal talks, and so avoids the resistance felt by patients at going to visit a psychiatric outpatient department (especially if this is, quite wrongly, seen as the first step to the mental hospital).

The conduct of the first interview has already been discussed (see p. 1) and its value in providing 'first aid' has been emphasized. It is possible that this may be enough to let the patient find his own readjustment. But a second interview must be arranged to check what has happened and it may well be that the GP needs to go further, so he will need more skill and more support. Recently, therefore, more systematic efforts have been made to teach the basis of this approach to students and to help GPs develop and assess their skills and attitudes.

It must be admitted, sadly, that many GPs and other doctors — and even some students — find themselves irritated by patients with psychiatric complaints; and it is easy to sympathize with anyone under pressure, confronted by a patient who is demanding, who 'doesn't really seem ill', or who can't explain what the matter is. Yet a display of impatience will certainly make the patient more demanding and less capable of expressing his real feelings and needs, either to this doctor or to the next one he sees; and thus the number of chronic psychiatric patients is increased. The doctor must therefore be prepared to look beneath the surface; to give himself a chance of doing so by fixing a time when he is less pressed himself; and to try to meet the underlying need.

There are two special examples of this. The first is that of the aggressive patient; if he behaves badly or irrationally it is easy enough to dismiss him as unhelpable, which only means someone else has to try with less hope of success. If his aggression is more subtly displayed, and, worse still, if he picks on points which are legitimate, the situation becomes more tense; the doctor is tempted in his turn to find some legitimate excuse for giving up. Yet this aggressive behaviour, like anxiety or pain, is generally a symptom of underlying illness and if the doctor can realise this and can school himself not to be counter-aggressive in return, his tolerance may be the first step towards resolving a long-standing conflict which has caused misery to the patient and his family for years. But aggression is less easy to tolerate than anxiety or pain (which arouse sympathy) for it naturally produces counter-attack, especially if directed against oneself or one's interest. It is therefore essential that doctors should learn to handle their own reactions when they are students, for it will be far more difficult to do so later in the pressures of general practice or hospital ward, and when exposed to the increased pride in one's position which a professional standing supplies.

Chronic aggressive behaviour on the part of many people – whether patients or not – is of course often due to long-standing grievances or resentments, which go back to childhood or adolescence and are only partly realized by their possessor and expressed indirectly if at all. The importance of this in various psychiatric conditions has already been emphasized (see pp. 78, 181, 193); much more could be done to prevent the development of the latter if doctors and other counsellors could help the individual deal with his feelings before vicious circles of social antagonism or personal ill-health have become established.

The second difficult problem is the dependent patient; every surgery, every psychiatric department, and all social services have many such regular attenders whose complaints are often physical, and often minor. Each tends to feel that he can help no more and that the patient should be someone else's responsibility, which of course increases the patient's insecurity still further. There are unfortunately many people, more women than men, who have always been dependent and who, when old, become more lonely, and frightened of death, of helplessness from chronic physical illness, of the risks of street violence, burglary or just being left alone to die, all with some justification. Paradoxically there is more loneliness and less support from neighbours in big cities than in country villages; no doubt then increasing urbanization and the breakdown of family support will make all this worse.

For such people the medical and social services are their only comfort and they attend with complaints which compel one to listen; these are often time-consuming and rambling. But they are really appeals for reassurance and support; once this is realized many people can be much helped (and so attend less often) by being assured that someone cares for them, will pay regular (but not necessarily frequent) visits and will be available in an emergency and will eventually provide terminal care. Much progress has been made by the psycho-geriatric services in this way; though they are already short of staff and likely to be more so as the average age of the population rises. If then the professional services can enlist the help of any relatives or volunteers in the community so much the better, but they too will need help with their own anxieties.

Thus, irritation of doctors and others with such patients is greatly diminished if the doctor understands that it stems from his own ignorance and impotence, and if he is prepared to do what he can, and accept that he can do no more, as he would in dealing with any physical ailment.

Undergraduate experience is being increased by providing supervision for medical students to take suitable cases on for psychotherapy (Ball and Wolff 1963, Wolff 1967).

If students are supervised in small groups, they not only learn more by taking part in discussion of other student's work with patients, but their own sensitivity and self-understanding is also increased, the group acting as a sensitivity-training group. Postgraduate teaching has been developing over a longer period and has become far more widespread in the formation of what are now known as 'Balint' groups in many countries of the world (see Balint, M. 1964, Balint, M. and E. 1961). The main emphasis here is on helping the GP to understand what is going on in his relationship to the patient and how to use this in a therapeutic manner; but these groups have also provided valuable knowledge on such subjects as asthma, unconsummated marriage, attitudes to impending death (see p. 304), 'repeat prescriptions', and the value of a 5-minute interview with the patient. No doubt the future will see on-going groups of this kind established in all areas where GPs are insistent enough to demand them.

The GP's treatment may follow several lines, sometimes simultaneously. He will listen, provide explicit or implicit reassurance and hope, and if possible, relieve or help to tolerate guilt on aggression and sexual problems. He may try to increase the patient's understanding (not necessarily directly) by exploration, explanation, 'reflection', and the removal of prejudices. He may also recommend action and distraction, which may help the patient to express his emotions constructively, or at least harmlessly, and may provide other interests to restore his sense of proportion. Besides this, he may prescribe drugs for symptoms (see those recommended under the various syndromes, but also see p. 316).

A thorny problem lies in some aspects of the doctor's relationships with his patients, which may risk becoming unprofessional. Stories of women patients falling in love with their male doctor are exaggerated; but some are true, and have indeed ruined the doctor's reputation or bank balance, or the patient's health, or even the life of either. The fear of these risks no doubt leads many doctors, especially GPs, to be very wary in their dealings with any woman patient who seems attracted by them, and even warier with anyone to whom they are attracted. As a result, as Asher (1972) points out, any patient who has the misfortune to fall in love with her doctor may get at best neglect, and at worst insult from the one person who might be expected to help her in her predicament. Possibly this leads many doctors to the general idea that they must be careful in showing any sort of warmth to their patients; though there are other reasons for this.

Yet as students in their first year see very clearly, warm sympathy and a sincere attempt to understand are exactly what many patients need, especially those with some psychiatric ailments, such as depression. Students also see only too often patients who complain that their GP does not 'care' for them — in any sense; they hear less of those that do, since these naturally send their patients less to psychiatric departments.

The conflict is very real; the only logical way of dealing with it seems to be to encourage students at this phase to learn more how to express their own feelings about patients, which means understanding and discussing the feelings, so that later they are more in control of them, and can use them according to their patients' needs. This indeed seems a very important point in the system of teaching students some skill in superficial psycho-therapy (see p. 350) which has unfortunately been neglected until recently.

SPECIALIST HELP

If the GP is dissatisfied with the progress, or feels out of his depth, he must consider the following:

1 He may need to discuss the case with a psychiatrist to advise on his handling; such opportunities nowadays exist in GP groups, e.g. at the Tavistock Clinic; but also he can talk it over at his local psychiatric clinic.
2 The patient may need more profound help direct from a psychiatrist either by an assessment interview, or by treatment (e.g. psychotherapy, or physical treatment or both combined).
3 The patient may need a change of environment, e.g. to a psychiatric unit. In many areas there are such units in general hospitals, as well as in a mental hospital.
4 The GP should consider the help available from psychiatric social workers based on the local authority.

THE RELATIVES

Most patients spend more time with their relatives than with their doctor and the former's influence may therefore outweigh the latter's. Then the doctor must try, without breaking confidence, to encourage the relatives to take the same line as he does; if uninformed, they may unwittingly oppose him.

Many relatives have problems of their own which are relevant to or directly connected with the patient's problems. The GP can offer help by seeing the relatives but sometimes it is wise to suggest another doctor, i.e. a partner or, if appropriate, a social worker or psychiatrist if the patient or his relatives prefer it. They may often have strong feelings towards the patient and it may be helpful to them to ventilate these to a doctor or social worker instead of to the patient and so relieve the antagonism which the patient's illness has created around him. Occasionally it is useful to offer a joint interview, e.g. to husband and wife but special skill is needed to conduct an interview without taking sides with one or other partner.

The GP's relationships with social workers and other potential allies are discussed below (see pp. 371 and 360).

FURTHER READING

Asher, R. J. (1972). In *Richard Asher Talking Sense*, edited by F. Avery Jones, London, 1972; a book cordially recommended to all students and doctors.

Balint, M. (1964). *The Doctor, his Patient and the Illness*. Pitman, London.

Balint, M. and E. (1961). *Psychotherapeutic Techniques in Medicine*. Tavistock Publications, London.

Ball, D. H. and Wolff H. H. (1963). 'An experiment in the teaching of psychotherapy to medical students'. *Lancet*, 1, 214.

Finlay, B. et al. (1956). 'The management of stress disorders in general practice'. *General Practitioner*, 177, 729.

Hopkins, P. (1955). 'The general practitioner and the psychosomatic approach'. In O'Neill, D. (ed.), *Modern Trends in Psychosomatic Medicine*. Butterworth, London.

Shepherd, M., Cooper, B., Brown, A. C. and Kalton, G. W. (1966). *Psychiatric Illness in General Practice*.

Wolff, H. H. (1967). 'Influencing students' attitudes towards the emotional aspects of illness'. *J. Psychosom. Res.*, ii 87.

57 Rehabilitation

Many of the symptoms of psychiatric illness interfere seriously with the patient's mental efficiency at work — and sometimes with his physical efficiency. They also lead to social disability. He cannot mix easily with his friends, cannot face new situations, loses confidence and may feel everyone is against him. His resulting suspiciousness and withdrawal do indeed sometimes provoke some hostility or withdrawal in others, which confirms his paranoid ideas. If depressed, he is inclined to resist offers of help; and to make his family and friends impatient and helpless in turn.

From all this develops a vicious circle of antagonism and increasing social isolation. To send a patient back into this situation after treatment would only provoke a serious relapse. It is, then, important to ensure that he regains enough mental efficiency and social skill to deal with whatever environment he meets; no doubt something can be done by discussion between GP, PSW or psychiatrist with the family and employers, to make the latter more tolerable; but their patience and consideration cannot be infinite and they themselves may have painful memories of the patient's previous behaviour.

The psychiatric patient in fact needs mental and social rehabilitation as much as anyone, long immobilized by physical injury, needs physical exercises to regain full use and confidence of his limbs. Unfortunately most staff are less interested in mental rehabilitation which is less visible and more difficult, and they may give the impression of working against the patient. In physical rehabilitation one feels one is working with the patient to overcome a weak part of himself; in mental and social rehabilitation one is of course doing the same but the patient may be resisting more strongly.

The patient is thus in need both of professional help and of a tolerant atmosphere if he is to understand his own feelings and to accept them, and to express them, if he can, usefully, or at least harmlessly. He will need to go step by step patiently and he may need also to gain confidence, achieving minor successes and consolidating them before he can undertake more. To go too fast may simply lead him to regress. Yet there are great pressures on a healthy looking person to make rapid progress. Schemes for industrial rehabilitation of long-stay psychiatric patients must start while they are in hospital.

To achieve rehabilitation at home or at work may be difficult; special conditions are needed under skilled supervision. This was not easy in mental hospitals when they had to cope with the stigma which surrounded them, and some unfortunately still have to do so. For this reason special rehabilitation centres have been set up, e.g. by Ling (1943) at Roffey Park, where graded exercises in social and mental skills were provided, e.g. by letting the patients do tasks for each other, taking part in entertainments, accepting responsibility for committee decisions and organizing individual activities, even handling visitors and newcomers. But this specialized unit has since had to revert to the functions of an ordinary psychiatric unit. Similar systems have been developed in special psychiatric units and great efforts have been made to create the atmosphere of a therapeutic community. Dunkley and Lewis (1963) described some of the difficulties. At the same time, certain firms, notably Vauxhall and Austin, worked on the same lines in providing rehabilitation units in their factories for workers who were physically or mentally disabled, or both. Graded activities were provided which were in fact of industrial value, and as great ingenuity was shown in adapting tools to exercise weak muscles as in promoting self-confidence and mutual tolerance.

Since then industrial rehabilitation units and centres for re-training have developed in many areas, but even so it is easier to deal with physcial problems than with mental or social ones. Placement into suitable jobs is also essential. The Disablement Resettlement Officers employed by the Ministry of Labour have this task and have achieved much with co-operative firms.

The local community has an enormous part to play too if it can be led to shoulder its responsibilities; an early example of this was provided at Bromley in a club, the Stepping Stones (Morgan and Tylden 1957), where many volunteers undertook to provide a great deal of care and activity for psychiatric patients out of hospital. Progressive local authorities have developed many services since then, where finance and staff have allowed. There is no doubt that these are valuable not only for rehabilitation, but also in preventing recurrent breakdowns. Besides this, local volunteers can create and maintain a framework of care for the emotional and physical needs of people at risk, which may appear more personal than official help. Church and social organisations play their part; good administration is essential, but, inevitably, success depends on the enthusiasm and patience of the workers involved.

REFERENCES

Dunkley, E. W. and Lewis, E. (1963). 'North Wing: a psychiatric unit in a general hospital'. *Lancet*, i, 156.

Ling, T. M. (1945). 'Roffey Park Rehabilitation Centre'. *Lancet*, 203.

Ling, T. M. and Wilson, V. W. 'A survey of occupational problems in a neurosis centre'. *Brit. Med. J.*, ii, 558.

Morgan, G. D. and Tylden, E. (1957). 'The Stepping Stones Club: a survey of occupational problems in a neurosis centre'. *Lancet*, i, 877.

Morgan, R. (1970). 'Industrial rehabilitation of long stay patients'. *Proc. Roy. Soc. Med.*, 63, 1332.

Wansborough, S. N. (1970). 'The patient's response'. *Proc. Roy. Soc. Med.*, 63, 1335.

Wing, J. (1971). 'Social psychiatry'. *Brit. J. Hosp. Med.*, 5, 53.

58 The community's attitude

HISTORICAL BACKGROUND

The idea of looking after patients suffering from mental illness in their own homes, as opposed to putting them into a mental hospital, is one which has only recently become a legal part of our Welfare State. Atypical forms of behaviour, including mental illness and mental deficiency, have always been present in human communities. Attitudes to these vary from time to time and from society to society. In medieval communities there was no clear differentiation between mental illness, epilepsy and mental deficiency. The victims of all these could be regarded as bewitched, or star crossed, or blessed. Depression, hallucinations and other manifestations of insanity were regarded as possession by devils and treated by torture or exorcism. Anti-social behaviour was punished by exclusion or imprisonment. The mentally ill whose symptoms were less socially destructive became jesters, or lived in some sort of social equilibrium as the village idiot. Religious orders sometimes provided institutional care for some mentally sick or inadequate; the treatment of kings, queens and nobles was at home in special apartments under the care of attendants who nursed, sedated, or flogged the patient under the supervision of the doctor.

It was not until 1793 that Pinel removed the chains from the inmates of the Bicêtre in Paris; and in England in 1796 the Quaker William Tuke opened the York Retreat where mental patients were treated with kindness instead of by restraint and flogging. The laws of the nineteenth century, however, continued to assume that not only mental deficiency, but all mental illnesses were conditions lasting a lifetime, making the patients socially irresponsible and sometimes actively antisocial. Hospitals (originally asyla) for mentally sick patients protected them (and other people). Patients were deprived of their rights as citizens: the right to vote, to work, to spend or bequeath money, to marry, to have children and to travel. This attitude to mental illness still persists in some doctors as well as much of the lay community.

Despite these drawbacks, the ideas of the reformers were very much in the mind of those Victorians responsible for the building and staffing of so many of our large mental hospitals in the middle of the nineteenth century. Every attempt was made to provide an environment of concern for the patients with more respect being paid to individual dignity and comfort. When they were first built, these hospitals were showplaces for visitors from abroad and efforts were made to prevent the decay of ties between patients and their families. Sadly, they were soon overwhelmed by a tide of overcrowding thrown up by the rapid rise in the population of the country, and in addition the advances of scientific medicine which did not extend into psychiatry left them behind as neglected backwaters for staff and patients alike. Overcrowded and understaffed, they encouraged sterile custodial attitudes to replace therapeutic concern. The effect on patients was to intensify the apathy and withdrawal already produced in many cases by the illnesses from which they suffered. Gradually this decline has been halted and then reversed. New physical treatments have played their part, but equally important have been changes in policy and attitudes to psychiatric care. An important landmark was the Mental Treatment Act (1930) which encouraged voluntary admission of psychiatric patients. The establishment of the National Health Service brought psychiatric and general hospitals under the same administration.

THE MENTAL HEALTH ACT

All previous mental health acts were repealed and a new Mental Health Act was passed in 1959. It reflects the progressive trends which have been taking place, not only in general administration of our hospitals, but also in regard to the admission of patients and to their care and treatment.

The broad principles on which the Act is based are:

1 To give maximum encouragement to patients suffering from any form of mental illness or disability to seek treatment promptly and informally.

2 To ensure adequate safeguards where patients, in the interest of safety, must be compulsorily treated and detained.
3 To encourage the care of psychiatric patients in the community, and to call upon local authorities to provide appropriate day care and residential facilities.

Thus it recognizes that mental illness is treatable and that many mentally retarded individuals are trainable. It abolishes the previous legal distinction which was made between these two conditions, though it designates special hospitals for different conditions. A minority of patients have to be compulsorily detained in hospital, but this can only be done when the application of a close relative or social worker is supported by medical recommendations. In all cases it must be certified that the patient is mentally ill *and* a potential danger to others or himself or both, *and* that informal admission is not possible. The procedures involved vary according to the nature of the emergency, as follows:

Section	Application made by	Medical recommendations	Duration
Urgent Admission, Sec 29	Any relative or approved Social Worker	Any doctor; if practicable, having previous acquaintance with patient	72 hours
Admission for Observation, Sec 25	Nearest relative or approved Social Worker	Two doctors, one of whom must be approved under Section 28 as having special psychiatric experience and one of whom should if practicable have previous acquaintance with the patient	28 days
Admission for Treatment, Sec 26: usually follows one of the above	Nearest relative or approved Social Worker in exceptional circumstances	As for 25	1 year renewable

The Act also recommends that the majority of mentally ill patients should be treated at home or in the community, and that many mentally retarded patients should live and work in the community. Implicit in these recommendations is that adequate facilities for community care should be provided by the Local Authorities. Some of these will be described in the next section, but failure to make necessary provisions has seriously impeded these proposals in many parts of the country.

FURTHER READING

Macrea, A. K. (1973). 'Forensic psychiatry'. In Forrest, A. (ed.), *Companion to Psychiatric Studies*, Vol. 2, Ch. 20. Churchill Livingstone, London.
Zilboorg, G. (1941). *A History of Medical Psychology*. Norton, New York.

59 Hospital and community services

COMMUNITY CARE

The legal changes that have been mentioned have played a part in the development of the policy of community care in psychiatry. Community care is not in fact a single idea, but rather a set of related and intervening ideas and policies aimed at providing more efficient, wide-ranging and flexible psychiatric care while avoiding wherever possible the isolation of the patient from his community. The NHS re-organisation which came into force in April 1974 has provided the framework on which these plans can continue to develop. As with other medical care, psychiatric treatment will be based on the district, with out-patients and the majority of in-patients being treated in the District General Hospital. There are many alternatives to hospital admission, and day centres. Day hospitals and hostels can all play their part. There is great emphasis in community care on collaboration between the different professionals involved. General practitioner, nurse, social worker, psychologist, occupational therapist, and psychiatrist can each have their role and can draw on one another's skills.

Schemes of community care have already been developing, although at different speeds, throughout the country. In general, experience has confirmed the value of these projects, and psychiatric care has been given an exciting new impetus. At the same time some of the more enthusiastic early claims for community care have proved over-optimistic. It has become clear that harm can be done both to patients and their families by a blinkered insistence on the dogma that it is bad for any patient to be in a psychiatric hospital.

The facilities that can go to make up a full range of community services will now be discussed.

INPATIENT UNITS

The psychiatric inpatient services provide some 40% of the total beds in the country's hospitals, and the bulk of these are in mental hospitals. Many of them are still occupied by chronic patients, who became so before any effective treatment was known, and by old people who cannot be cared for elsewhere. But the majority of acute admissions today can expect only a short stay in hospital and a discharge back to their home.

Admission units

Patients admitted to hospital now go either to a growing number of District General Hospital Units, or to specially designated admission wards in mental hospitals, which will gradually be closed as new units open. The Department of Health has suggested that a district of 200,000 population will need about 100 beds of this kind, but many psychiatrists believe that more will be required. There is also a danger that these units will become filled up with chronic patients because other community facilities have lagged behind the provision of hospital beds.

Long-stay mental hospital beds

The present population of chronic patients in mental hospitals will decline by discharge and death. Some very optimistic views of community care have held that in future no patients will become chronic and no long stay beds will be needed. However, there is a growing evidence that a small number of 'new chronic' patients are going to need long admissions, and so slow the rundown of mental hospitals. It is very important not to allow these hospitals to become second-rate dumping-grounds, which would discourage staff and patients alike. Instead, it is essential to integrate their facilities into local services; where rehabilitation skills are concerned, they have much to offer the community.

Services for the elderly

Psychiatric illness is very common in the elderly, and many acute patients who require hospital admission can be successfully treated in ordinary admission units. Severely demented patients still go to chronic wards in the mental hospital. About 80 beds will be necessary to cover both needs for a district of 200,000 population. But since, in many cases, acute psychiatric and physical disorders co-exist, there are plans to set up special psycho-geriatric assessment units where psychiatrist and geriatrician work together. 10-20 beds are probably necessary in each district.

Special centres for neurotics

In the past, mental hospitals took mostly psychotic patients, and there was very little inpatient accomodation for neurotics. Certain pioneer units were developed for their special needs, notably the Cassel Hospital at Richmond (Surrey), a centre for psychoanalytic treatment and research; Roffey Park, Horsham, originally a centre for rehabilitation of cases of industrial neurosis, on a short-term basis; and Belmont Hospital, at Sutton, Surrey, where war experiences of acute neuroses were turned to use for similar states, due to industrial or domestic stress.

Many neurotics can, and certainly should, be treated as outpatients, but these units have demonstrated in their various ways that some need special inpatient facilities, either to allow a temporary escape from domestic pressures, or, more importantly to provide more intensive group, individual and physical treatment than can be given outside. Moreover, these units need special facilities which are not easy to provide in a general hospital, in the shape of occupational and social treatment; so that they need to be separate, though obviously closely linked to the general and mental hospitals.

Special units for psychopaths and delinquents

A pioneer centre for psychopaths was set up at Belmont, and later became a separate unit under the direction of Maxwell Jones (1952) known as the Henderson Hospital (see p. 68). In this most difficult type of patient, some results, which would not have been possible for outpatients, have been achieved by specially trained staff in an environment which can tolerate 'acting-out'.

Hospitals for the mentally subnormal

Originally, these were largely built by local authorities: some were well provided with facilities for occupation, and training: and considerable work was done in this, and in finding work locally, under sheltered conditions. They were also taken over by the NHS and became for a time clogged by extra patients referred from the community, and gravely hampered by shortage of staff. More recent research on the causes of retardation, and on the possibilities of training, and a more encouraging attitude in the community now allows more hope for the useful employment of the retarded, who can either live at home, or in hostels under some supervision.

Day hospitals

Admission to day hospital allows most psychiatric treatment to take place while preserving the position of the patient in family and community as well as saving hospital staff. Day hospitals are also useful as a half-way stage in the discharge of inpatients. For a district of 200,000, the Department of Health recommends about 120 day hospital places.

OUTPATIENT CLINICS

Adult and special units

Adult outpatient clinics were greatly increased at the start of the NHS and now exist in most general hospitals. Outside London, they are mostly staffed by the local mental hospital consultants. The need for adequate outpatient facilities is illustrated by the fact that between 1961 and 1971, the number of new outpatient referrals increased by 30% (Bransby 1974).

The treatment available naturally varies a great deal. Some clinics attempt to provide a full range of physical and psychological treatment, but owing to shortage of psychotherapeutic facilities in the NHS there is nearly always a long waiting list for the latter. Elsewhere only physical treatment is possible and occasional short interviews; the lack of adequate facilities for psychological treatment is particularly serious in view of the high proportion of patients with psychoneuroses, personality disorders and psychosomatic symptoms.

Special units exist for various problems, e.g. marital, adolescent, delinquent (e.g. the Portman Clinic), alcoholic or other addictions; but these are few. Patients can be referred by their GP, by other specialists, or by social workers.

Child guidance clinics

Though some have existed for years, the number was much increased after the Education Act in 1944; they are sometimes run by hospital staff, sometimes by local authorities, sometimes jointly. They see children with developmental and learning difficulties as well as those who are frankly ill, who may be referred by their GP, or by the school service.

A few special counselling services in mental subnormality exist. Obviously in both, counselling of parents and teachers is to be considered as much as direct treatment of the child.

Domiciliary visiting

Domiciliary visiting by psychiatrists is a valuable extension of out-patient assessment. It caters for patients who are afraid to come to hospital, spares the elderly a tiresome and possibly confusing journey, gives the psychiatrist an impression of family relationships and living conditions, and allows closer contact with the GP. Crises can be met by immediate intervention and support.

SOCIAL AGENCIES

Social services departments

Psychiatric illness rarely occurs without associated social diffi-culties, whether these be cause or effect. Social services departments serve the same populations as Area Health Authorities, although they are administered separately, and can provide services and facilities which are crucial to the successful development of community care. Although some of these services are required by law, others are only recommendations in the Act. This discrepancy has led to uneven development of care across the country.

Social workers

The community social worker is often the lynch-pin of community care. She may be the first person to contact the patient and family in distress, and can then provide a range of services from intensive personal case work to practical advice on social security benefits. She has knowledge and access to the various other departmental services, and has an important role in guiding the patient through the system of care. She can make a referral to a psychiatrist or draw the patient to the attention of the GP to whose practice she may in fact have an attachment.

The social worker may also be involved in the process of admission to hospital, whether this be informal or compulsory, and in the latter case may be one of those approved for the statutary duty of making applications for orders under the Mental Health Act, a function of the old Mental Welfare Officer. She may have special qualifications (see pp. 358, 372).

Day centres

Day centres run by the social services departments differ from day hospitals in that they provide no nursing or medical care. Their main aim is to build up or restore social skills, and they do so by a range of measures including work training, general social activities and group discussions. They also relieve loneliness in the socially isolated. The Department of Health recommends about 120 places for a district.

Hostels

The Mental Health Act recommended that local authorities set up hostels for the after care of patients discharged from hospital, but for various reasons, including lack of funds, hostels have been slow to develop.

The original idea was that these places would provide six months to one year of 'half-way house' care to assist patients to recover their place in the community. As more and more chronic patients are discharged from mental hospitals and fewer of the disabled are admitted for long-term care, a glaring need has been demonstrated for many more long-term hostel places. One of the most disquieting consequences of the implementation of community care policies has been the rapid rise in the number of psychiatrically ill people in prison, in doss-houses and living rough. This is because the rate of the closure of hospital beds has been allowed to run ahead of the provision of proper community facilities. The Department of Health suggests about 50 hostel places for a district.

The whole problem of the organisation of the social and community services has been the subject of the recent Government Report of the Committee on Local Authority and Allied Personal Services (Seebohm Report) published by HMSO, 1969.

Summary of Department of Health's guideline recommendations for community care facilities for a population of 200,000 (a district)

Admission beds	100
Beds for senile dementia	80
Psychogeriatric assessment	10-20
Long stay beds for adult mental illness	none (?)
Day hospital	130
Day centre	120
Hostel	50

NURSES

Nurses are likely to meet psychiatric patients in three places; psychiatric units, wards of general hospitals, and in their own homes. Those who work in the former have generally been specifically trained and are members of a psychiatric team taking an active part in the day to day treatment of the inpatient or day patient, and (in many places) following them up when discharged. All of this is a great advance from the custodial role of the mental nurse in the old mental hospital.

It is often not realised by the staff of general hospitals, or by medical students who work in them, that the general nurse, even in training, can be of inestimable value in helping the neurotic or psychosomatic patient. She is often the recipient of confidences from an anxious or depressed person; she can do much by sympathetic listening, though even today this is sometimes regarded as a waste of time by the nursing hierarchy, and she may thus have valuable information to pass onto the doctor. For all this she clearly needs teaching and a chance to voice her anxieties about particular patients and on special subjects such as the dying patient, or, say, abortion.

The nurse in the district, either attached to a general practice, or to the MOH, undertakes very much the same role as the case worker for psychiatric patients. But she has another one too: to handle emotional problems at a very early stage, for she often sees the patient first when he has some physical complaint and her attitude then can do much to allay (or sadly sometimes to increase) any anxiety which he has about it.

OTHER SOCIAL SERVICES

There are many other social agencies, each of which may at times be most helpful to the GP. They include infant welfare departments, housing departments, the children's department, the services of the Ministry of Labour, Industrial Rehabilitation and Government Training Centres, Disablement Resettlement Officers, and Ministry of Social Security. There are also many voluntary bodies, e.g. the National Association for Mental Health, the Mental After-care Association and many local groups. These services are well described in the Family Welfare Association's guide to the social services.

OTHER PROFESSIONS

There are other professions who are natural allies of the psychiatrist or the general practitioner concerned with mental illness, e.g. the clergy, probation officers, personnel managers in industry. All these are asked for advice and help by patients, and have their own special skills, as well as an ability to provide 'first-aid' by listening and counselling. Collaboration between them, the medical profession and the social services is growing. In particular, the clergy and doctors are bridging the gulf which has separated them for centuries, and learning to collaborate in case-work, as well as in education. The Institute of Religion and Medicine exists to further this collaboration.

It is useful when working in an area to get to know and to respect anyone concerned in the welfare services. NSPCC inspectors, called in on alleged cases of child cruelty, rarely prosecute and often give help and support to the families in difficulties. Ambulance drivers transporting patients to and from hospitals or occupation centres often notice and report deterioration, and in some cases lives have been saved because a milkman, or neighbour, takes the trouble to report uncollected milk bottles. Shop stewards often act as very successful counsellors for fellow-workers who would not seek a doctor's advice.

In many areas the police behave as skilled and very patient social workers, even for drug addicts.

THE GP's ROLE

The above account describes the hospital services, social agencies and other people who may help the GP treat his psychiatric patients. In some circumstances, they may take over his responsibilities, at least temporarily. But the GP should be the key figure in the patient's continuing treatment, and he should maintain this position wherever he can. He will be greatly helped in doing so if he seeks the collaboration of his colleagues listed above, and does not 'pass the buck'. His own methods and opportunities are described elsewhere (see p. 347). He may benefit from regular discussions with a psychiatrist visiting his surgery (Holmes 1974).

Group meetings of patients

But directing people to social agencies is not, of course, the whole answer, as there are a very large number who continue to require help for a considerable period of time, particularly those patients who find it difficult to get on with other people. Where a number of patients share a common problem a great deal of help can be given through the medium of regular group discussions, where there is a pooling of the knowledge of all members of the group to help one another. The doctor, or social worker, working in such a group, often finds that there is a clarification of his or her own problems as well as those of the patients, and group therapy can be very effective when the members of the group feel that they are all working to a common end.

Groups of parents of disturbed children meeting in Bromley discovered that the district lacked special educational facilities, child minding services and playgroups for the under-fives. Groups of patients discharged from mental hospitals discovered at the Stepping Stones in Bromley that they needed various recreational outlets such as carpentry, drama, handicrafts and art, and as a result of this they formed a club which has 800 members and provides these facilities for patients within the district (see p. 355). Through the medium of such group activities it is possible to keep in touch with far more patients than could possibly be supervised individually. It is essential that professional people should be available in these contexts as they can cope with patients' relapses.

TEAM-WORK

In all these services, team-work is vital if the patient is not to suffer; in hospital, treatment is directed by the consultant psychiatrist, but carried out by many different people, any one of whom may have a leading part to play in any particular patient's recovery: sister and nurse, psychiatric social worker, occupational therapist or physiotherapist, psychologist may all be involved, as may the student in a teaching hospital. All must communicate on the patient's progress and their plans. The atmosphere of a therapeutic community, aimed at in any psychiatric unit, must depend on communication and harmony in the staff, if 'acting-out' is to be tolerated, let alone used constructively; and the collaboration of any other medical or surgical colleagues involved, unused perhaps to such behaviour, must be obtained.

Team-work is equally essential between workers in the community, of whatever profession (and more may be concerned). And above all, collaboration between hospital and community and GP is vital. In this respect the PSW can do untold good, whichever of these three she is officially attached to (see below).

REFERENCES

Holmes, S. M. (1974). Personal communication.
Kearns, J. L. (1973). *Stress at Work*. London, The Priory Press.
Scott, J. (1974). Personal communication.

FURTHER READING

Bransby, E. R. (1974). 'The extent of mental illness in England and Wales'. *Health Trends*, 6, 56.
Cawley, R. and McLachlan, G. (eds.) (1973). *Policy for Action: A symposium on the planning of a comprehensive district psychiatric service*. OUP, London.

Clark, D. H. (1964). *Administrative Therapy*. Tavistock, London.
Jones, M. (1952). *Social Psychiatry*. Tavistock, London.
Wing, J. K. and Hailey, A. M. (eds.) (1972). *Evaluating a Community Psychiatric Service*, OUP, London.

60 The psychiatric social worker

The work of the social worker has already been discussed (p. 365). Even more important is her colleague with specialized training, the psychiatric social worker (PSW), a key-member of any psychiatric team. In particular she* works with the social and emotional problems which arise in connection with mental illness. They may be connected with the material circumstances of the patient's life or with his personal relationships with his family, at work, or in some other sphere. She may work in the hospital, or the community.

The reorganization of the social services in Britain after the Seebohm report included the transfer of all social workers, including PSWs, to the social service departments. But as there is obviously a special need for PSWs in hospitals, and adult and children's psychiatric departments, it was in general agreed that they should continue their work there, by being seconded from the official responsibility of the directors of social service.

The situation is more complicated outside hospital, for the role of the psychiatric social worker in the community is by no means universally agreed upon; and opinions differ too about the precise skills she must learn and tasks she must undertake. This is not surprising, for no general agreement exists about what the community needs from any social worker, and indeed neighbouring communities may have totally different views about deviant behaviour — which to one is 'mad', to the other 'bad'. Hence it is essential that before she can help

---

* The psychiatric social worker is referred to as 'she' throughout this section; most of the members of the profession are women though the number of men has increased considerably in recent years.

at all the social worker must assess as accurately as possible what the community expects from her and what it does in fact need from her (Tredgold 1974). Her training and skills must be understood by those who collaborate with her.

Professional social work is now based on one- or two-year professional courses, in which the content is generic, but the student's special interests (e.g. psychiatry, probation work) receive supervision. Further needs which are becoming more recognised, are met by in-service training.

FUNCTIONS OF THE PSW

Diagnosis and plans for treatment

Psychiatric social workers may be asked to investigate the interaction of the patient's illness and his environment, and to obtain the information needed to understand the relevant social and emotional factors in his life and family. They must be able to make realistic assessment of the weaknesses and assist in the total situation, in order to help the psychiatrist make a diagnosis. The team then works out a treatment plan. The important role of the PSW in such teamwork, especially in the community has been stressed by Maxwell Jones (1968).

Information and advice

Some patients need information and advice on how to use the social services. The PSW needs to keep herself informed of changes in social legislation and in other social resources, so that she can make them fully available to patients when necessary, either directly or through the doctor concerned.

Casework

Many patients will require casework help. This is a method of giving individual help to people who have social and emotional problems they cannot deal with by themselves.

The PSW may be asked to work directly with the patient, or

with relatives and other people in his life. If the patient is a child, the PSW normally works with the parent.

The help is given within a personal relationship which is professionally defined and in many respects resembles a psychotherapeutic relationship. The practice of social casework involves the following principles:

1 The aim is to help the person reach his own decisions rather than to direct his actions. He has a right to govern his own life and this right is in no way affected by the fact that he is seeking another's help.

2 Respect for the individual is one of the fundamental principles of casework and the PSW must accept and value each person for what he is. The PSW may have to help the person concerned to realize the implications of his attitude and behaviour but a non-judgmental attitude is needed to achieve this.

3 Sometimes the actual problem presented may mask the person's real need and his real feelings about his life situation. The PSW needs to understand how his feeling and fantasies affect the realities of life as he experiences it. Feelings are facts which must be dealt with.

4 The PSW tries also to understand herself and her own biases and prejudices. Her personal needs and reactions should not affect the relationship. For example, she may be tempted to respond to a need by giving advice, which may not be in the best interests of the patient. He may need to be helped to take responsibility for his own decisions and to explore the real need behind the request. Similarly the PSW must not be discouraged or antagonized if her advice is ignored.

Psychiatric social workers also take part in the running of therapeutic groups, and are likely to do so increasingly.

The use of psychiatric and other social workers varies a great deal in different countries, according to the needs of the community, and the way in which the social services have developed there. A useful description of this in Europe is given in a WHO report (1974).

REFERENCES

Jones, M. (1952). *Social Psychiatry*. Tavistock Publications, London.
Jones, M. (1968). *Social Psychiatry in Practice*. Penguin.
Tredgold, R. V. C., (1974). *Mental Health in the Community*. Forthcoming.
WHO Regional Office for Europe. *The Role of the Social Worker in the Psychiatric Services*. WHO, Copenhagen.

61 Choice

Students are generally taught to put their whole interest and care on the patient in hospital in front of them, and this is very right. But it has one disadvantage, that they forget the waiting list, and get no experience of having to decide between the needs of several competing patients. This need to choose may hit them in resident house jobs, insofar as they may have to decide the priority of patients awaiting admission. But even here their feelings are cushioned, since their contact with demanding patients or relatives is more often by telephone, or through a secretary, than face to face.

The GP is in a much less protected position. Small wonder if his own anxiety spills over at times on to his patients and colleagues, and indicates his lack of confidence and experience in this field.

Yet he is likely to meet more and more situations where he has to choose, and his choice may literally mean life to one patient, death to another. Dramatically this can happen to a surgeon dealing with casualties after battle or train crashes; to a service officer deciding whom to evacuate, whom to leave behind to be cared for (or not) by the enemy; and to a physician deciding to whom to give a kidney machine, or a transplanted organ. These questions may seldom arise in general practice, but the less spectacular decisions are many; for example, whether to spend time listening to one patient's account of his neurosis, or to another's of his enuretic child. Psychotherapeutic facilities in general are very limited and GPs and psychiatrists often have to decide for whom to provide long-term psychotherapy, whom to refuse, and to whom to give what they can in the way of support, if only to prevent deterioration; circumstances may press them hard, and the 'demanding' patient may receive treatment before the more conscientious and independent — with unfortunate social implications.

A wider question still is only considered by few: whether to work in an already well-doctored area or hospital, or in Africa where many people have no doctor at all. There is no easy answer to any of these questions. There is all the more reason for them to be discussed before qualification.

Some sort of ethical choice will have to be made whenever a new development in medicine or social custom exceeds the capacity of the existing services. Transplantation surgery may provoke many in the future. Two problems have already caused much concern: that of the drug addicts (see p. 139) and the steep rise in unwanted pregnancies, which, under the new Abortion Law, threatened to be more than gynaecologists could cope with. This is discussed in detail below.

The balance of the doctor's judgment must therefore be preserved in all his dealings with his patients and their relatives: this has been very well expressed in the 'litany' attributed to the late Sir Robert Hutchison:

'From inability to leave well alone, from too much zeal for what is new and contempt for what is old, from putting knowledge before wisdom, service before art, cleverness before common sense, from treating patients as cases, and from making cure of a disease more grievous than its endurance, Good Lord, deliver us.'

FURTHER READING

Fox, Sir T. F. (1965). Purposes of Medicine (Harveian Oration). *Lancet*, ii, 801.

62 *Termination of pregnancy*

THE DOCTOR'S REACTIONS

Although abortion was in fact legal in Britain on several grounds before the Abortion Act 1967, the number of women referred to clinics with unwanted pregnancies has since increased.

Many patients are referred with extremely distressing stories and very mixed feelings. A few come simply because they do not want their child. The doctors concerned, GPs and psychiatrists alike, may naturally feel pity for the first, and some resentment and moral indignation at the second. Obviously, either feeling tends to influence their judgment and subsequent behaviour. The doctor's training should enable him to understand and allow for his own reactions, even if he cannot fully control them. This will be easier if he remembers that the first question is a legal one, and that the woman's present and future mental health is the issue rather than his personal moral or religious convictions.

THE LAW

The law is that termination is permissible (1) if continuance of the pregnancy is a greater risk than abortion to the life or health of the pregnant woman herself or of any existing children of her family (account may be taken of her actual or foreseeable environment), or (2) if there is a substantial risk that the child to be born will be seriously handicapped physically or mentally.

Any two medical practitioners (or one in an emergency), acting in good faith, can make a legally valid decision. Neither need be a gynaecologist or a psychiatrist, but if the psychiatrist is asked by the GP implicitly or explicitly for his opinion on this point his first duty is to give it. Once this is done he will advise on how best to help the patient.

It seems illogical to draw any distinction between physical indications for termination and psychological ones, and the law does not do so. Presumably, a desire to distinguish the two is based either on the feeling that psychiatric signs are less definite or that psychiatric cases are always blameworthy. Experience should remedy both misconceptions.

THE ASSESSMENT

A psychiatric opinion must be formed on one's own judgment of the evidence supplied. This consists of two parts:

1 The history from patient and relatives, and a full report from

the patient's regular GP, with details in particular of the mental changes which have occurred in her since she knew she was pregnant; of her previous response to similar stress; and of the stresses she will have to meet during the remainder of the pregnancy and subsequently if she goes to full term. For this reason the regular GP must always be fully in the picture, and attempts to side-step him must be resisted.

2 The examination, which must elicit mental signs. These must be recorded as objectively as are physical signs in, say, heart disease. Beware of the patient who seems far better than reported. This may well be because she has been explicitly or implicitly led to believe that a termination will be recommended. Beware also of the rarer patient and/or husband or sexual partner who consciously exaggerate or even invent symptoms.

An important point is generally the risk of suicide in a depressive, and there is often a harrowing decision to be made between recommending that the foetus or infant (and there seems no logical distinction) should be destroyed and risking a suicide and the possible break-up of a happy home. It has been said that pregnant women do not commit suicide. This is untrue. On the other hand, the psychiatrist must realize that, in some patients — notably those who have been brought up with strong religious views — termination may provoke guilt and further depression. This is rare in practice.

Before the Abortion Act was passed, and soon afterwards, it was usual, though not necessary legally, to get a psychiatric opinion on all women who sought termination on psychiatric grounds; but now more gynaecologists act on their own judgment and experience, which has naturally grown steadily. It seems that an increasing number see no reason to oppose the wishes of a patient who wishes her pregnancy to be terminated; and although abortion on demand is not the law, many cases can be regarded as coming within the criteria of the Act; and to insist on any woman bearing a child she· does not want is coming to be regarded as uncivilized by more doctors. Changes in technique cast less strain on the surgeon, though sometimes more on the nurses. For these reasons, psychiatrists now tend to be asked only to see patients whose real wishes are in doubt, to try to unravel them, and to say if they find any contra-indication to termination; and of course to provide any treatment possible.

Unwanted pregnancies very often indicate a psychological crisis in the woman, generally in her relationship to her husband or friend. If the opportunity of the pregnancy can be used to resolve this crisis, much good may come, whether termination is advised or not. But this is difficult and needs immediate and' intensive psychotherapy. It is probable that if more psychiatric sessions were available at ante-natal clinics, some patients now recommended for termination could safely be got through their pregnancy. But in fact, there are very few psychiatrists working in this way. With the present pressure of work, it is extremely difficult to arrange intensive treatment at an ordinary clinic for what always presents as an emergency. But if psychotherapeutic help is available and the woman is prepared to accept it, it should be provided, either to deal with her guilt feelings and other anxieties associated with the termination, if this is recommended, or to help her with her problems during the pregnancy and afterwards if she has agreed to let it continue; and again antidepressant drugs and electro-convulsive therapy may be successful at times.

AFTER-CARE AND FOLLOW-UP

A phase of remorse and some guilt does, however, occur as a temporary reaction in many women after termination. It is important that this should be helped by the attitude of the surgeon and nurse at this stage. Both the latter may have their own emotional problems, in that termination is naturally repugnant to them. Full information from the psychiatrist or PSW may help them as well as the patient at this stage. Longer-term support should be offered to the patient.

Assessment would be easier were there more evidence on the follow-up of depression through pregnancy, whether terminated or not. This is as yet inadequate, though several Scandinavian studies by Höök suggest that few women suffer from more than temporary depression after termination. This is supported by Clark et al. (1968), and Hamill and Ingram (1974). Chronic depression is especially likely to follow a termination which the woman really did not want, but was persuaded to have.

Psychiatric assessment is essential if this is in doubt. Follow-up studies (Pare and Raven, 1970) have also shown that serious psychiatric disability can follow refusal of termination in women who are determined not to have the baby; after termination serious disability is rare if the woman wanted it done (Lask, 1975).

ADOPTION

Continuance of an unwanted pregnancy and adoption of the child is a logical solution, which naturally is preferable in that it saves the infant's life. But in practice in Britain, adoption is not easy; and even where this course had been taken, the mother has experienced as much, or more distress; her own views on the possibility of having the child adopted must therefore be fully taken into account.

EMOTIONAL OBJECTIONS

At present some psychiatrists and some gynaecologists, on religious or on medical grounds, hold that termination is never permissible. Their sincere opinions must be respected but it logically follows that the specialists who hold them must undertake to cope with the consequence of continued pregnancy; and it is possible that if they did so some would change their views. But, instead of this, it often happens that the GP and/or patient seek a specialist's help outside the consultant they normally use for other problems. This means that in a short space of time specialists who are known to be ready to judge each case on its own merits are grossly overworked, while those whose minds are already set against termination avoid the unpleasant task.

The law now includes a conscience clause for those unwilling to be party to an abortion, with the burden of proof on the person who claims he is genuinely conscientiously against it. This has not yet been tested. But, in any case, a gynaecologist or psychiatrist or GP disliking abortion can still say he believes it is against the woman's interests. With many doctors disliking an inherently horrible task, and yet with demands for abortion increasing, the crisis on this subject is by no means over. Hence, the Departments of Obstetrics and Psychiatry in some hospitals have agreed on a policy of accepting only cases from within their own district, or from GPs who regularly use them, and insist on a full report from the latter with, if possible, a discussion. In practice this may often be very difficult.

Attempts were made by The Abortion Law Reform Association to include in the law rape or incest as legal grounds for abortion. At present these apply if it is held that these have affected or are likely seriously to affect the mother's health. Similarly, even the fact of a suicidal father does not appear to be legal grounds unless (as is likely) the mother would break down as a result.

Sterilization is a separate issue, but certainly should not be recommended while patient, and perhaps husband, are under considerable emotional tension (see Section 63). It must be discussed after the question of termination has been decided. Contraceptive advice must, however, be given after termination to prevent further unwanted pregnancies.

It is important to note that the Report of the Committee on the Working of the Abortion Act (Lane Report, 1974) considers that in general the humane recommendations of the Act are fulfilling their purpose, and that every pregnant woman considering a termination should have access to the medical profession under the NHS for unprejudiced help and advice. But opponents of abortion are still pressing for changes.

REFERENCES

Clark, M., Forster, I., Pond, D.A. and Tredgold, R. F. (1968). 'Sequels of unwanted pregnancy'. *Lancet*, ii, 501.

Cunningham, L. *et al.* (1975). 'Studies of adoptees'. *Brit. J. Psychiat.*, 126, 534.

Hamill, E. and Ingram, I. M. (1974). 'Psychiatric and social factors in the abortion decision'. *Brit. Med. J.*, i, 229.

Höök, K. (1963). *Act. Psych. Neurol.*, Scand. Sup., 168.

Lane Report (1974). *Report of the Committee on the Working of the Abortion Act.* HMSO, London.

Lask, B. (1975). 'Short-term psychiatric sequelae to therapeutic termination of pregnancy'. *Brit. J. Psychiat.*, 126, 173.

Pare, C. M. B. and Raven, H. (1970). 'Follow-up of patients referred for termination of pregnancy'. *Lancet*, 1, 635.

Tredgold, R. F. (1964). 'Psychiatric indications for termination of pregnancy'. *Lancet*, ii, 1251.

FURTHER READING

Church Assembly Board for Social Responsibility (1965). *Abortion: an Ethical Discussion.*
Williams, G. (1958). *The Sanctity of Life and the Criminal Law* (esp. Chapters 5 and 6).

63 Sterilization

Not infrequently a patient is sent to a psychiatrist for advice as to (1) whether sterilization on psychiatric grounds is legal and (2) if so, whether it is advisable and (3) whether such a patient needs psychiatric help. These decisions are only one degree less difficult than that of termination of pregnancy.

There is no English statute law and no test case; and the general opinion of counsel (e.g. when asked by medical defence organizations) has been that sterilization with the patient's consent would be upheld by an English court if it were (a) therapeutic, i.e. to save health being damaged by a further pregnancy, or (b) based on well founded eugenic grounds, but not simply for personal (or professional) convenience.

THERAPEUTIC AND SOCIAL GROUNDS

Therapeutic grounds exist if there would be a threat of death or permanent damage to health from another pregnancy, either from physical disease (not considered here), or psychological, where the danger is in practice either that of suicide from acute depression, or a breakdown into a chronic schizophrenic or depressive state, or the likelihood of severe, chronic psycho-neurotic illness; for example if a woman, perhaps in her late thirties, already has a large family so that for psychological and social reasons she finds it an increasing strain to look after them. But clearly the decision is one to be taken reluctantly in a young woman without children and even in a young married woman with children who might, against all present expectations, want to get re-married later. It should be very carefully explained to both patient and her husband that it is irreversible. It is wise to get their signed consent.

The decision should not be taken by the consultant or patient under pressure. Although it is understandable that some gynaecologists who are asked to terminate wish to insist on sterilization as well, it seems to be the wrong moment to decide, when the woman is in distress from an unwanted pregnancy and the husband's opinion may also be biased. Once the decision to terminate has been accepted by all concerned, and when it is agreed that the woman's state of mind has become stable (which *may* occur before termination), then sterilization can be considered as a separate issue and an objective decision taken.

It must be remembered that, rarely, a man's or a woman's request to be sterilized is a symptom of a psychiatric illness in which case the latter should be treated rather than a sterilization carried out.

EUGENIC GROUNDS

If husband or wife is thought likely to transmit a genetic disease or defect, they may feel that one of them should be *voluntarily* sterilized to avoid the risk of transmitting it. This obviously deserves sympathetic help. Certain types of mental defect are known to be genetic, and in theory sterilization would be logical. But defectives unfortunately are less socially responsible, less controlled and less far-sighted in this way — and less reliable in using contraceptives: also the question arises whether any consent they give is valid. For these reasons some reformers and doctors in hospitals for subnormals have felt that sterilization should be *compulsory* for all defectives, and their responsibilities to the public, in fact have led them sometimes to offer their patients the chance of liberty with sterilization or segregation.

As can be imagined, this suggestion of compulsory sterilization aroused antagonism on religious grounds and moral grounds in those concerned with the rights of the individual to propagate his kind, regardless of the possibilities of caring for them. Their antagonism gained wider popular support when Hitler sponsored mass sterilization on allegedly scientific grounds.

Moreover it became realized that only certain types of defect were genetic and that general sterilization would achieve little. For these reasons the question is now restricted to these types, though research may increase the number.

Sterilization has been viewed with sympathy by leaders of the Church of England (see below) who have themselves modified the opinions of their committee held in 1949-50. Roman Catholic opinion still appears to be firmly against eugenic sterilization.

METHOD

Sterilization may be performed on either the female or the male, by ligation of the Fallopian tube or vas deferens respectively. Which partner is chosen must depend on an assessment of the likely reaction of either, and of their long-term future, and also on the practical possibilities. In certain countries male sterilization has been favoured as the only practicable means of population control for the masses, as in India.

SEQUELS

It must be recalled that fears of castration or other mutilation are not uncommon fantasies of adolescents — though often unconscious later. If so they may well be activated by sterilization, and depression may follow this operation, though it is generally temporary. Ekblad's Survey (1961) found that 175 out of his 225 women were wholly satisfied with their sterilization; 15 had regretted it and were moderately (but not severely) disturbed; 25 had temporarily regretted it, and 10 were 'troubled but did not regret it'. Serious guilt, regret and depression afterwards, are much more likely in young women even though they themselves had demanded it originally. On the whole it is likely that if sexual activity has been inhibited in the past by fear of another pregnancy, it will be less inhibited — and happier now. Ekblad found sexual satisfaction improved in 75, unchanged in 121 and reduced in 29 women.

Vasectomy in the male carries less physical risk than sterilization in women: but depression and impotence may be the psychological sequels. The husband who offers himself for the operation to save his wife should be carefully assessed. But Ferber's (1967) study of 73 men showed 72 satisfied with their decision and 55 with more sexual enjoyment. Wolfers (1970) on the other hand observed that psychological problems had developed in a significant proportion (12%) of men who had undergone voluntary vasectomy. Clearly psychotherapy may be required either at once to help husband or wife find objectivity in their decision, or later to help either deal with any remorse, guilt or depression which occur.

REFERENCES

Blacker, C. P. (1962). *The Eugenics Review*, 54.

Ekblad, M. (1961). 'The prognosis after sterilization on social grounds'. *Acta Psych. Neurol., Scand.*, Supplement 161.

Ferber, A. S., Tieltze, C. and Lewit, S. (1967). 'Men with vasectomies: a study of medical, sexual and psychosocial changes'. *Psychosomatic Medicine*, 29, 354.

Wolfers, H. (1970). 'Psychological aspects of vasectomy'. *Brit. Med. J.*, 2, 297.

FURTHER READING

Blandy, J. (1973). 'Vasectomy'. *Brit. J. Hosp. Med.*, 9, 319.

Church Assembly Board for Social Responsibility (1962). *Sterilization: an Ethical Enquiry*.

Williams, G. (1958). *The Sanctity of Life and the Criminal Law*. Faber, London.

64 Euthanasia

Euthanasia has already been mentioned in the discussion on death and dying (see p. 306). To the doctor the problem is likely to increase as modern science extends life without making it more enjoyable — certainly old age is seldom pleasant.

Two very different questions are often confused, for the term 'euthanasia' is used in two senses: the first, 'voluntary' euthanasia is to assist the patient who wants to die to do so peacefully and speedily: the second, 'involuntary' euthanasia, is to kill (or not 'to strive officiously to keep alive') the patient who can express no wish one way or the other, but whom the doctor feels would be better dead, e.g. a patient in coma, or an inarticulate idiot. Unfortunately, in the reports of any statement or any public debate, it is likely that these two questions will be confused, and much emotion engendered.

VOLUNTARY EUTHANASIA

It is only voluntary euthanasia which the Euthanasia Society seeks to legalize. The doctor may be asked to help here by providing an easier means of death, e.g. by an overdose for a patient who could, if he preferred, cut his throat, or by providing the only means of death for, say, a paralysed patient.

Opinions as to the morality of voluntary euthanasia have swung from side to side in history. Some governments have accepted the responsibility for this decision. In Sybaris, for example, a city noted for its pursuit of pleasure, any citizen who wished could apply to the government for a dose of hemlock. No doubt social pressures have influenced opinion, e.g. the burden of old people, and religious views about the after life. Today liberal opinion backed by leading clergy is more concerned with the quality of life than with the precise moment of death; and the resolute prohibition on euthanasia enjoined by a previous generation is disappearing. This indeed is logical, both for those who believe that the next life is inevitably and eternally pleasanter than this, and for those who believe that it does not exist and that death is pleasanter than suffering.

Voluntary euthanasia is at present not legal; if it becomes so, the doctor must judge each case on its merits. He must be as certain as he can what the patient's real desires are, distinguishing a temporary phase of depression. He must consider the reactions of relatives and of his other patients. He must also somehow cling above all to his major duty, namely his patient's welfare — in its widest sense.

INVOLUNTARY EUTHANASIA

Involuntary euthanasia is a very different matter. It would clearly be most undesirable if patients considered that their doctor was — at any time however distant — inclined and empowered to end their life, against their will. Involuntary euthanasia is therefore generally still opposed, in principle. It must have happened in practice in cases such as either of the two examples quoted, and could be defended on the grounds that an idiot baby has no hope of any personality (if this can be proved) or that an adult would not have wished to be kept alive if comatose (if evidence of his previous personality is available).

Hard cases, perhaps, make bad law: and the Euthanasia Society is not pressing for this form of euthanasia. Nor is it supported by many doctors yet, though advances in medical techniques may raise the issue more acutely in the future. For if this type of euthanasia is illegal, the question follows: who is to be resuscitated, and for how long should the doctor try, for example in the case of unconscious patients being kept alive by means of a respirator for months on end. Frantic procedures to defer physical death may do no more than remove the dignity of death, an outrage to nurses and relatives. Conversely, neglect of chances may waste a valuable life. No rule can be laid down, except that as ever the doctor's conscience, sense of proportion and duty to his patients' real interest must lead him to his decision.

FURTHER READING

Church Assembly Board for Social Responsibility (1965). *Decisions about Life and Death.* London Church Information Office.
Williams, G. (1958). *The Sancity of Life and the Criminal Law.* Faber, London.

65 *Giving evidence*

A doctor is often asked for an opinion on a matter with legal consequences on which he may therefore later be called to give evidence for one side. In the existing habits of court procedure, he is examined by counsel, and cross-examined by opposing counsel, whose job (some bitter victims have felt) is not only to question and discredit his evidence, but to question and discredit himself.

Some even think that the emotional atmosphere of a major trial is not the best environment for discovering the truth of facts or feelings. Misunderstandings are common, because of three major points: the language used by doctors may be incomprehensible to lawyers, and vice versa; lawyers necessarily tend to think of black and white, while to a doctor there are many shades of grey; and a doctor is inevitably, at present, representing his patient's interest (so that one judge made the notorious comment that the doctor was always a biased witness). Consequently, we often have the sad sight of doctors on different sides, at cross-purposes with each other and with the court.

Much medical opinion therefore favours the policy, adopted in several other European countries, of the doctor giving evidence to the court rather than for either side: legal opinion in this country seems, more slowly, also to be moving in this direction.

PRIVILEGE

The doctor may object to giving evidence. But once involved he may be subpoenaed and have to go to court. He need not object to speaking of matters which his patient has agreed to, but he may also be asked to divulge, without the patient's consent, matters told in confidence. He can refuse, but if the judge then directs him to answer he has no professional privilege to protect him, and he can be imprisoned if he refuses. This has happened to journalists, but not, so far, to a doctor, and a judge in a case recently made it plain that he did not intend to insist on a doctor speaking against her conscience.

All the above applies to any medical evidence: the difficulties about psychiatric evidence are greater, and confusion occurs even more easily. Eminent psychiatrists before now have been entirely tangled up in cross-examination. A young doctor is very earnestly advised not to use psychiatric terms without great caution, and without being sure he can define them if asked to do so by counsel.

RESPONSIBILITY

In particular, questions of responsibility arise. The so-called McNaughton rules, for use in murder trials, set out to determine whether the accused knew what he was doing (the nature and quality of his act) and, if so, whether he knew it was wrong. There are of course conditions, e.g. paranoid schizophrenia, when murder could be committed in response to a persecutory delusion, which made it seem to the patient justifiable self-defence. There are other occasions when a patient may deny all memory of his act. If this is genuine it could indicate either a rare state of post-epileptic automatism, in which he was not responsible for violence, or a hysterical amnesia, occurring as a result of horror for an act for which he was at the time responsible.

The concept of diminished responsibility is now accepted in English law, and a doctor may well be asked to express his view as to whether the emotional strain on a patient prevents him exercising full responsibility. The suggestion of an overmastering impulse, being open to abuse, is still looked at askance by many judges.

FITNESS TO PLEAD

The patient may be regarded by a doctor as unfit to plead, since he could not understand court procedure, e.g. in a case again of schizophrenia, or severe subnormality. If his unfitness to plead is thought to be only temporary he is likely to be detained until he is fit.

FURTHER READING

Gibbens, T. C. N. (1974). 'Preparing psychiatric court reports'. *Brit. J. Hosp. Med.*, 12, 278.
Mayer-Gross, W., Slater, E. and Roth, M. (1969). *Clinical Psychiatry.* Chapter 13: 'Administrative and legal psychiatry'. Baillière, Tindall and Cassell, London.

66 Compulsory treatment

Some notoriety has been given to the subject by reports of compulsory admission to psychiatric hospitals in Russia and compulsory treatment therein of people whose political views differed from the Government's. The suggestion that any psychiatrist should take part in such a procedure has been condemned by many, including the Royal College of Psychiatrists. An outcry has also been heard in the United States, where, it was alleged, compulsory psychiatric treatment, including surgery, was being performed on prisoners in civil prisons, to diminish their aggressive or anti-social tendencies (by leucotomy): while in Denmark Stürüp (1971) has reported on castration to reduce the drive of sexual offenders. To do so compulsively seems quite unethical. However, some prisoners have consented, influenced by a promise of liberty if their impulses can be thus brought under control: though it has been objected that consent so obtained is really consent under duress. Certainly if long imprisonment can be avoided, so much the better for all — for that too has undoubtedly a damaging effect on personality.

As to admission, many people in many countries have been compulsorily detained in psychiatric hospitals because of antisocial behaviour, and the law still allows this to be done if the behaviour constitutes a danger to the individual or to others; and besides this in an acutely disturbed or violent patient, the only means of quieting him, and so diminishing these dangers, may be by injecting drugs (see p. 316) to which he has not consented, and could not consent because of his mental state. Obviously, all this should be for as short a period as possible, but may be regarded under those circumstances as clinically justifiable; every effort should be made to persuade the patient to accept treatment if it is at all possible to do so.

It would, however, seem to be wrong to give ECT or surgery, or any drugs which may have lasting effects, without discussing these with the patient; and of course it would be quite illegal to do so for patients who are not compulsorily detained (and today in Britain approximately 83% are admitted of their own free will). In any case, besides being unethical to attempt to do so, it could hardly fail to undermine a patient's confidence in his doctor, on which the success of future treatment might well depend.

FURTHER READING

Stürüp, G. K. (1971). 'Sex offenders in Denmark'. In Ramsey, I. T. and Porter, R. (eds.), *Personality and Science.* Edinburgh.

67 The future

THE NEED FOR PSYCHIATRIC SERVICES

There is no doubt that the attitude of most people to psychiatric illness has become more tolerant and more humane. This is partly because modern treatment, both physical and psychological, has shown that it is no longer incurable nor incomprehensible. Many people have recovered from illness and returned happily to their homes and efficiently to their jobs. Further progress is to be expected in research and in treatment and so in popular attitudes.

It may therefore seem that psychiatric illness will diminish a great deal in the next decade and the number of psychiatrists with it. But this is most unlikely; and the reasons why are various. There are at present chronic patients still in hospital and outside it who are not getting the treatment they need. Mental hospital staff are far too few, psychiatric outpatient departments in general hospitals have long waiting lists and there is little sign of economic improvement which would allow the money to be provided for more staff. Drugs may be found to cure more conditions; but even if so, it is probable that a great number of people will still grow up with personality weaknesses and unhealthy reactions to stress for which some form of psychotherapy or support is required, and an increasing number of people, not necessarily seriously mentally ill, are themselves asking for psychotherapeutic help. Each rise in industrialization in developing countries has been accompanied by a rise in neurotic behaviour which has smothered the existing medical services. Increased standards of living do not remedy this; they may even create a more competitive atmosphere which makes it worse.

It is doubtful if any National Health Service can afford to pay for a full psychiatric service; only the most successful citizens and their dependents can afford to pay for it privately.

It is far easier and quicker to produce neurosis in a child than to train a psychotherapist and probably it always will be.

PREVENTION

Prevention must be considered even more seriously. Our understanding of mental development and of the effects of stress has increased far faster than it has been applied. In the field of physical health vitamin deficiencies are rare in civilized countries; but the mental symptoms of lack of emotional 'vitamins' are still wide-spread and our knowledge is only beginning to be systematically disseminated. Research into how to apply the findings of research is still a priority. Parents go on making appalling psychological errors in bringing up their children; industrial sickness costs more in productivity than strikes, and much of it is neurosis and psychosomatic illness. Frustration in work and life finds an outlet in racial prejudice and violence. If war begins in the minds of men, we must ask how close we are to race suicide.

Education offers hope of preventing some disasters — if it can produce understanding of the causes and some acceptance of emotional tension, especially of aggression, and allow some control of their direction, with some sense of social responsibilities. This entails knowledge of defence mechanisms which are built in; has psychiatry a part to play in assisting education here?

Research by sociologists, anthropologists, psychologists, psychoanalysts, psychiatrists and biologists on the sources of human behaviour and on methods of teaching may be increasingly applied. Education on sex is being put into practice against considerable opposition. Can education on aggression become equally widespread? It may be that education in Western culture has gone too far in stimulating competitiveness, too little in teaching collaboration. Certainly the former may lead the bright child to develop his gifts more, which indeed is essential to the community: it may also lead to too much self-centredness, and prevent the balance between the individual and the group's needs being found, and may also prevent duller people from giving of their best by making them feel guilty and disgruntled that they have not been top of the class.

Further, mental sickness in individuals is often the result of living in a sick society; can psychiatry contribute to creating a healthier society?

TREATMENT

Psychiatric patients will still be with us and will need treatment. How then can psychiatry be best employed for this in the future? Long-term psychotherapy will always be required for selected cases and as a tool in research; but it can never be applied comprehensively. Short-term methods of treatment must be developed further, especially briefer forms of psychotherapy; and research into the process of psychotherapy and the psychology of learning on the one hand, and into psychopharmacology and the physiology of emotion and thought on the other, may lead to more effective psychological and physical treatment – especially if patients can be selected more effectively. In this the general practitioner is the central figure. He has opportunities for early diagnosis and treatment which may well deal with mildly unhealthy reactions and minor stress disorders and prevent more severe illness. The psychiatrist will still have the more severe, acute and long-term cases to treat himself; but his equally important role will be to help the general practitioner with a far larger group of patients, by increasing his knowledge and skill; and also to help others with similar responsibilities (see p. 350).

TRAINING OF MEDICAL STUDENTS
AND DOCTORS

The need for better training of medical students in all aspects of psychiatry has been stressed by all those who are concerned with medical education. Psychiatry can no longer be regarded as a narrow specialty but, as we have tried to show in this book it affects a great deal, if not most, of medical practice. The Report of the Royal Commission on Medical Education (1968) has emphasized the need for more intensive training of students in human psychology, sociology, the psychological aspects of medicine, and of psychiatric illness at all stages of medical training; as well as of post-graduates and especially of general practitioners. It seems likely that as these recommendations are being put into practice many more, if not most doctors, in whatever branch of medicine they may be working, will become more competent in recognizing and handling the psychological and psycho-social problems of their patients.

The challenge before those responsible for undergraduate and postgraduate training is how to provide teaching programmes in which the biological, psychological and social aspects of medical and psychiatric practice are properly integrated. At the undergraduate level this means that students need to be shown the relevance of all those aspects to every patient, not only the psychiatric but also the general medical, surgical and obstetric patient. They need to learn how to interview patients as people and how to relate to them. They need to be taught how to understand and handle their patients' physical and emotional disorders in terms of their knowledge of organic and psychological disease processes; they need to understand the nature of psychotherapeutic procedures; and lastly they need to become familiar with the dynamics involved in family interaction and wider social relationships, and with the place of the individual in the community. At our hospital, special provision is made for this, firstly by weekly teaching sessions on medical and obstetric patients by a psychiatrist; and secondly by allowing students to volunteer to take on a patient each for regular psychotherapy under weekly supervision in small groups. In this way such students (about a third of the total) not only learn how to conduct psychotherapy but also understand themselves and their own reactions more closely (Ball and Wolff 1963) (see p. 350).

Training in psychiatry must be continued at the postgraduate level; general practitioners in particular need to be given more opportunity to attend refresher courses so that they can keep in touch with advances in the diagnosis and treatment of mental and psychosomatic illness, and even more important to attend seminars and discussion groups so that they can improve their ability to understand and handle their patients' psychosocial problems (Balint 1964). This has been outlined previously (see p. 350).

As psychiatrists will play a central role in all such training programmes it is essential that in their own training the biological, psychological and social aspects are given equal emphasis, so that a trained psychiatrist can combine all these approaches in the diagnosis, treatment and prevention of psychiatric illness. No doubt the increasing complexity and scope of psychiatry will make it more and more essential for psychiatrists to specialise within their own speciality, and especially when doing research. Some perhaps are more interested in the organic, others in the psychotherapeutic, and yet others in the community aspects of their field; but these are not alternative approaches — all must be integrated and applied to every patient according to his particular need. That has been the aim of this book.

FURTHER READING

Balint, M. (1964). *The Doctor, his Patient and the Illness.* Pitman, London.

Ball, D. H. and Wolff, H. H. (1963). 'An experiment in the teaching of psychotherapy to medical students'. *Lancet*, i, 214.

Russell, G. F. M. and Walton, H. J. (eds.) (1970). 'The training of psychiatrists'. *Brit. J. Psychiat.*, Special Publ. No. 5.

Wolff, H. H. (1967). 'Influencing students' attitudes towards the emotional aspects of illness'. *J. Psychosom. Res.*, 2, 87.